THE ENCYCLOPEDIA OF

ENDOCRINE DISEASES AND DISORDERS

THE ENCYCLOPEDIA OF

ENDOCRINE DISEASES AND DISORDERS

William Petit Jr., M.D.
Christine Adamec

Facts On File, Inc.

The Encyclopedia of Endocrine Diseases and Disorders

Facts On File, Inc.
132 West 31st Street
New York NY 10001

Library of Congress Cataloging-in-Publication Data

Petit, William.
The encyclopedia of endocrine diseases and disorders / William Petit Jr., Christine Adamec.
p. ; cm.
Includes bibliographical references and index.
ISBN 0-8160-5135-6 (hc : alk. paper)
1. Endocrine glands—Diseases—Encyclopedias. [DNLM: 1. Endocrine Diseases—Encyclopedias—English.
WK 13 P489ea 2005] I. Adamec, Christine A., 1949– II. Title.
RC649.P48 2005
616.4′003—dc22   2004004916

Facts On File books are available at special discounts when purchased in bulk quantities for businesses, associations, institutions, or sales promotions. Please call our Special Sales Department in New York at (212) 967-8800 or (800) 322-8755.

You can find Facts On File on the World Wide Web at http://www.factsonfile.com.

Text and cover design by Cathy Rincon

Printed in the United States of America

VB FOF 10 9 8 7 6 5 4 3 2 1

This book is printed on acid-free paper.

CONTENTS

FOREWORD

As an endocrinologist, I am very familiar with the importance of the endocrine glands to human functioning. These glands work continuously to maintain the health of all individuals as we move through each and every day of our lives. In fact, when one or more of the endocrine glands malfunction, the person's entire system is often thrown into disarray. For example, if a person develops Hashimoto's thyroiditis, an autoimmune disorder that causes hypothyroidism, the person's once-normal thyroid levels will drop. He or she may become lethargic and show a variety of symptoms. These range from annoying to severe and affect many activities of daily living. Due to lethargy, the patient's physical activity level will usually decrease. Thus the patient may gain weight, even though he or she eats about the same amount of food as they had before becoming hypothyroid. The individual with hypothyroidism may also appear apathetic and depressed, sometimes leading the patient to seek treatment for these symptoms rather than for the underlying cause.

There are many other examples of endocrine diseases that manifest profound effects on those who live with these illnesses, especially if their endocrine disorder is not identified and treated. For example, diabetes mellitus has a major health impact on millions of people. Sadly, many people who have diabetes, and particularly Type 2 diabetes which usually can be treated with oral medications, are undiagnosed and untreated. These people risk suffering severe complications from their long-term untreated illness.

Other, less common endocrine diseases and disorders also have an impact. Some patients face cancer of their endocrine glands, such as cancer of the pancreas, thyroid, ovaries, testes, and the other organs that comprise the endocrine system. These cancers are not as commonly diagnosed as are cancers of the lung, breast, prostate, or colon. However, they are equally as devastating to those who experience them.

Some people develop very rare diseases of the endocrine system. One such disease, gigantism, causes extremely tall height due to a malfunction of the pituitary gland. Other individuals have unusually short stature, or dwarfism, often due to genetic mutations they have inherited from their parents and sometimes from deficiencies of growth hormone.

In this volume, we have attempted to cover the gamut of endocrine diseases and disorders, ranging from the more common diseases, such as thyroid disease and diabetes, to the rarer medical problems. Our goal is to provide readers with a broad overview of the endocrine system, illustrating how the endocrine glands function when they work normally as well as describing what happens when the endocrine glands malfunction and discussing what can be done in the case of the latter.

We must also point out that although doctors cannot cure all diseases and disorders, many illnesses that were not treated years ago—because the medical tools were not available at that time—can now be treated by endocrinologists. For example, if infertility is caused by an endocrine disorder, the problem can often be identified and treated, enabling an anxious couple to become transformed into happy parents.

If the illness is potentially fatal, such as cancer, many treatments are available that can help patients resolve their cancer or extend their life for many years. We doctors still do not have all the answers, of course, but we are learning more all the time. Continuing research will enable us to discover much more about endocrine diseases and disorders and how to treat them more effectively.

In the meantime, we also know that patients can take many actions to increase the probability of their good health. For example, eating a healthy diet and exercising regularly will not only help many patients avert the scourge of obesity but will also significantly reduce their risk of developing diseases such as diabetes or hypertension.

Such healthy habits are very important. Recent studies have shown that the prevalence of both obesity and severe obesity has greatly increased. For example, a study reported in a 2003 issue of *Archives of Internal Medicine* reported that the prevalence of people with a body mass index (BMI) of 40 or greater and who were about 100 pounds or more overweight (and thus considered severely obese) increased from one in 200 Americans in 1986 to one in 50 by the year 2000.

In addition, over the same time period, the number of people who were obese (with a BMI of 30 or greater) increased from one in 10 to one in five Americans—another dramatic change. Clearly, obesity is a major problem in the United States. It is also one that needs to be addressed by both patients and their doctors.

Patients also bear other responsibilities in managing their health. For example, they should have annual checkups and should see their doctors more frequently if they are ill. Doctors are not mind readers. They need to see their patients regularly.

Doctors also need to be given complete and accurate information by their patients. When patients withhold information from their doctors, such as facts about smoking habits, intake of alcohol, and use of alternative remedies, they may be compromising their health.

In summary, when doctors and patients work together in a healthy partnership, many endocrine diseases and disorders, as well as many other medical problems, can often be successfully resolved or managed.

—William Petit Jr., M.D.

ACKNOWLEDGMENTS

Dr. Petit and Christine Adamec would both like to thank the following individuals: Marie Mercer, reference librarian at the DeGroodt Public Library in Palm Bay, Florida, for her assistance in locating hard-to-find journal articles and books. In addition, they would like to thank Mary Jordan, interlibrary loan librarian at the Central Library Facility in Cocoa, Florida, for her research assistance. Thanks also to Stuart Moss, librarian at the Nathan Kline Institute for Psychiatric Research in Orangeburg, New York, for helping to locate documents that were difficult to find.

Dr. Petit would like to thank his wife, Jennifer Hawke-Petit, and his daughters, Hayley Elizabeth and Michaela Rose, for allowing him to monopolize the computer to trade electronic mails and files with his coauthor. He would like to thank his coauthor, Mrs. Adamec, for her unwavering support and hard work and for continuing to push him as he continued his usual clinical and speaking duties, leaving only nights and weekends to write.

Dr. Petit would also like to thank all his patients over the years who continue to teach him clinical endocrinology. These include, among many others, his first patient with diabetes mellitus and pancreatic cancer when Dr. Petit was a third-year student; a patient in his clinic in Rochester, New York, with a very rare combination of empty sella syndrome and isolated adrenocorticotropic hormone (ACTH) deficiency; and his patients with immobilization hypercalcemia during his years at the Clinical Research Center at Yale University, involved with the Diabetes Control and Complications Trial (DCCT). He would also like to thank the nurses of Hunter 5.

Dr. Petit would also like to thank the following: his team members in his offices, including Doreen Rackliffe, PA-C, Doreen Akehurst, Milagros Cruz, Cheryl Dunphy, Mona Huggard, and Michelle Rodriguez; his team members at the Joslin Diabetes Center at New Britain General Hospital, including Mary Armetta, Sue Bennett, Lynne Blais, Linda Ciarcia, Carole Demarest, Lynn Diaz, Tracy Dube, Cindy Edwards, Jen Kostak, Linda Krikawa, Marc Levesque, Karen McAvoy, Terri McInnis, Pat O'Connell, Denise Otero, Robin Romero, Kate Simoneau, Ursula Szczepanski, and Sue Zailskas; and his physician colleagues at New Britain General Hospital in New Britain, Connecticut, including Jim Bernene, M.D., Latha Dulipsingh, M.D., Joe Khawaja, M.D., Tom Lane, M.D., Ray LeFranc, M.D., Joe Rosenblatt, M.D., and Mubashir Shah, M.D.

Christine Adamec would like to thank her husband, John Adamec, for his support and patience throughout the project.

Special thanks to James Chambers, editor in chief, Arts & Humanities, Facts On File, Inc., for his support of this project.

INTRODUCTION

Endocrinology is the study of normal and abnormal hormonal function. The endocrine glands are vitally important organs that are necessary to sustain all human functions as well as life itself. The glands that comprise the endocrine system affect the ability to become pregnant and successfully carry the pregnancy, the ability to breast-feed an infant, and the ability of a child to grow and develop normally, including sexual differentiation. On a minute-to-minute and a day-by-day basis, the endocrine system helps to regulate an individual's basic functions, such as heart rate, blood pressure, cognitive processes, appetite, energy storage and utilization levels, tissue growth and rejuvenation, sleep, sexuality, bone health, fertility, overall body metabolism, masculinity and femininity, and virtually every aspect of continued life.

The endocrine glands comprise an elegant and complex system. This system is basically the brain that orchestrates and monitors numerous vital bodily functions through the release of a cascade of hormones. These hormones send chemical messages to other parts of the body, enabling actions to start or end as well as to speed up or slow down.

Some important hormones that are released exert their primary effect on other hormones, and they, in turn, either trigger or inhibit the release of yet other hormones. For example, the hypothalamus releases growth hormone-releasing hormone, which triggers the pituitary to release growth hormone. The effects of growth hormone are mediated throughout the body by insulin-like growth factor 1 (IGF-1). The hypothalamus can also release a compound that inhibits the release of prolactin.

By using sophisticated and complex feedback loop systems that are somewhat comparable to the sensors of a thermostat and yet are also far more complicated than the most sophisticated computer, the endocrine glands and the other systems of the body work together. They sense and respond to the numerous minor and major changes in the person's daily environment and the resulting bodily needs.

If a person is in danger, for example, the adrenal glands increase the production of adrenaline (also known as epinephrine), so that the individual is more alert and ready either to take action or to seek escape. (This is also known as the fight-or-flight reaction.) The person's blood pressure and heart rate both increase, enabling the individual to respond with an attack or by running away. When the perceived danger is over, the endocrine glands signal the body to move to a lower and normal level of alertness. Adrenaline levels drop, and the person's heart rate and blood pressure stabilize to normal. In addition, the generalized feeling of fear, panic, or anxiety subsides as the catecholamines that were released are metabolized and return back to their basal levels.

This is only one example of the numerous feedback loops that are constantly operating in the human body, internal sentinels that are always on duty, ready to react to an individual's particular needs. Of course, most modern situations do not actually require any physical battles to occur between people. However, contemporary humans still have the same basic physical anatomy and the same endocrine system as people had during the earliest times when they needed to survive by either standing up to threats and fighting or by running away from them as fast as possible.

The Endocrine System Works Around the Clock

The endocrine system is comprised of the following key organs: the hypothalamus, the pituitary gland, the pineal gland, the thyroid gland, the parathyroids, the thymus gland, the pancreas, the adrenal glands, the ovaries, and the testes. All these glands are actively involved in both major and minor daily life processes. Researchers have also found that certain organs that were previously not believed to have endocrine functions do, in fact, secrete hormones. Examples include atrial natriutetic factor from the left atrium in the heart, leptin from the fat cells, and angiotensin from the blood vessels.

For example, before people wake up in the morning, the blood levels of many hormones, including cortisol, begin to rise, facilitating the awakening. Cortisol is secreted by the adrenal glands. Its effect is to help to maintain normal blood pressure and blood glucose levels, to maintain a normal level of electrolytes, and also to help people to maintain their vigilance and alertness. Later in the day and during sleep, the cortisol levels will drop to lower yet appropriate levels.

Another hormone, growth hormone, is released in a pulsatile fashion while people sleep. This hormone mediates growth as well as helps to repair the often microscopic damage that has occurred to the tissues, whether a person is eight or 88 years old.

Both cortisol and growth hormone operate in part on a biological cycle, sometimes known as the circadian cycle. They are affected by whether the person is asleep or awake. Other hormones are released fairly continuously, such as thyroid hormone and parathyroid hormone.

After the individual awakes and consumes her breakfast, the pancreas works to keep her blood sugar stable and within a very tight range by producing insulin as needed. How much insulin is needed, though, varies with whether she eats a bran muffin, a Danish, a piece of fruit or, as occurs in some cases, skips breakfast altogether, depleting her energy stores for the morning. Thus, the pancreas is directly affected by, and also affects, the digestive system. In other words, eating food and the type of food that is eaten will trigger changes to the pancreas and the digestive system.

While the person travels to her job, the endocrine glands are still actively functioning, with some glands on standby alert. For example, if another car suddenly darts into the driver's path, the surge of adrenaline released by the adrenal glands (as well as by the sympathetic nervous system) will often enable the driver to react quickly and, one hopes, to allow her to avert a car crash. After the danger subsides, the individual's adrenaline levels will drop back down again as they are no longer needed to keep her at such a high level of alertness.

When an individual arrives at work, her endocrine glands continue to pump out hormones, regulating her blood pressure, blood sugar, calcium transfers from her bones to the blood, and so on. Assuming that she is a healthy woman, her thyroid gland enables her to have normal energy levels. Her pancreas maintains a normal blood sugar level, unless she has diabetes and needs to take medications on a regular basis to attain a normal or near-normal rate of blood sugar. The endocrine glands continue their vigilance with a constant unconscious and involuntary monitoring of the body throughout the day. They adjust the output of hormones as needed. If it is a slow and easy day for the owner of the endocrine glands, they generally need not be as active as when she has difficult physical (or emotional) problems that need to be resolved.

Endocrine Glands Over the Life Span

Endocrine glands affect people over the entire course of their lives. They enable women to achieve pregnancies (or to suffer from problems with infertility), to breast-feed their babies (or to have difficulty with breast-feeding), to respond to crises, and to sleep well or poorly. For example, from the age of puberty until about the age of 50, a woman's ovaries will produce increased and fluctuating levels of estrogen and progesterone hormones, which will affect many aspects of her life.

Estrogen levels will vary during the menstrual cycle. Prior to menstruation, some women develop bloating, headaches, and other symptoms until the onset of their periods. The ovaries also produce eggs that will enable a woman to ovulate and also often to achieve a pregnancy if she has unprotected sex with a fertile man.

Similarly, the testosterone that is produced by the man's testes (also known as the testicles) increases the male libido and contributes to the man's ability to have an erection, enabling intercourse. Testosterone, in conjunction with follicle-stimulating hormone (FSH) and other hormones, allows the development of spermatozoa. Testosterone and other hormones also later facilitate the release of sperm into the man's ejaculate, which can then combine with a fertile woman's egg to create a pregnancy. Low levels of testosterone may result in problems with a male's sexual development, libido, and erectile function as well as his fertility.

Of course, fertility is affected by many different factors, and the key one is age. Fertility declines with age. Women over age 35 are significantly less fertile than women who are younger. Fertility also declines for men as they age, although it does not appear to decline as precipitously or at as young an age in men as in women. Elderly men can father children, although this is not common.

If a woman becomes pregnant, her endocrine glands will adapt to that major body change as well. Once the woman becomes pregnant, the body senses this change and, consequently, ovulation ceases. Prolactin levels may begin to rise during pregnancy. They particularly increase after childbirth, enabling the woman to breast-feed her child. The dopamine that normally inhibits the release of prolactin is not released and thus breast milk can be produced.

Most women are healthy during their pregnancies, but some women experience endocrine difficulties. For example, a small percentage of women develop gestational diabetes that is triggered by the pregnancy. Gestational diabetes is controlled by diet, exercise, and insulin, depending on the severity of the gestational diabetes. Women with gestational diabetes will need to test their blood and monitor their diet closely. They will also need to consult with an endocrinologist as well as with their obstetrician.

Once the woman with gestational diabetes has delivered the baby, her glucose levels will usually return to normal again, although she is at risk for developing gestational diabetes at every subsequent pregnancy. All women with gestational diabetes should have an oral glucose tolerance test six weeks after giving birth. Women who have had gestational diabetes also have an increased risk of developing diabetes mellitus later in life, usually during middle age.

Women who have had Type 1 or Type 2 diabetes prior to their pregnancy will need to monitor their glucose levels closely and carefully watch their diet and exercise levels. In addition, they may need to change their dosages and/or the medications that they take during pregnancy. Women who formerly took oral agents for their Type 2 diabetes may need to take insulin during the pregnancy. Postpartum levels will also need to be checked.

Some pregnant women develop abnormalities of their thyroid levels, becoming hypothyroid or hyperthyroid, although hypothyroidism is more common. The thyroid levels may normalize after delivery or they could also worsen considerably. Pregnant women with even minor thyroid abnormalities should consult with an endocrinologist about their own health and the health of their infants.

After menopause, a woman's estrogen levels drop. Some women experience difficult symptoms, such as hot flashes, insomnia, and mood swings. Some women decide to combat these symptoms by using hormone replacement therapy (HRT), which is a combination of estrogen and progesterone. Those who have had a hysterectomy can safely use only estrogen replacement therapy (ERT). Studies have shown that HRT may be dangerous for some women, particularly those with a family history of breast cancer. ERT has been associated with an increased risk for developing ovarian cancer. Each woman who is considering using hormones (HRT) after menopause must consider the pros and cons of their use and discuss the issue with her gynecologist.

Testosterone levels in men also decline with aging, although few men use testosterone on a regular basis as a hormone therapy in the same way that menopausal women use HRT. Perhaps in the future, testosterone use will become a more standard and accepted medical practice for men, and they will take their TRT (testosterone replacement therapy) every day, along with their morning coffee.

The Endocrine Glands Affect Every Other System in the Body

The endocrine glands affect all other systems in the body. The parathyroid glands, for example, are integral to the health and maintenance of the skeletal system. They utilize both calcium and vitamin D to help with the process of maintaining healthy bones. Illnesses such as osteoporosis or Paget's disease impair the normal production of bone tissue. Patients with hypoparathyroidism, a rare disease of the parathyroid glands that is caused by damage or trauma to the parathyroid glands, develop hypocalcemia, and they need to take supplements of calcium and vitamin D. Malnourished children with rickets also have abnormally mineralized bones, with bowed legs and other abnormal features of the skeleton.

The digestive system is also impacted by the endocrine system in many ways, affecting the individual's overall metabolism, the degree of appetite, and the speed and efficiency of digestion. For example, diabetes mellitus can slow down the stomach emptying and thus slow digestion (a condition called gastroparesis).

Some diseases greatly affect an individual's appetite and feeling of fullness (satiety). The best example of this effect is Prader-Willi syndrome, an endocrine disorder that causes patients to have enormous appetites. The parents or caregivers of children with Prader-Willi syndrome will literally lock up the refrigerator because the children with Prader-Willi syndrome will eat themselves sick.

Such children and adults have severe and continuing problems with obesity, and researchers are seeking a way to help them. The key to resolving Prader-Willi syndrome may also help many people without the disorder but who nonetheless have problems with chronic obesity.

In the circulatory system, the blood and heart are kept healthy by a normal metabolic rate maintained by the thyroid gland. The nervous system and the brain are also affected by the endocrine glands, particularly by the thyroid gland. The skin is affected by the endocrine system. Excessive levels of androgens (male hormones) in a woman can cause severe acne, excessive hair growth (hirsutism), depression, and infertility. These problems, once identified, are usually treatable.

When Problems Occur with the Endocrine System

Sometimes the functioning of one or more of the endocrine glands goes awry. If the highly complex system of feedback loops that tells the body when and how much of certain hormones should be secreted seriously malfunctions, diseases and occasionally even death can result. Yet many different life-threatening malfunctions of the endocrine system are often manageable when competent and caring physicians treat the person.

For example, diabetes mellitus is a common disorder of the endocrine system, affecting an estimated 18 million individuals in the United States. Type 1 diabetes, which affects about 1 million people in the United States, is an autoimmune disorder of the endocrine system caused by the destruction of beta cells in the pancreas. The beta cells within the pancreas make insulin, and without insulin, people die. Fortunately, people who have Type 1 diabetes can inject insulin, enabling most people with this type of diabetes to live long and healthy lives. However, even with insulin injections, people with Type 1 diabetes must still make many accommodations in order to maintain their health and to help avoid the many complications that can occur with diabetes, such as diabetic nephropathy (a kidney disease), diabetic neuropathy (a nerve disease), and diabetic retinopathy (an eye disease) as well as heart attack, strokes, and other health risks.

One major accommodation that people with both Type 1 and Type 2 diabetes must make is to perform daily blood testing of their glucose levels, with subsequent adjustments of their medication and diet based on the blood test findings. For example, if their blood sugar is low (hypoglycemia), these patients need to ingest some glucose in the form of a glucose tablet or fruit. If no better choices are available to them, then sugary food or fluids can provide the needed blood sugar boost.

Type 2 diabetes is a far more common problem than Type 1 diabetes. In those with Type 2 diabetes, the beta cells of the pancreas produce some insulin, although inadequate levels to maintain normal blood glucose levels (euglycemia). These patients need to take oral medications and also test their blood at least several times each day so they can make needed adjustments to their diet, exercise plans, and medications.

Having too much circulating hormone is also possible, whether the hormone is testosterone, estrogen, thyroxine, or any other hormone that the endocrine glands produce. For example, all females produce a small amount of testosterone. However, if too much testosterone is generated by the ovaries, this leads to a virilizing effect, causing the woman's breasts to flatten, increased body hair to grow on the chest and face, and infertility. Fortunately physicians can seek the cause of this condition and then act to treat it.

Endocrine Disorders and Development in Children and Adolescents

Adults are not the only people affected by endocrine diseases; children and adolescents are susceptible as well. For example, if a child or an adolescent develops a tumor of the pituitary that secretes excess growth hormone, he or she may develop gigantism, causing the child or adolescent to grow to very tall heights. Occasionally, the child can exceed seven feet in height. Conversely, a deficiency of growth hormone, due to a malfunction of either the pituitary or the hypothalamus, will lead to growth failure. As a result, the person will be significantly shorter than his or her peers.

Yet these are also conditions that physicians have begun to correct by administering specific medications or growth hormone treatments. Although such treatments may help children tremendously, both physically and psychologically, these treatments continue to be controversial among some physicians. Some experts do not want to alter nature and their philosophical view is that, for example, if a person is biologically destined to be very tall, then he or she *should* be very tall. Others argue that height will affect a person for the rest of his or her life and thus they feel that it is a parent's right to choose to do what is in the best interests of the child, including actions to limit height.

Children and adolescents with suspected or diagnosed endocrine disorders should be treated by pediatric endocrinologists, physicians who specialize in both pediatrics and endocrinology. The father of pediatric endocrinology is regarded by many as Lawson Wilkins, a physician in Baltimore, Maryland, who is said to have established the first endocrine clinic for children at Johns Hopkins in 1935. Other clinics were created, and the specialty evolved further in the mid 1950s and 1960s. By 2002, there were 65 training programs in the United States for pediatric endocrinologists.

The American Board of Pediatrics has an endocrinology board that certifies the training and competence of pediatric endocrinologists in endocrinological diseases, including diabetes. According to a 2004 article in *Pediatric Research*, 927 pediatric endocrinologists have been certified by the board since 1978.

Although most children and adolescents do not experience any disorders of the endocrine system, their endocrine systems do affect normal life changes as they grow. Such life changes include the onset of puberty and, in a female, the onset of menstruation (menarche), the growth of breasts (thelarche), the appearance of underarm hair (adrenarche) and pubic hair (pubarche), and so forth. Boys experience typical male signs of puberty, such as facial and body hair and maturing changes in the testes and penis, as described by Dr. Tanner in 1962 and subsequently called Tanner stages.

The amazing transformation of a child into a man or woman is a major achievement orchestrated by the endocrine system, as is the decline of the hormones, no longer needed after the childbearing years are over. In some cases, however, children develop disorders that may cause either an early puberty (precocious puberty) or a delayed puberty or another growth disorder. Pediatric endocrinologists should be consulted to evaluate and treat such illnesses.

Endocrine Disorders and the Elderly

As individuals age into their senior years, they face an increased risk for developing certain endocrine disorders. These include thyroid disease, particularly hypothyroidism, and bone disorders such as osteoporosis and osteopenia. Elderly individuals also face a greater risk of developing some dangerous and often fatal forms of cancer, particularly tumors of the ovary and the pancreas. Older individuals are also more likely to develop below-normal levels of calcium in the blood (hypocalcemia), a condition that is treatable with both calcium and vitamin D supplements.

In addition, seniors face an increased risk of developing Type 2 diabetes. They urgently need treatment to help avoid the many complications that can occur with untreated diabetes mellitus, such as diabetic retinopathy, diabetic neuropathy, and diabetic nephropathy as well as heart attack and stroke. Elderly men are prone to developing erectile dysfunction (ED), often a treatable condition.

Genetics and the Endocrine System

Sometimes genetic diseases or other influences impair a person's normal sexuality. For example, in Turner syndrome, a medical problem found only in females, one of the X chromosomes is either missing or impaired. Thus the female does not develop normally. As a result, women with this disorder experience a broad variety of medical problems. With Klinefelter syndrome, a genetic condition inherited only by males, the male has two or more X chromosomes in addition to the Y chromosome. This condition causes small testes and infertility.

Many other endocrine diseases and disorders have an underlying genetic element. For example, the children of parents with diabetes mellitus have an increased risk for development of diabetes. Autoimmune disorders, such as thyroid diseases, often have a familial link. An example of just a few other endocrine diseases with a strong genetic component include adrenal leukodystrophy, Carney complex, congenital adrenal hyperplasia, Graves' disease, and McCune-Albright syndrome.

Of course, having a genetic predisposition to develop an endocrine disease or disorder does not mean that a person is doomed to develop the illness. Instead, it means that the risk for developing such a disorder is increased when a family member (such as a parent or sibling) has that disorder, compared with other individuals whose family members do not have the disorder.

Most doctors take careful family medical histories from patients because they want to take note of potential health problems. That way, they can be vigilant about the problem and administer periodic tests, as appropriate. For example, if a person has parents with diabetes mellitus, the physician is likely to watch for diabetes in this person, particularly if the person begins to exhibit any symptoms of the disease.

Psychological Effects of Endocrine Disorders

Endocrine disease can have a profound impact on the emotional and mental health of those afflicted. For example, people who are hyperthyroid can sometimes seem almost manic in their behavior, while those who are hypothyroid may appear depressed and lethargic. Psychiatric drugs will not resolve these problems. Only a proper diagnosis can lead to effective treatment.

Ironically, sometimes the treatment for existing psychiatric illnesses can result in endocrine disorders. For example, lithium is a medication that is often given to treat individuals with bipolar disorder (manic depression). Lithium can induce a form of diabetes insipidus (nephrogenic DI) as well as induce hypercalcemia, hyperparathyroidism, hyperthyroidism, hypothyroidism, and thyroiditis.

As a result, patients who are exhibiting new psychiatric symptoms should be screened for an endocrine disorder. In addition, if patients have both psychiatric problems and endocrine diseases, psychiatrists and endocrinologists should work together to provide the best treatment for the patient.

Cancer and the Endocrine System

Sometimes cancer strikes the endocrine organs. The prognosis for patients who develop such cancers ranges from good, with forms of cancer such as testicular cancer and thyroid cancer, to very poor, as with ovarian cancer or pancreatic cancer. The reason for the high death rates among most people diagnosed with ovarian cancer or pancreatic cancer is that symptoms usually do not appear until the disease has spread to other organs and is no longer curable.

Researchers are actively seeking better ways to diagnose and treat cancers of the ovaries and the pancreas. Research breakthroughs with earlier diagnoses and better treatments are anticipated in the years ahead. As of this writing, for example, scientists are evaluating a test that may indicate a marker for early ovarian cancer. If the test works, the disease would be far more treatable than at later stages, when the disease is now usually discovered.

Yet there is considerable hope for the future, even in cases of ovarian cancer and pancreatic cancer, as research continues. Of importance is that as recently as the 1970s, a diagnosis of testicular cancer was essentially a death sentence for the men who developed the disease. However, research and advances that have occurred since then have made most cases of testicular cancer not only treatable but also frequently curable.

Zeroing in on the Endocrine Glands

Each gland of the endocrine system has at least one (and usually more than one) distinctively important function. In a healthy person, the glands in the endocrine system work together smoothly. Sometimes, though, medical problems and conditions occur that can impair the endocrine system as well as the overall harmony of the body. The individual glands themselves may malfunction due to disease, an autoimmune disorder, or another reason. In addition, external factors may impair the endocrine glands, such as when a person is in a car crash or other accident and the pituitary or other glands are damaged.

In addition to the known hormones that are released by the endocrine glands, more than 40 different hormones are produced within the gastrointestinal tract. Many of their functions are still unknown. Other organs such as the heart (specifically, the left atrium) produce hormones such as peptides.

The following are some examples of the glands in the endocrine system as well as potential medical problems that may occur in these glands. These topics are also discussed in the entries throughout this encyclopedia.

The Hypothalamus and the Pituitary Gland

The hypothalamus is a complex gland. It controls the function of the pituitary gland and also directly affects the release of the seven pituitary hormones. Corticotropin-releasing hormone (CRH) factor stimulates the release of adrenocorticotropic hormone (ACTH). Thyrotropin-releasing hormone (TRH)

stimulates the release of thyroid-stimulating hormone (TSH). Growth hormone-releasing hormone (GHRH) stimulates the release of growth hormone (GH). Gonadotropin-releasing hormone (GNRH) stimulates the release of both luteinizing hormone (LH) and follicle-stimulating hormone (FSH). Dopamine inhibits the release of prolactin (PRL). Desmopressin acetate (DDAVP) is relayed via neurons to the posterior pituitary gland to help regulate fluid and also salt and water balance in the body.

In addition, the hypothalamus also includes centers that directly affect the libido, the individual's appetite (the desire to eat), as well as the feeling of fullness after eating (satiety). Malfunctions of the hypothalamus can sometimes be minor, but they can also become severe and even life threatening.

The hypothalamus and the pituitary glands together control the overall growth and development of a child, but they continue to be important for people of all ages. Even elderly people secrete small levels of growth hormone.

The hypothalamus also helps to maintain both a normal body temperature and blood pressure.

When the hypothalamus or pituitary glands malfunction, they can cause extremely large or extremely small size in children and adults. Andre the Giant was an example of a person whose pituitary gland caused him to develop gigantism as a child. If the pituitary gland malfunctions in a similar way in an adult, as with acromegaly, it will not cause increased height because the bones are already fused and completed (longitudinal growth). However, the cartilage and tissue can still grow and can also overgrow. This results in a much distorted personal appearance, causing a person to suffer from facial or other physical deformities. Acromegaly is treatable with surgery, radiation therapy, and medications.

A malfunctioning pituitary gland may result in a person with a moon-faced appearance who suffers from obesity, hypertension, and diabetes. Harvey Williams Cushing discovered this medical problem, stemming from excessive ACTH secretion from the pituitary, in 1932. It was subsequently named Cushing's disease.

An excess of cortisol (hypercortisolism) can also initiate from a cause other than the pituitary gland,

ENDOCRINE SYSTEM

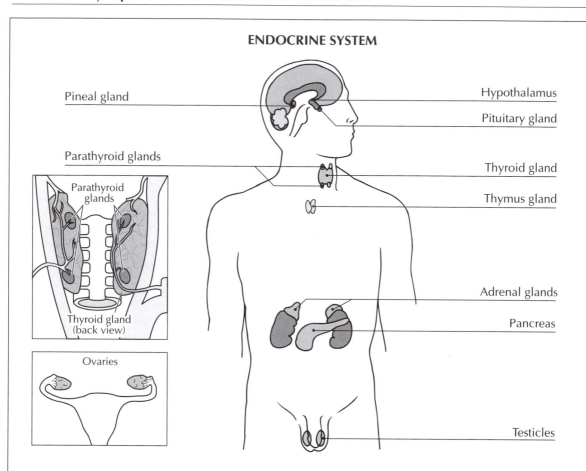

Pineal gland

Hypothalamus

Pituitary gland

Parathyroid glands

Thyroid gland

Thymus gland

Parathyroid glands

Adrenal glands

Pancreas

Thyroid gland (back view)

Ovaries

Testicles

Your endocrine system is a collection of glands that produce hormones that regulate your body's growth, metabolism, and sexual development and function. The hormones are released into the bloodstream and transported to tissues and organs throughout your body. The table below describes the function of these glands.

Adrenal glands	Divided into 2 regions; secrete hormones that influence the body's metabolism, blood chemicals, and body characteristics, as well as influence the part of the nervous system that is involved in the response and defense against stress
Hypothalamus	Activates and controls the part of the nervous system that controls involuntary body functions, the hormonal system, and many body functions, such as regulating sleep and stimulating appetite
Ovaries and testicles	Secrete hormones that influence female and male characteristics, respectively
Pancreas	Secretes a hormone (insulin) that controls the use of glucose by the body
Parathyroid glands	Secrete a hormone that maintains the calcium level in the blood
Pineal body	Involved with daily biological cycles
Pituitary gland	Produces a number of different hormones that influence various other endocrine glands
Thymus gland	Plays a role in the body's immune system
Thyroid gland	Produces hormones that stimulate body heat production, bone growth, and the body's metabolism

(CREDIT: American Medical Association)

and in such a case, the disease is known as Cushing's syndrome rather than Cushing's disease. Both Cushing's syndrome and Cushing's disease include the same array of medical problems: obesity, diabetes, hypertension, and other illnesses.

The Thyroid Gland

The thyroid gland is a very important butterfly-shaped organ situated in the neck. It controls the basic metabolism of the body and affects an individual's energy levels, sleep cycles, hair growth, skin texture, and even fertility. Hypothyroidism, or an underactive thyroid gland, is a type of thyroid malfunction that results in patients becoming lethargic and apathetic. The individual may also suffer from widespread aches and body pains. Sometimes the patient may be misdiagnosed with another medical problem altogether, such as arthritis or fibromyalgia.

Simple blood tests, along with clinical observations of a patient and a thorough evaluation of the patient's signs and symptoms, can usually determine whether the patient's thyroid levels are within the normal range. In the mid-20th century, doctors determined that a patient had abnormal thyroid levels by measuring the patient's basal metabolic rate (BMR) upon awakening using special hospital equipment that measured oxygen consumption. The BMR test, however, was proven to be an extremely inefficient and imprecise way to ascertain the presence of thyroid disease. Another test, the radioactive iodine uptake scan, used equipment to determine the biological activity of the gland as well as its size and contour.

In the mid-20th century, researchers also developed a blood test to measure thyroid hormone in the blood, using protein-bound iodine (PBI) measurements to diagnose thyroid disease. In the latter part of the 20th century, the more sophisticated thyroid-stimulating hormone (TSH) blood test was developed. As of this writing, the TSH test is still considered the gold standard for diagnosing most thyroid diseases.

The thyroid gland can go into overdrive, becoming hyperthyroid or overactive. The gland may enlarge and develop a goiter, which is sometimes visible even to a layperson. Medications can often dampen the overactive effect of hyperthyroidism, but surgery or radioactive iodine may also be required to manage this illness.

Thyroid surgery has been used on patients since the late 19th century when surgeon Theodor Kocher developed procedures to remove the thyroid gland to treat patients who had tumors and goiters. Kocher received the Nobel Prize in 1909 for his successful work with the thyroid gland. However, doctors also found that removing too much thyroid tissue left patients very ill. Kocher himself noted that the total thyroidectomy caused patients to suffer serious consequences.

In 1891, British physician George Murray isolated thyroid extracts from sheep. He provided them to a severely hypothyroid patient who subsequently improved and took the thyroid supplements for 28 more years. In 1927, researchers first synthesized thyroid hormones and found that the synthetic form of thyroid was as effective as the thyroid hormone extracted from animals.

Today, most people in the United States who need thyroid hormones take levothyroxine, a synthetic form of thyroid hormone. In fact, Synthroid, a form of levothyroxine, is one of the top 10 best-selling medications of all types in the United States.

Some people suffer from autoimmune thyroid diseases in which the body mistakenly perceives the thyroid gland as if it were a bacterial invasion. In such cases, the immune system actively seeks to destroy the thyroid gland.

In one syndrome, the antibodies actually stimulate the gland to enlarge and to become overactive. The symptomatology of hyperactivity, an enlarged thyroid gland and bulbous eyes, was first identified by Irish physician Robert James Graves in 1835 and was subsequently named after him. Graves' disease is an autoimmune hyperthyroid disorder that has been experienced by many people, including former President George H. W. Bush and his wife Barbara Bush, as well as by the late John F. Kennedy Jr. The comedian Marty Feldman, recognizable by his very bulging eyes, also had Graves' disease. For most patients, Graves' disease is treatable with medications and surgery.

Hashimoto's thyroiditis, an autoimmune disorder that was first described by Japanese physician Dr. H. Hashimoto in 1912, is the most common cause of hypothyroidism in the United States. It may initially cause individuals to become transiently hyperthyroid. Then, as the gland is further destroyed by the disease, patients develop hypothyroidism.

In rare cases, infants are born with congenital hypothyroidism, which would, if left untreated, cause severe developmental delays and retardation. Fortunately, all newborn infants in the United States are screened for thyroid disease. If it is detected, they are immediately treated with iodine, thyroid drugs, or other medications and are carefully followed by their pediatricians.

The thyroid may also develop cancer. Fortunately, in many cases it is a slow-growing cancer that is identifiable and treatable. Sometimes the thyroid gland develops nodules, which may be solid, cystic, or a combination of solid and cystic. Thyroid nodules are often biopsied for cancer, although they are often benign.

The Pancreas

The pancreas is a critical organ that maintains and fuels the body in the process of digestion and the assimilation of nutrients. Its functions are essential to life. If the pancreas fails, the insulin and the digestive enzymes that it normally produces must be replaced for the person to survive. This is achieved through medication or, in the most extreme case, through a pancreatic transplant from a recently deceased person. In many cases, it is achieved through the administration of insulin.

Insulin was discovered in 1921 by Canadian doctor Frederick Banting and then–medical student Charles Best, who first tested insulin on diabetic dogs. When the dogs' health improved, Banting and Best went on to test insulin on diabetic children and adults, with success.

Before this discovery of insulin, every person with Type 1 diabetes died from the disease. They often succumbed in their childhood, teens, or early adulthood. Insulin has been synthesized and considerably improved upon since then. However, this remarkable early discovery has enabled millions of people worldwide to lead normal lives. People with Type 1 diabetes today stay alive only because they inject insulin.

In some cases, the pancreas produces a subnormal amount of insulin or even an amount that would usually be sufficient for survival, but the person's body is unable to use the insulin because of insulin resistance. Such patients have Type 2 diabetes, which is a major endocrine disease affecting millions of people in the United States and other countries.

People who are alcoholics often experience damage to their pancreas caused by excessive drinking and poor nutrition. This may lead to pancreatitis, a severely painful and dangerous inflammation of the pancreas.

Pancreatic cancer is another malfunction of the pancreas. As of this writing, few people survive this deadly form of cancer, because it is rarely detectable in its early stages. As a result, once the characteristic jaundice (yellowing of the skin) of pancreatic cancer is clearly visible, death typically follows. (The presence of jaundice alone does not always indicate that a person has pancreatic cancer. Hepatitis and other diseases may also cause jaundice. However, whenever a person of any age is jaundiced, physicians should actively seek to identify the cause so that treatment may begin.)

The pancreas is an unusual organ in that it is both an endocrine gland and an exocrine gland. An endocrine gland is ductless, while an exocrine gland contains ducts. Depending on which function is being considered, the pancreas is an endocrine gland or an exocrine gland. For example, the islets cells of the pancreas produce insulin, which is an endocrine function. However, the pancreas also produces digestive enzymes, which is an exocrine function. Even people with diabetes who depend on insulin have pancreases that produce digestive enzymes.

The Parathyroid Glands

Although most people have never heard of the parathyroid glands, they are very important glands. The parathyroids are tiny glands that are embedded in and around the thyroid gland. They are directly responsible for regulating the flow of calcium from the blood and into the bones and then back again as needed throughout the day and night. The parathyroid glands directly affect the healthy functioning of an individual's bones, kidneys, and gut.

Calcium is necessary for life. Without it, a person will eventually go into seizures (tetany) and, if the condition continues uncorrected, will die.

Fortunately, severe hypocalcemia is rare. When it does occur (such as with the accidental removal of or injury to the parathyroids during thyroid surgery), it is nearly always easily treatable with intravenous calcium followed by maintenance doses of oral calcium and vitamin D after the patient recovers from the surgery.

Having too much calcium is also possible, a condition called hypercalcemia. This can lead to kidney stones, malaise, decreased cognitive function, osteoporosis, and a host of other serious medical problems. Hypercalcemia often stems from either hyperparathyroidism or cancer.

The parathyroid glands can also become cancerous.

The Adrenal Glands

The adrenal glands are two glands located adjacent to the kidneys and close to the pancreas. They are organs essential to healthy growth and development and also sustain normal life. The adrenal glands produce adrenaline, cortisol, and aldosterone as well as androgens, and deficiencies of these hormones can lead to serious diseases. Hypofunctioning adrenal glands can lead to Addison's disease, while hyperfunctioning leads to Cushing's syndrome and adrenal hyperplasia. The adrenal glands also affect the overall metabolism of the body.

Addison's disease, a malfunction of the adrenal glands causing inadequate levels of circulating cortisol, is a dangerous and sometimes life-threatening condition that requires lifelong monitoring by physicians and the patients themselves. Thomas Addison first described this disorder of the adrenal glands, which caused skin darkening and was life threatening, to the South London Medical Society in 1855. The disease was subsequently named after him, although Dr. Addison reportedly received no acknowledgment for his important discovery within his lifetime. Cushing's syndrome and Addison's disease are both diseases that, once identified, are treatable. Patients and their physicians must continue to be alert to changes in cortisol levels and treat them accordingly.

The adrenal glands can also develop a cancerous tumor. Adrenocortical carcinoma is a rare and highly malignant tumor, more commonly found among middle-aged females. Tumors called pheochromocytomas can also occur in the adrenal medulla.

The Pineal Gland

The pineal gland is a somewhat mysterious gland with functions that are yet to be fully explored. Scientists do know that the pineal gland produces natural melatonin, which is the hormone that helps people to fall asleep. It is also involved in the daily sleep/wake cycles. Some experts suspect that melatonin may be more important than has been previously realized, and they have begun studying the relationship of melatonin to other hormones such as testosterone.

Some early studies indicate that low levels of melatonin are linked to low levels of testosterone. By increasing testosterone levels (by administering testosterone to males with low blood levels of this hormone), researchers have found that melatonin levels will also increase. In addition, if administering supplements of melatonin to raise a man's melatonin levels, his testosterone levels will apparently increase as well. Further studies may bring important new information about melatonin and the pineal gland.

The Ovaries

The ovaries are the source of female sexual characteristics as well as of female fertility. The ovaries produce hormones, such as estrogen, that lead to female sexual characteristics, such as soft skin and hair, healthy breasts, and a functioning reproductive system. Estrogen was isolated as a hormone by researchers in the early 20th century, as was testosterone. The ovaries also release an egg each month that can unite with a sperm to create an ovum and, ultimately, a pregnancy.

Because many women throughout time have wished to avoid or delay pregnancy, many women and their partners were extremely pleased when the first oral contraceptive was developed and sold in the United States in 1960. This drug was based on studies by such researchers as Gregory Pincus, who showed that progesterone prevented ovulation.

When ovaries malfunction, they can become extremely disruptive, causing pain, excessive menstrual bleeding (or the lack of menstrual periods, which is known as amenorrhea), infertility, extreme hair growth, and other medical problems.

Polycystic ovary syndrome (PCOS) is a medical condition that causes great distress to some women. It may cause moderate to extreme hairiness (hirsutism), anovulation (failure to ovulate), infertility, and other serious medical problems. If PCOS is left untreated, women may develop Type 2 diabetes and cardiovascular diseases.

Another disease of the ovaries is ovarian cancer, a disease that is extremely dangerous and one that is not usually detected until it is inoperable, as with pancreatic cancer. Researchers have recently developed a blood test for early ovarian cancer, and experts are evaluating this test as of this writing. It may have the potential to save the lives of thousands of women each year by allowing ovarian cancer to be treated in the early stages.

Sometimes women develop ovarian cysts, which are fluid-filled and usually benign growths on the ovaries. These cysts can become large and extremely painful. They may require surgery. However, some women have cysts that cause no pain or any other symptoms for years or even ever. These ovarian cysts are detected only during a routine ultrasound or other imaging test that is performed for another purpose.

The Testes

Just as the ovaries are responsible for female sexuality and fertility, the testes are vitally important to male sexuality. The testes control both the male sex drive and the ability to reproduce. Testosterone, a hormone released by the testes, creates and drives male sexual characteristics, such as muscle mass, body hair, and sexuality. If a male loses his testes before puberty, he will not develop a deepened voice or body hair. If one or even both testes are lost after puberty, however (for example, because of testicular cancer), the man's deep male voice will not change nor will his basic adult male characteristics.

The most common malfunction of the testes is an underproduction of testosterone (hypogonadism), which is a problem that men of all ages may experience, although it is far more commonly seen among older men. Testicular cancer is another medical problem of the testes that may also

occur, and it is diagnosed most frequently among men in their 20s–40s. Fortunately, testicular cancer is usually detectable and treatable, and the survival rate is high. In addition, if the man loses one of his two testes, he will usually retain normal sexual function and will remain fertile.

The Thymus

The thymus is a very small endocrine organ located in the chest. As far as is known, it does little except contribute to some immune functions. Future research may reveal a more important role for the thymus than is currently known.

Newer Hormones and Endocrine Discoveries

As research continues, scientists are discovering many more key hormones that are directly linked to the endocrine system. For example, in the late 20th century, scientists in Japan discovered that the stomach produces a hormone called ghrelin, which is intimately associated with both appetite and satiety. Because obesity is a major problem in North America, Europe, and other parts of the globe, researchers are attempting to determine if obesity can possibly be resolved by manipulating the appetite, perhaps by creating an antighrelin kind of medication. In fact, researchers are currently seeking to develop such a medication.

Major Breakthroughs in Treatments of Endocrine Diseases and Disorders

Probably the greatest recent breakthroughs in treating endocrine diseases have come with startling advances in treating diabetes mellitus. For example, physicians have successfully implanted insulin-producing cells from the pancreases of deceased individuals into patients with Type 1 diabetes, and these individuals no longer need to take any insulin.

In another recent success, in 2003, scientists at Massachusetts General Hospital found that injecting spleen cells into the pancreas of diabetic rats somehow caused the pancreatic cells of the rats to regenerate. This treatment actually cured the laboratory animals of their diabetes. Researchers were not expecting this result at all. As of this writing, they are not clear on how or why it happened; for years, the spleen has been regarded by experts as an expendable organ.

This research finding is potentially a huge breakthrough for people with diabetes mellitus. Human clinical trials will be performed to test whether the same results can be found in people. If so, this may lead to what so many patients and doctors have dreamed of for so long: a cure for diabetes.

Breakthroughs have also been made with the testing equipment used by patients with diabetes to determine their own blood sugar levels. Because many patients with diabetes are resistant to testing their blood because of the pain and the inconvenience, researchers have developed devices that can nearly painlessly extract a tiny amount of subcutaneous fluid from the forearm, and a display readout will show the patient the results of the test within minutes.

Some patients have enormous difficulty maintaining normal insulin levels. Researchers have recently developed implantable insulin pumps that dole out regular amounts of insulin and can be ordered to provide extra doses on an as-needed basis. These are only two examples of devices that have been created to encourage patients with diabetes to test their blood and to act upon the findings.

Future Advances

Many medical advances in the diagnosis and treatment of endocrine diseases are anticipated over the next decade and even earlier. Scientists hope to discover how to use hormones in newer and more innovative ways. For example, peptide hormones will likely be created as a therapy for many patients. In addition, experts anticipate that hormonal therapies will be used not only to kill abnormal cells but also to grow beneficial and healthy cells. Monoclonal antibodies will be developed for early detection of cancers and detection of cancer spread, as well as to create better therapies for treating cancer.

Conclusion

Most people never realize the importance of their endocrine glands to their continued survival or even that they have such glands working actively to keep them alive and healthy. Yet these under-appreciated glands and the entire endocrine system itself can greatly enhance life as well as cause extremely serious and even life-threatening medical problems.

This encyclopedia provides basic information about how the glands and hormones within the endocrine system function when the system works normally. It also helps explain what happens when serious medical problems occur and offers information on how physicians work to help their patients resolve these problems.

Fisher, D. A. "A Short History of Pediatric Endocrinology in North America." *Pediatric Research* 55 (2004): 716–726.

Gardner, Lytt I., M.D., ed. *Endocrine and Genetic Diseases of Childhood and Adolescence,* 2d ed. Philadelphia, Pa.: W. B. Saunders Company, 1975.

Gordon, Richard. *The Alarming History of Medicine.* New York: St Martin's Griffin, 1993.

Kodama, Shohta, et al. "Islet Regeneration During the Reversal of Autoimmune Diabetes in NOD Mice," *Science* 302 (November 14, 2003): 1,223–1,227.

McDermott, Michael T., M.D. *Endocrine Secrets.* Philadelphia, Pa.: Hanley & Belfus, Inc., 2002.

Neal, J. Matthew, M.D. *How the Endocrine System Works.* Williston, Vt.: Blackwell Publishing, 2002.

Niewoehner, Catherine B., M.D. *Endocrine Pathophysiology.* Madison, Conn.: Fence Creek Publishing, 1998.

Petit, William, Jr., M.D., and Christine Adamec. *The Encyclopedia of Diabetes.* New York: Facts On File, Inc., 2002.

Porter, Roy, ed. *The Cambridge Illustrated History of Medicine.* Cambridge, England: Cambridge University Press, 1996.

Porterfield, Susan P. *Endocrine Physiology,* 2d ed. St. Louis, Mo.: Mosby, Inc., 2001.

Stanbury, John B., M.D. *A Constant Ferment: A History of the Thyroid Clinic and Laboratory at the Massachusetts General Hospital: 1913–1990.* Ipswich, Mass.: The Ipswich Press, 1991.

Tanner, J. M., M.D. *Growth at Adolescence with a General Consideration of the Effects of Hereditary and Environmental Factors Upon Growth and Maturation from* *Birth to Maturity,* 2d ed. Springfield, Ill.: Charles C. Thomas, 1962.

ENTRIES A–Z

acanthosis nigricans   A hereditary skin condition that is commonly found among patients with severe INSULIN RESISTANCE (a condition in which the body is not able to use the insulin produced efficiently and, thus, attempts to overcome this problem by synthesizing more insulin). In rare cases, acanthosis nigricans is a marker for an aggressive form of internal cancer (malignant acanthosis nigricans). In particular, it indicates cancers of the liver or gastrointestinal tract (hepatocellular cancer and gastric cancer).

With the exception of malignant acanthosis nigricans, the condition is more common among people of African descent, followed by those of Hispanic descent, although individuals of any race may develop acanthosis nigricans. Some medications, such as corticosteroids, ORAL CONTRACEPTIVES, niacin, or GROWTH HORMONES, may sometimes induce the development of acanthosis nigricans. Physicians have been aware of acanthosis nigricans since the 19th century.

The incidence of acanthosis nigricans in the population is unknown. Both men and women may develop this condition. It is also found among children and adolescents.

Signs and Symptoms

Acanthosis nigricans is characterized both by its appearance on the skin and its texture. The skin is often described as having a soft and velvety texture. The skin has gray or black patches that give it an overall burned appearance and that cause it to appear dirty in these areas. The dark areas are caused by an excessive amount of melanin, a hormone that increases natural skin color. If the skin becomes thick enough, it may become malodorous and macerated.

When present, acanthosis nigricans is usually found on the neck. However, it may also appear on the elbows, knees, groin, underarms, knuckles, and even around the thighs and the anus. The patient may also have many papillomas (benign skin tumors or skin tags) as well as a generalized thickening of the skin (hyperkeratosis). The skin areas affected by acanthosis nigricans are often hairless.

Diagnosis and Associated Medical Conditions

Acanthosis nigricans may be diagnosed in infancy or early childhood but generally does not appear until adolescence or adulthood. Unless it is related to a malignancy, acanthosis nigricans is typically associated with insulin resistance syndrome.

The presence of acanthosis nigricans may be a risk factor for the development of TYPE 2 DIABETES. In one study of 89 African Americans with acanthosis nigricans, 21 percent of the patients were found to have Type 2 diabetes. Acanthosis nigricans is also found in some patients who have been diagnosed with ACROMEGALY and CUSHING'S SYNDROME. In addition, it may also be associated with OBESITY and/or POLYCYSTIC OVARY SYNDROME (PCOS) as well as with HYPOTHYROIDISM.

As of this writing, there is no cure for acanthosis nigricans: however, identifying the underlying cause of this condition is important so that it can be treated.

The agents used to lighten skin coloration have limited success in the treatment of acanthosis nigricans.

See also DWARFISM; SKIN.

Levine, Norman, M.D. "Acanthosis Nigricans," Available online. URL: http://www.emedicine.com/DERM/topic1.htm Downloaded on June 14, 2002.
Stuart, C. A., et al. "Hyperinsulinemia and Acanthosis Nigricans in African Americans." *Journal of the National Medical Association* 89, no. 8 (August 1997): 523–527.

Wynbrandt, James, and Mark D. Ludman. *The Encyclopedia of Genetic Disorders and Birth Defects,* 2d ed. New York: Facts On File, Inc., 2000.

achondroplasia   See DWARFISM; GROWTH HORMONE.

ACTH (adrenocorticotropic hormone)   A protein hormone that is synthesized and secreted from the anterior pituitary gland in a pulsatile manner following a specific circadian rhythm (biological cycle). In most people, their ACTH production is at its highest level in the morning when they wake up and at its lowest level in the late afternoon. ACTH stimulates the adrenal glands to cause growth and the production of steroid hormones, especially CORTISOL. ACTH is initially secreted as a prohormone called PMOC (pro-opiomelanocortin), which contains lipotropins, endorphin, and melanocyte-stimulating hormone (MSH) that can lead to hyperpigmentation.

This excessive skin pigmentation can be seen in diseases such as ADDISON'S DISEASE or primary adrenal insufficiency. In these cases, inadequate cortisol is produced, thus decreasing the inhibition of the hypothalamus on cortisol release (CR) and the anterior pituitary for ACTH. In Cushing's disease, in which ACTH is overproduced, hyperpigmentation can also be seen. With some cancers, such as small cell carcinoma of the lung, ectopic ACTH may be produced in very large amounts, leading to hyperpigmentation and a Cushing's-like syndrome.

Stress, such as that from a trauma, serious infection, or surgery, can cause higher than normal levels of ACTH to be secreted. HYPOGLYCEMIA (low blood sugar) leads to appropriate physiological increase in ACTH levels. Some emotional states, such as anxiety or depression, can raise the levels of ACTH. In contrast, cortisol is a hormone that inhibits the release of ACTH.

See also ADRENAL GLANDS; CUSHING'S SYNDROME/ CUSHING'S DISEASE; HORMONES; PITUITARY GLAND.

acromegaly   A rare endocrine disorder generally caused by a benign pituitary tumor that secretes excessive amounts of growth hormone. These growth hormone-secreting pituitary tumors or adenomas account for about one-third of all pituitary tumors. Rarely, the tumor leading to acromegaly may be cancerous.

Acromegaly is also called GIGANTISM if it presents before puberty because the excessive levels of growth hormone cause individuals to attain unusual heights. If the disorder presents after puberty, the individual does not grow taller but will likely present with characteristic abnormalities that may significantly alter his or her appearance. It will flatten both the nose and face and will cause the enlargement of any bones that have not yet completed their growth, such as the jaw, hands, and feet.

An overgrowth of tissue in the nasopharyngeal area (nose/tongue/throat) may cause hoarseness and may even cause sleep apnea, a potentially dangerous condition in which the person stops breathing for frequent, short periods during sleep. Snoring is also quite common among patients with acromegaly.

Causes of Acromegaly

Acromegaly occurs in only about three to four people per million. About 20–30 percent of patients with acromegaly also have DIABETES MELLITUS. In other rare cases, tumors of the pancreas, lungs, or adrenal glands (commonly carcinoid tumors) may cause acromegaly by secreting growth hormone. Acromegaly may also be caused by the secretion of another hormone: growth hormone-releasing hormone (GHRH). This hormone stimulates the secretion of growth hormone from the pituitary. The hypothalamus, an area of the brain just above the pituitary that secretes many hormones that help regulate the pituitary's function, may also secrete excessive GHRH, and this secretion may cause acromegaly.

Signs and Symptoms of Acromegaly

There are many different indicators of the presence of acromegaly. Some signs and symptoms of this disorder are as follows:

- Oily skin
- Headaches (in 60 percent of patients)
- Achy joints (arthralgias)
- Back pain (which may be secondary due to

fractures from OSTEOPOROSIS stemming from decreased estrogen or testosterone levels)

- Extreme sweating (hyperhydrosis)
- Generalized weakness/malaise
- Skin tags (achrochordons)
- Hypertension (high blood pressure)
- Thickened skin
- Excess enlargement of the mouth, nose, and tongue (acral growth, leading to deformities of the face and teeth)
- Deepening voice
- Irregular menstrual cycles with lowered estrogen levels leading to vaginal dryness and hot flashes
- ERECTILE DYSFUNCTION/lowered libido/decreased beard growth/testicular atrophy (due to decreased levels of testosterone)
- Increased prolactin levels, causing galactorrhea (breast milk production in non-nursing females) and hirsutism (excessive hair growth in women)
- Carpal tunnel syndrome (compressed median nerve, accompanied by numbness, tingling, and weakness in the wrist, thumb, index, or middle finger)

Diagnosis of Acromegaly

The diagnosis of acromegaly is usually delayed a long time in adults—by as long as 15 to 20 years. This occurs because the onset of this medical problem is slow and insidious. Additionally, the signs and symptoms of acromegaly are not immediately obvious.

In fact, the changes in the person's facial features usually occur so slowly that many patients and their own family members do not notice them. Awareness of these changes often occurs only due to the observation from someone who is outside the family or who has not seen the person for years. As a result, a person may not be diagnosed with acromegaly until 35–50 years old, even though the problem may have begun many years before then. In contrast, however, gigantism is very noticeable and it is diagnosed in the individual during or prior to adolescence.

Physicians who suspect a patient may have acromegaly will often ask the patient to bring in photographs from 10–20 years before in order to check these photographs for the typical facial changes of the disease. The physician who suspects acromegaly/gigantism may also order a fasting blood test (impaired glucose fasting level) of growth hormone and/or insulin-like growth factor 1 (IGF-1). These levels are both increased in people with acromegaly/gigantism.

Patients suspected of having acromegaly may also be tested simultaneously for diabetes with an ORAL GLUCOSE TOLERANCE TEST. This test can serve a dual purpose. For patients with normal GROWTH HORMONE secretion, the ingestion of glucose will lead to decreased levels of growth hormone. In contrast, the abnormal secretion of growth hormone found in acromegaly is not suppressible and will not decrease after giving glucose. As a result, if the growth hormone levels have not dropped, then acromegaly is likely. In addition, the patient's blood glucose levels can be measured to determine if the patient has normal glucose tolerance, impaired glucose tolerance, or overt diabetes mellitus.

Imaging tests such as COMPUTERIZED TOMOGRAPHY (CT) scans or MAGNETIC RESONANCE IMAGING (MRI) scans of the pituitary gland are also ordered. These help to identify tumors that may be causing the acromegaly.

Medical Problems Caused By or Associated With Acromegaly

Patients with acromegaly have an increased risk of developing thyroid disorders, such as GOITERS and HASHIMOTO'S THYROIDITIS. In one study that was reported in a 2002 issue of the *Journal of Endocrinology Investigation*, 78 percent of the patients with acromegaly also had thyroid abnormalities.

In addition to causing thyroid disease in the majority of patients and causing diabetes in about a third of them, acromegaly may be the cause of other medical problems. These include hypertension (about 25 percent of acromegaly patients are hypertensive), cardiomyopathy (abnormal heart pumping action), arthritis, HYPOTHYROIDISM, HYPOGONADISM (the decreased ability to make sex steroid hormones due to damage to the pituitary cells that control TESTOSTERONE and ESTRADIOL synthesis), and kidney stones.

Patients with acromegaly may also experience visual problems, especially visual field abnormalities. These occur because the tumor can grow into the optic chiasm (the major cranial nerve to the eyes that lies just above the pituitary gland).

In addition, individuals with acromegaly are at a greater risk for developing polyps in the colon as well as for developing colorectal cancer. As a result, experts recommend that for patients with acromegaly, a colonoscopy should be performed every two to four years, depending on the recommendation of the treating physician.

Individuals with acromegaly also face an increased risk for developing other forms of cancer. Dr. D. Baris and colleagues studied the outcomes for patients with acromegaly in Sweden (1965–93) and Denmark (1977–93) and reported their findings in a 2002 issue of *Cancer Causes and Control.* They found that patients with acromegaly had a significantly increased risk of developing various forms of cancer, particularly cancer of the small intestine, colon, and rectum. The patients also faced increased risks for developing cancers of the brain, thyroid, kidney, and bone.

The death rate for patients with acromegaly is two to four times the normal rate. Death typically results from cancer or heart disease unless the growth hormone and IGF-1 levels can be brought back into the normal range.

Treatment of Acromegaly

All patients with acromegaly should be treated due to the multiple complications and high mortality caused by this medical problem. Acromegaly is often treated with pituitary surgery (usually through the sphenoid sinuses, with a technique called transsphenoidal surgery). This procedure is successful in about 80–90 percent of the cases.

Neurosurgery is performed if the physician identifies a microadenoma (a pituitary tumor less than 10 millimeters in size) or a macroadenoma (a tumor greater than 10 millimeters in size) that is pushing into the optic nerve or into the cavernous sinuses (the very large veins found on both sides of the pituitary that contain several cranial nerves, the carotid artery, and the jugular vein). The neurosurgeon will perform surgery only if he or she thinks the patient can be cured or significantly helped. Remission of many of the patient's symptoms, particularly the facial abnormalities, will gen-

erally occur within days after surgery. Some patients are treated with radiation therapy, either as the primary treatment or as a supplemental treatment after having surgery.

Medications are also a common form of treatment for patients with acromegaly. BROMOCRIPTINE (Parlodel), pergolide (Permax), and CABERGOLINE (Dostinex) are medications that have been successful in improving the quality of life of many patients with acromegaly. These drugs have some side effects, such as gastrointestinal upset, nausea and vomiting, and nasal congestion. These side effects can be reduced in patients by starting with a very low dose and increasing the dose very slowly. The physician may also advise lowering the dose and having the patient take the medication with a meal. These drugs are less effective than octreotide (Sandostatin), and they will normalize growth hormone levels in only about 15 percent of patients.

Sandostatin or lanreotide (a synthetic form of the pancreatic hormone SOMATOSTATIN, which decreases the production of growth hormone) are both injectable drugs and are effective in many cases of acromegaly. This medication is usually given after surgery and before dopamine agonists are used. Injections must be performed frequently, up to every eight hours. However, there is a depot (long-lasting) form of the drug (Sandostatin Lar) that can be given as infrequently as one to four times per month.

These drugs may cause nausea, discomfort at the injection site, and gas and loose stools in some patients. About 25 percent of the patients who receive Sandostatin or lanreotide will also develop asymptomatic gallstones. More significantly, patients with diabetes mellitus may be able to reduce their insulin dosage because the acromegaly drug can improve glucose control. (Conversely, Sandostatin or lanreotide can also worsen diabetes symptoms in some patients.)

Other drugs that block the action of growth hormone may also be given to patients with acromegaly. One such drug is pegvisomant, an oral growth hormone antagonist medication that blocks the binding of growth hormone to its receptor. This drug has been effective in reducing soft tissue swelling and other symptoms in some patients, although its long-term safety is not known as of this writing.

In one study of 112 patients with acromegaly, reported in a 2000 issue of the *New England Journal of Medicine*, the patients were treated with differing daily doses of pegvisomant (Somavert) over 12 weeks. (A placebo group received a pill with no medication.) A majority of the patients, 93, had previously received pituitary surgery. Of these, 57 had also been treated with radiation therapy. (Four patients withdrew from the study for varying reasons.)

The researchers found that pegvisomant worked well in most patients, successfully reducing IGF-1 concentrations within about two weeks of starting taking the drug. However, because the study was conducted for only 12 weeks, the researchers stated that further study and longer periods of treatment would be needed to determine the continued safety and effectiveness of the drug.

Because pegvisomant blocks the binding of growth hormone to the receptor, some patients begin to synthesize more growth hormone. Some reports have discussed the growth of the tumor and of visual field changes that necessitated a change in the patient's medication therapy.

Radiation therapy is often used to treat acromegaly. In most cases, 4,000–5,000 rads (40–50 Gy) are given over five weeks. The growth of the tumors is often slowed or stopped by radiation therapy. However, the effects on the secretion of growth hormone are very slow and will decrease only about 10–20 percent per year, thus making the patient's symptomatic response very slow.

A variety of helpful imaging techniques (CT and MRI) have been used to try to focus the radiation directly on the tumor and thus to limit the damage to the surrounding normal brain tissue. Proton bean therapy has also been helpful for some patients; however, it is not widely available as of this writing. Stereotactic gammaknife therapy is now also being used on some tumors.

All forms of radiation therapy can lead to the loss of other pituitary functions over the course of many years and can also increase the patient's risk of developing an intracranial malignancy. In addition, radiation may cause changes in both visual and cognitive functions, depending on the type and amount of radiation used as well as the size of the radiated field.

See also AMENORRHEA; BLOOD PRESSURE/HYPERTENSION; BONE DISEASES; CARNEY COMPLEX; DWARFISM; HYPERPHOSPHATEMIA/HYPOPHOSPHATEMIA; PITUITARY ADENOMAS; PITUITARY GLAND; PREDIABETES.

For further information about acromegaly, contact the following organization:

Pituitary Network Association
223 East Thousand Oaks Boulevard
Number 320
Thousand Oaks, CA 91360
(805) 496-4932

Baris, D., et al. "Acromegaly and Cancer Risk: A Cohort Study in Sweden and Denmark." *Cancer Causes and Control* 13, no. 5 (2002): 395–400.

Gasperi, M., et al. "Nodular Goiter Is Common in Patients with Acromegaly." *Journal of Endocrinological Investigation* 25, no. 3 (2002): 240–245.

Larsen, P. Reed, et al. *Williams Textbook of Endocrinology.* New York: W. B. Saunders Company, 2001.

LeRoux, Carel, Abeda Mulla, and Karim Meeran. "Pituitary Carcinoma as a Cause of Acromegaly." *New England Journal of Medicine* 345, no. 22 (November 29, 2001): 1,645–1,646.

Trainer, Peter J., M.D., et al. "Treatment of Acromegaly with the Growth Hormone-Receptor Antagonist Pegvisomant." *New England Journal of Medicine* 342, no. 16 (April 20, 2000): 1,171–1,177.

Addison's disease   A rare endocrine disease in which the adrenal glands do not produce enough CORTISOL (hypocortisolism or primary adrenal insufficiency). Cortisol is a key hormone that helps the body respond to stress in many different ways. It regulates blood pressure, maintains adequate blood glucose levels for energy, regulates electrolytes, such as potassium and sodium, and performs many other key functions within the body. Addison's disease is also known as chronic primary adrenal insufficiency. Sometimes patients with Addison's disease are also deficient in the hormone ALDOSTERONE, which is also produced by the adrenal glands.

The disease may be first diagnosed when it is life threatening because most patients have few or no symptoms in the early stages. Addison's disease occurs in about one in 100,000 people, and it affects both males and females equally. President John F. Kennedy suffered from Addison's disease.

The average patient with Addison's disease is diagnosed at about 40 years of age. Periods of stress, caused by illness, work, or family problems, worsen the already-existing condition.

Causes of Addison's Disease

The cause of Addison's disease is the destruction of the adrenal cortex. In most cases (about 80 percent), the disease appears to stem from an autoimmune reaction of the body to an unknown stimulus. In some cases, the condition may be a hereditary one, particularly when diagnosed in males.

In rare cases, patients with acquired immune deficiency syndrome (AIDS) develop Addison's disease as a result of the destruction of their adrenal glands caused by infections that the patient's body could not fight off. Tuberculosis can also lead to the development of Addison's disease, although this problem is not usually seen in patients in developed countries such as the United States, Canada, and western Europe. Rarely, Addison's disease can be caused by a systemic fungal infection. Adrenal hemorrhage and destruction by tumors are additional causes of Addison's disease.

Signs and Symptoms

In addition to hypocortisolism, Addison's disease is also characterized by an extreme weight loss and a coppery skin tone. All patients with Addison's disease experience a significant weight loss before diagnosis, and about 90 percent evince a darker skin coloration than is normal for the patient. The skin color change is a key diagnostic indicator if the disease is advanced.

Sometimes the symptoms of Addison's disease are confused with those of ANOREXIA NERVOSA, a severe eating disorder in which the patient engages in voluntary self-starvation. Some patients with Addison's disease have actually been misdiagnosed with anorexia nervosa. However, patients with anorexia nervosa typically have yellowish skin, rather than copper-colored skin. In addition, patients with anorexia nervosa are more likely to have high levels of cortisol rather than low levels (hypocortisolism).

Patients with anorexia nervosa may be hyperglycemic. In contrast, patients with Addison's disease are more likely to be hypoglycemic. Last, patients with anorexia nervosa are often low in potassium blood levels, while patients with Addison's disease are hyperkalemic (with excessively high levels of potassium in the blood).

Other signs and symptoms of Addison's disease may include the following:

- Chronic fatigue
- Dizziness/light-headedness
- Cold intolerance
- Nausea and vomiting
- Malaise
- Depression
- Hypotension (low blood pressure)
- Loss of underarm (axillary) and pubic hair in adult women
- Elevated levels of blood urea nitrogen (BUN)
- Anemia
- Poor concentration
- Mood swings
- Hypoglycemia (low blood sugar)
- Thyroid disease
- Craving for salt

If a Medical Crisis Occurs

Individuals diagnosed with Addison's disease should always wear a medical identification bracelet. In the event of an emergency, they will urgently need to receive glucocorticoid injections, typically given as hydrocortisone, CORTISONE, prednisone, dexamethasone, or methylprednisone. They also require fluid resuscitation, usually administered as normal saline (salt water) and dextrose if needed. In a crisis situation, a patient's blood pressure may fall to extremely low levels (hypotension). He or she may also experience problems with severe hypoglycemia (low blood sugar) and excessively high levels of potassium. When experienced in combination, these three symptoms may be life threatening. In fact, if the condition is left untreated, it is fatal. When patients with Addison's disease plan to travel, they should be sure to bring with them needles, syringes, and an injectable form of cortisol for emergency use.

Diagnosis and Treatment

If physicians suspect that a patient has Addison's disease, they will perform a variety of laboratory tests, including the adrenocorticotropic hormone (ACTH) or Cortrosyn stimulation test. In this test, synthetic ACTH in the form of Cortrosyn is injected intravenously after a baseline cortisol level is measured in the blood. Cortisol levels are then measured in the blood after 30 minutes from the time of the injection and, on occasion, after 60 minutes.

The insulin tolerance test is considered the gold standard test for the diagnosis of Addison's disease, but it is used less frequently due to the risk of severe hypoglycemia. In this test, a graded amount of rapid-acting insulin is administered intravenously to the patient in order to induce hypoglycemia purposely, and cortisol levels are measured at specific times. Cortisol is a counterregulatory hormone. Thus, cortisol levels should increase appropriately when the body develops hypoglycemia. If they do not increase, the test indicates a problem and the presence of Addison's disease.

After the biochemical diagnosis is made, an imaging test can be used to help determine the cause of the adrenal insufficiency. In most cases, a COMPUTERIZED TOMOGRAPHY (CT) scan of the adrenals is the first test used. With autoimmune Addison's disease, the adrenal glands may appear normal sized, but they are often atrophic. If there has been a destructive lesion such as hemorrhage or tumor, the glands will appear enlarged. If the possibility exists of secondary or tertiary adrenal insufficiency, CT or MAGNETIC RESONANCE IMAGING (MRI) of the pituitary is often valuable.

Patients diagnosed with Addison's disease are treated with replacement glucocorticoids and, on occasion, mineralocorticoids. Prednisone, cortisone acetate, methylprednisone, dexamethasone, or hydrocortisone can be used. The dose may be given once daily. However, it is typically split with 50–65 percent being given in the morning and the remainder in the afternoon, thus attempting to mimic the body's own circadian pattern.

No one specific test allows the endocrinologist to monitor a patient's response to therapy. Most important are the patient's sense of well-being, blood pressure, appetite, and energy. Serum electrolytes in the form of potassium and sodium, as well as the renal function tests (blood urea nitrogen and creatinine), are monitored. Renin and ACTH levels are sometimes helpful in guiding dose changes.

Monitoring of patients with Addison's disease is crucial. If too much glucocorticoid replacement is used, the excessive medication will cause such symptoms as weight gain, HYPERGLYCEMIA, hypertension, and other problems in a medically induced form of Cushing's syndrome.

Patients found to be deficient in aldosterone may need mineralocorticoid replacement in the form of fludrocortisone (Florinef).

If patients with Addison's disease become ill or feverish, they may need to double or even triple their glucocorticoid dosage. Doctors should discuss this issue ahead of time with all patients who have Addison's disease. If these patients become acutely ill, they will need an emergency intravenous dosage of glucocorticoids and may also require hospitalization. Most patients will recover in a day or two.

See also ACTH; ADRENAL CRISIS/ADDISONIAN CRISIS; ADRENAL FATIGUE; ADRENAL GLANDS; CACHEXIA; SKIN.

For further information, contact the following organization:

National Adrenal Disease Foundation
505 Northern Boulevard
Suite 200
Great Neck, NY 11021
(516) 487-4992

Adams, Robert, M.D., et al. "Prompt Differentiation of Addison's Disease From Anorexia Nervosa During Weight Loss and Vomiting." *Southern Medical Journal* 91, no. 2 (February 1998): 208–211.

Oelkers, Wolfgang, M.D. "Adrenal Insufficiency." *New England Journal of Medicine* 335, no. 16 (October 17, 1996): 1,208–1,212.

Ten, Svetlana, Maria New, and Noel MacLaren. "Addison's Disease 2001." *Journal of Clinical Endocrinology & Metabolism* 86, no. 7 (2001): 2,909–2,922.

adolescents Individuals who are either undergoing or who have recently undergone puberty, usually in the age range of about 12–17 years.

Adolescents are prone to many of the same endocrine diseases as children or adults. However, they are at risk for some diseases more specific to their age group (although the risk is still low). Examples of such diseases are MATURITY ONSET DIABETES OF YOUTH (MODY) and DELAYED PUBERTY. EARLY PUBERTY (precocious puberty) is a less frequently occurring problem. Adolescents are more prone to developing ANOREXIA NERVOSA than adults, although the illness may persist into adulthood. TYPE 1 DIABETES, formerly called juvenile diabetes, may present in early adolescence and will persist throughout life. However, some patients with Type 1 diabetes are not diagnosed until early adulthood or even later.

Menstruation and Adolescents

The onset of menstruation can be difficult for some adolescent girls, who may find it painful and/or embarrassing.

Interestingly, the presence of secondary sexual characteristics and the onset of menstruation among girls in the United States have apparent racial and ethnic differences. This is based on information from the Third National Health and Nutrition Examination Study of 1988–94, reported by Dr. Wu and her colleagues in a 2002 issue of *Pediatrics*.

According to this report, the study of 1,168 girls ages 10–16 revealed that Mexican-American and African-American girls developed pubic hair and experienced their first menstrual cycle earlier than the Caucasian girls in the study. Nearly half (49.4 percent) of the African-American girls had breast development at the age of nine years, compared with 24.5 percent of the Mexican-American girls and 15.8 percent of the Caucasian girls of the same age. In addition, the average (mean) age of the appearance of pubic hair was 9.5 years for African-American girls, 9.8 years for Mexican-American girls, and 10.3 years for Caucasian girls.

The onset of menstruation was closer for all three groups. However, it still occurred earlier for African Americans and Mexican Americans than for Caucasians. The mean age for the onset of the first menstruation was 12.1 for black girls, 12.2 for Mexican-American girls and 12.7 for white girls. It is unclear why black and Mexican-American girls experience earlier signs of puberty than white girls. When physicians are considering diagnosing a girl with an early puberty, they may wish to take into account racial factors that may indicate that she is on track compared to other girls of the same race.

Males and Adolescents

Males may find adolescence difficult, particularly if they have a delayed puberty, causing them to be smaller and less mature than other males of the same age. Some parents ask their doctors for GROWTH HORMONE to speed the development of puberty and growth. This use is controversial. In general, parents are more likely to ask for growth hormone for boys than girls.

See also TANNER STAGES.

Wu, Tiejian, M.D., Pauline Mendola, and Germaien M. Buck. "Ethnic Differences in the Presence of Secondary Sex Characteristics and Menarche Among US Girls: The Third National Health and Nutrition Examination Survey: 1988–1994." *Pediatrics* 110, no. 4 (October 2002): 752–757.

adrenal cortical cancer A malignant tumor of the cortex of the adrenal gland, also known as an adrenocortical carcinoma or adrenal cancer. Only about one or two people in a million develop this very rare form of cancer. When it occurs, it is usually found among adults who are in their 40s or 50s, although adrenal cortical cancer also can be seen in children under the age of five years. It more commonly occurs in females. Sometimes adrenal cortical cancer is found among patients diagnosed with MULTIPLE ENDOCRINE NEOPLASIA, type 1 (MEN 1). A tumor found in the adrenal medulla or in an area other than the adrenal cortex is known as a PHEOCHROMOCYTOMA.

Some tumors actively secrete hormones, while others do not. Different studies have shown variable percentages of patients with actively secreting tumors. Patients with actively secreting hormones are discovered upon a physical evaluation of the patient, who typically presents with signs and symptoms of CUSHING'S SYNDROME or virilization (male symptoms in females). This includes hair where it is not typically seen in females, such as on the chest, face, and so forth.

In the case of patients who have a nonsecreting tumor, the tumor is usually identified because of symptoms caused by its large size. In other cases, the tumor is found serendipitously when the patient has had an imaging study for an unrelated issue. An inactive tumor is more commonly seen in older patients. This type often progresses at a faster rate than those that are hormonally active.

An adrenocortical tumor is usually curable only when it is identified in an early stage, when the tumor is still confined to the adrenal gland. At this point, that particular adrenal gland can be surgically removed. Patients can then live a normal life, with the other adrenal gland taking over full duty to make the appropriate levels of hormones needed by the body. However, discovering this tumor at an early stage is not common. In fact, an early tumor, if discovered, is usually found accidentally. By the time adrenal cortical cancer is usually identified, it has often metastasized (spread to other organs), typically to the lung, liver, lymph nodes, and bones.

Diagnosis and Treatment

Physicians consider the diagnosis of adrenal cancer when the patient presents with rapidly progressive symptoms of Cushing's disease or with virilization. In contrast, cancers that secrete feminizing hormones or aldosterone are very rare.

A basic tenet of endocrinology is that a medical syndrome should be clearly characterized biochemically through laboratory studies prior to obtaining imaging studies. Doing so avoids unnecessary testing and also helps the physician pinpoint the problem. As a result, laboratory tests may be ordered to help make a diagnosis.

When imaging tests are ordered, a COMPUTERIZED TOMOGRAPHY (CT) scan and MAGNETIC RESONANCE IMAGING (MRI) can identify the presence of a tumor. These tests are also used to define the size of the tumor as well as to determine whether there is any local spread or more distant spread to the liver or the lymph nodes. When an enlargement of an adrenal gland is found on a CT that was performed

for other reasons, endocrinologists suspect the presence of a malignant tumor, especially if the tumor is greater than five centimeters at its greatest dimension.

Treatment for adrenal cortical cancer is usually surgery. If the cancer is advanced, the patient may be treated instead with chemotherapy. Mitotane, a chemical related to DDT, has been the mainstay of chemotherapy for years. It is used initially in treatment, as well as later in treatment, in an attempt to prolong the patient's survival. When the tumor is responding poorly, other agents, such as cisplatin, etoposide, doxorubicin, cyclophosphamide, 5-fluorouracil (5-FU), and vincristine are added to the mitotane.

Because mitotane damages and destroys both malignant and healthy adrenal cortical cells, patients treated with mitotane must also be treated with glucocorticoid and mineralocorticoid medications in order to replace their endogenous cortisol and aldosterone.

Radiation therapy is rarely used to treat adrenocortical cancer. Percutaneous radio frequency tumor ablation has been used for patients with small tumors and early disease, with mixed results.

See also ADRENAL GLANDS; AMENNORHEA; CANCER; EARLY PUBERTY; HIRSUTISM IN WOMEN.

Abraham, Jame, and Tito Fojo. "Endocrine Tumors," in *Bethesda Handbook of Clinical Oncology.* Philadelphia, Pa.: Lippincott Williams & Wilkins, 2001, 419–440.

Hsing, Ann W., et al. "Risk Factors for Adrenal Cancer: An Exploratory Study." *International Journal of Cancer* 65, no. 4 (1996): 432–436.

Ng, L., and J. M. Libertino. "Adrenocortical Carcinoma: Diagnosis, Evaluation, and Treatment." *Journal of Urology* 169, no. 1 (2003): 5–11.

Vassilopoulou-Sellin, R., and P. M. Schwartz. "Adrenocortical Carcinoma: Clinical Outcome at the End of the 20th Century." *Cancer* 92, no. 5 (2001): 1,113–1,121.

adrenal crisis/addisonian crisis A term usually used to describe a life-threatening problem due to a lack of adequate cortisol. Individuals in an adrenal crisis present with severe hypotension (low blood pressure), malaise, fatigue, and dehydration and may actually fall into a coma. They often have severe electrolyte abnormalities with profound hyperkalemia (high potassium levels) that can cause a lethal heart arrhythmia and severe HYPONATREMIA (low sodium levels).

Often the clinical picture is clouded by the acute illness that induced the crisis, such as urosepsis, pneumonia, or heart attack. Adrenal crisis can often occur in postoperative patients who develop a bilateral adrenal hemorrhage that destroys both adrenal glands.

Individuals in an adrenal crisis need immediate emergency care with fluid and electrolyte resuscitation in addition to intravenous stress doses of steroids. Typically, 100 mg of hydrocortisone are given and then repeated every six hours for the first 24–48 hours. In addition, the underlying illness must be diagnosed and treated.

When a patient has a known case of ADDISON'S DISEASE or another cause of adrenal insufficiency, the treatment is clearer. However, when a patient presents for the first time with these symptoms, the doctor must be astute enough to consider the diagnosis of adrenal crisis and to begin therapy as soon as possible.

Individuals with Addison's disease (hypocortisolism) are the patients most likely to experience an adrenal crisis. People with Addison's disease must be educated about the appropriate stress doses of glucocorticoids they need when ill. In addition, they may need a prescription for intramuscular steroids, to be given at home, if they are unable to keep down their oral steroids due to nausea and/or vomiting. Keeping intramuscular steroids at home is also a good idea if patients live a long distance from medical care. In addition, patients need to know that they must make sure they drink fluids and consume extra salt when they begin to get ill to prevent the syndrome from progressing further. They also need to have a medical identification bracelet or necklace that identifies them as a steroid-using or Addisonian patient.

Emergency doses of cortisone or hydrocortisone are required to counteract an adrenal crisis and to meet the individual's urgent need for cortisol. If the patient remains untreated, an adrenal crisis may be fatal.

See also ADRENAL GLANDS; CORTISOL.

adrenalectomy Removal of an adrenal gland. This procedure is usually necessary because of a cancerous tumor, trauma with hemorrhage (severe bleeding), or a benign tumor (such as a PHEOCHROMOCYTOMA or aldosteronoma) that has caused the patient to experience serious physiological consequences, such as hypertension.

Some physicians have developed a means to remove the adrenal glands laparoscopically, through a small incision in the abdomen. This technique is safer than an open adrenalectomy, and it also costs less money, although it can be a longer procedure for the surgeon to perform. In addition, there is less blood loss with a laparoscopic adrenalectomy. In one published study, the length of the patient stay decreased from 7.4 days to 2.7 days with a laparoscopic adrenalectomy. However, the tumors must be small (less than six to seven centimeters in size) in order to perform this procedure. Laparoscopic surgery is more technically difficult than using a large incision to remove the adrenal gland and should be performed only by experienced surgeons.

If patients have both of their adrenal glands removed, they will develop adrenal insufficiency and require lifelong treatment with steroids in order to avoid an ADRENAL CRISIS. If only one adrenal gland is removed, patients may require only temporary treatment until the other adrenal gland begins functioning properly and handling the task of the body's entire adrenal needs.

See also ADRENAL CORTICAL CANCER; ADRENAL GLANDS; ALDOSTERONISM; CANCER.

Hansen, P., T. Bax, and L. Swanstrom. "Laparoscopic Adrenalectomy: History, Indications, and Current Techniques for a Minimally Invasive Approach to Adrenal Pathology." *Endoscopy* 29, no. 4 (1997): 309–314.

Soulie, Michel, et al. "Retroperitoneal Laparoscopic Adrenalectomy: Clinical Experience in 52 Procedures." *Urology* 56, no. 6 (2000): 921–925.

adrenal fatigue A condition of impaired adrenal function that is not severe enough to reach the level of ADDISON'S DISEASE or ADRENAL INSUFFICIENCY.

Adrenal fatigue is rare. However, some naturopaths and other unscrupulous or uneducated individuals have actively promoted the condition as an extremely common one that will resolve only with massive doses of vitamins (which they often sell), sometimes after administering unscientific tests that purportedly "prove" that the condition is present. In addition, some unscrupulous practitioners place patients on dangerously high dosages of prednisone.

Any person who is told that he or she has adrenal fatigue should be sure to consult with an ENDOCRINOLOGIST before pursuing any course of prescribed or over-the-counter medications or before taking massive dosages of vitamins or minerals.

See also ADRENAL CRISIS/ADDISONIAN CRISIS; ADRENAL GLANDS.

adrenal glands Endocrine glands located in a very posterior position in the abdomen. Unless they are extremely enlarged, as with an adrenal adenoma, they cannot be felt by hand. Adrenal hormones must be synthesized and secreted in very specific concentrations to ensure normal health.

The adrenal glands produce three key hormones: ADRENALINE (a catecholamine hormone), ALDOSTERONE, (a mineralocorticoid), and CORTISOL (a glucocorticoid hormone). The adrenal glands also produce some TESTOSTERONE and other ANDROGENS (male hormones). Malfunctions of the adrenal glands can lead to such serious endocrine disorders as ADDISON'S DISEASE, CUSHING'S SYNDROME, and adrenal hyperplasia. The adrenal glands directly affect the METABOLISM of every person.

The adrenal glands are best imaged using a COMPUTERIZED TOMOGRAPHY (CT) scan, and often the initial scan is performed without intravenous contrast. The CT scan is particularly helpful in patients with adrenal adenomas or adrenal incidentalomas (nodules found with a CT scan, ultrasound, MAGNETIC RESONANCE IMAGING (MRI) scan or other techniques that were performed for another purpose). The Hounsfield units (essentially, a measure of water content) that can be measured from CT scans of the adrenal glands can help determine if further evaluation is indicated.

If a mass is present, a cutoff size of five to six centimeters is typically used to determine whether a further evaluation, such as a biopsy, should be done, as the risk of malignancy increases as the size of a tumor increases. Large adrenal masses are often surgically approached via a very large posterior to anterior flank incision. However, the ability to do many surgeries using much smaller laparoscopic techniques are readily becoming the norm.

If an adrenal hemorrhage (heavy bleeding) occurs, the patient may develop ecchymoses (evidence of bruises) in the flank area of the body.

See also ADRENAL CRISIS/ADDISONIAN CRISIS; ADRENALECTOMY; ADRENAL FATIGUE; ADRENAL HORMONES; ADRENAL INSUFFICIENCY; ADRENAL LEUKODYSTROPHY; SKIN.

adrenal hormones The adrenal glands produce several hormones, including ADRENALINE, ALDOSTERONE, and CORTISOL.

Cortisol is the primary hormone secreted by the cortex of the adrenal glands. Cortisol is necessary for life. In many systems of the body, it functions as a permissive hormone, allowing that organ or system to function at an optimal level. Cortisol is needed to balance basic functions, such as blood pressure, alertness, blood glucose levels, and the salt and water balance of the body. Excessive levels of cortisol result in CUSHING'S SYNDROME or disease, while insufficient levels lead to ADDISON'S DISEASE.

Aldosterone is a hormone that helps to maintain a good electrolyte (primarily sodium and potassium) balance in the body. It also maintains normal blood pressure. People with Addison's disease may also be deficient in aldosterone and require supplementation. Hyperaldosteronism is a disease that usually involves small, benign tumors of the adrenal glands, which may require an ADRENALECTOMY.

Adrenaline (also known as epinephrine) is the fight-or-flight hormone that enables people to become hypervigilant and alert in the event of either real or perceived danger or times of high stress. Both adrenaline and cortisol are counterregulatory hormones. In other words, they counterbalance the effects of insulin and tend to increase the level of blood glucose. Thus, tumors that secrete excessive amounts of adrenaline, such as PHEOCHROMOCYTOMAS, may lead to increases in the blood glucose level and overt DIABETES MELLITUS.

adrenaline A hormone produced in the adrenal cortex of the adrenal gland. Adrenaline is also known as epinephrine. Adrenaline, which is also referred to as the fight-or-flight hormone, is very important. It enables individuals to become highly alert on an as-needed basis. This ability allows individuals to cope more effectively in the event of real or perceived danger or during periods of high stress. Adrenaline may also be administered on an emergency basis for individuals experiencing a life-threatening allergic reaction.

Adrenaline, which is synthesized in small amounts on a regular basis, also helps individuals to maintain stable blood pressure. It increases blood pressure when people arise from a sitting position by causing the smooth muscles in blood vessels to tighten (vasoconstriction).

Adrenaline is also produced by the autonomic nervous system in both the peripheral nerves and ganglia as well as in the brain. It is one of the counterregulatory hormones that rise rapidly when blood glucose levels fall. Adrenaline travels to the liver to counteract the effects of any insulin in the system. By increasing the pulse and causing sweating, jitteriness, and other symptoms, it alerts individuals that there is a problem that requires attention. Adrenaline also helps to break down preformed glucose that is stored in the liver in the form of glycogen.

Although measuring adrenaline can be difficult, it is possible. A laboratory test can measure the adrenaline level in the blood. Additionally, its metabolites can be measured in the urine. These lab tests are helpful in diagnosing PHEOCHROMOCYTOMA, a benign tumor of the adrenal gland that can cause fatal paroxysms of blood pressure.

See also ADDISON'S DISEASE; ADRENAL GLANDS; ADRENAL HORMONES.

adrenal insufficiency The condition that occurs when the adrenal glands make inadequate cortisol for proper health. Complete adrenal insufficiency is typically synonymous with ADDISON'S DISEASE. However, there may be degrees of adrenal insufficiency, ranging from minimal or partial to complete.

The most common causes of primary adrenal insufficiency are autoimmune destruction of the adrenal glands, tuberculosis, and hemorrhage. Adrenal insufficiency may also be caused by acquired immunodeficiency syndrome (AIDS), fungal infections, or the destruction of the adrenal cortex by cancers that have spread (metastasized) to that area.

In addition, adrenal insufficiency may be secondary to HYPOPITUITARISM. This problem with the pituitary gland produces inadequate adrenocorticotropic (ACTH) hormone. Adrenal insufficiency may also be tertiary due to a hypothalamic disorder in which inadequate levels of corticotropin releasing hormone (CRH) are generated, and consequently, inadequate levels of ACTH are also produced.

The most common form of secondary adrenal insufficiency is caused by the use of exogenous steroids in the treatment of another ailments. Exogenous steroids are frequently used to treat conditions such as asthma, rheumatoid arthritis, or organ transplantations and are often lifelong treatments.

This use of exogenous steroids leads to the suppression of the pituitary gland and the hypothalamus. The adrenal glands become atrophic or dormant as they are not needed to make adequate cortisol since the patient now has an external steroid supply. If these steroids are stopped suddenly or tapered off too quickly, the patient will develop acute adrenal insufficiency or an acute adrenal crisis. Patients may develop signs and symptoms of steroid withdrawal syndrome.

Patients with adrenal insufficiency, whether they have the primary, secondary, or tertiary forms of the condition, will feel extremely weak and tired. They may also have the following signs and symptoms:

- Loss of appetite and unintended weight loss
- Nausea and vomiting
- Diarrhea
- Dizziness

HYPONATREMIA (low sodium in the blood) and hyperkalemia (high potassium in the blood) are both signs of adrenal insufficiency that are found only with the primary form of the condition.

Patients with primary adrenal insufficiency also often present with hyperpigmentation of the skin and thus their skin appears darker. In the most extreme case, and if patients are left untreated, they will die. In addition, the hyponatremia may become life threatening. Individuals should be treated with intravenous normal saline (a sodium chloride solution) and glucocorticoid steroid infusions (hydrocortisone).

Diagnosis and Treatment

Adrenal insufficiency is often difficult to diagnose. Doctors take a careful medical history and perform a physical examination. If adrenal insufficiency is suspected, the Cortrosyn (cosyntropin) stimulation test should be performed. The patient's blood CORTISOL level is measured and then Cortrosyn (synthetic ACTH) is given intramuscularly or intravenously. The patient's cortisol blood levels are again measured in 30 minutes and, on occasion, in 60 minutes.

There is some debate about what constitutes a normal response. However, most experts think that the 30-minute level should be greater than 20 mcg/dl or the difference between the baseline test and the 30-minute levels should be greater than 12 mcg/dl. This level of response indicates that the HYPOTHALAMIC-PITUITARY-ADRENAL AXIS (HPA axis) is intact. In some cases, the test must be repeated, such as when the results are equivocal. Other tests must then be ordered to determine exactly what the adrenal function is like.

Patients with adrenal insufficiency are treated with glucocorticoid steroids and, on occasion, mineralocorticoid replacement with medications such as hydrocortisone or cortisone. Patients should also wear a medical identification bracelet identifying them as individuals with adrenal insufficiency in the event of a medical emergency.

They will also need to take maintenance doses of medication and be followed by physicians for the rest of their lives, with at least twice-yearly follow-up visits with their endocrinologist. Should these patients become very ill and/or feverish, they will usually need to increase the dosage of their hydrocortisone. Typically, a doubling of the dose is done for a minor illness and a tripling of the dose is recommended for a major illness. However, patients with adrenal insufficiency should consult with their own physicians about dosage needs should an illness occur.

Patients need to have an emergency dose of intramuscular medication available to them if they travel. This medication can also be used if patients have an illness accompanied by nausea and vomiting and, consequently, they are unable to keep their usual doses of medication down. If patients are unable to keep up with their body's fluid needs and are also unable to keep their steroids down, they will need emergency treatment with intravenous steroids and normal saline.

See also ADRENAL GLANDS; ADRENAL HORMONES.

Oelkers, Wolfgang, M.D. "Adrenal Insufficiency." *New England Journal of Medicine* 335, no. 16 (October 17, 1996): 1,206–1,212.

adrenal leukodystrophy (ALD) A very rare X-linked genetic disease that primarily affects males between the ages of six and 10 years old. Also known as adrenoleukodystrophy, ALD affects one in 20,000 males. Some female carriers of the disease may have a milder adult-onset form of ALD, which usually presents after age 35. There is also an adult-onset form of ALD among males. This type is not as severe as the childhood form and usually presents between the ages of 21 and 35, according to the National Institute of Neurological Disorders and Stroke. There is also a neonatal form of ALD. Most patients with ALD die within one to 10 years after first exhibiting the symptoms of the disease. ALD is also a rare cause of ADRENAL INSUFFICIENCY.

Genetic Issues

The ALD gene was first discovered in 1993. It is located on the *ABDC1* gene. Genetic counseling is available if it is suspected that the female may be a carrier of the disease. (If the male has ALD, he will exhibit obvious symptoms of illness.) If the family has a son who inherits the genetic defect, he will have the disease. A daughter, however, may inherit the defect but will usually be a carrier only. However, about 20 percent of female carriers will also develop a mild form of ALD.

Effects of ALD

Adrenal leukodystrophy affects the nervous system and the adrenal cortex. It causes a progressive and severe deterioration to the myelin sheath that insulates the nerve cells in the brain and also causes the adrenal glands to deteriorate. Patients with ALD amass large amounts of unbranched, very long chain fatty acids (VLCFA), particularly hexacosanoate (C26:0), in their brains and adrenal cortex. Because patients with ALD lack an enzyme to break down these fatty chains, the chains accumulate even further and cause severe damage. ALD is also classified as a peroxisomal disorder, with peroxisomes being the intracellular organelles located where this enzyme is deficient.

Background on Lorenzo's Oil

ALD became more prominently known to the general public with the success of the movie *Lorenzo's Oil*. It was based on a true story of parents who sought and found a treatment (not a cure) for their son who was diagnosed with adrenal leukodystrophy when he was a small boy in the early 1980s. In 2003, Lorenzo was 25 years old, according to information posted on The Myelin Project (http://www.myelin.org). At that time, he could communicate only by eye blinks and by wiggling his fingers.

Lorenzo's oil, which combines oleic acid and euric acid, is not approved by the Food and Drug Administration (FDA) as a treatment for ALD. However, at the time of this writing, it reportedly can be obtained by patients with ALD who participate in a clinical trial at the Kennedy Krieger Institute in Baltimore, Maryland. Experts report that Lorenzo's oil is usually not effective if the neurological impairment has already begun. Some insurance companies will reimburse patients for the medication, but many will not. As of 2003, a two-month supply of Lorenzo's oil costs about $440.

Signs and Symptoms of ALD

Boys with ALD exhibit poor memory, are withdrawn, and perform poorly in school. They may also have learning disabilities, seizures, poor muscle coordination, vision problems, deafness, difficulty walking (gait disorders), increased skin pigmentation, and progressively worsening dementia.

The symptoms and signs of adult-onset ALD progress much more slowly than the childhood form of the disease. However, this form of ALD can also cause worsening brain deterioration.

With neonatal ALD, the signs and symptoms are mental development delays, seizures, adrenal dysfunction, and an enlarged liver.

Women who are carriers of ALD and who have mild symptoms of ALD may experience urinary problems, worsening stiffness, and weakness in their lower legs.

Diagnosis and Treatment

The diagnosis of ALD is initially made based on the presenting symptoms and signs. A laboratory test is available for VLCFA. It is a highly accurate test for males who have ALD. The laboratory test is not widely available, however, and it can be performed only at a few specialized laboratories.

ALD can cause adrenal insufficiency in male patients, which is a possible indicator of the disease. Blood tests will also show abnormalities of the HYPOTHALAMIC-PITUITARY-ADRENAL AXIS (HPA axis), such as high levels of the adrenocorticotropic hormone (ACTH). Female carriers typically do not develop adrenal insufficiency, although they may on rare occasion develop mineralocorticoid insufficiency (hypoaldosteronism).

A MAGNETIC RESONANCE IMAGING (MRI) test may reveal classic patterns of the presence of ALD. However, correctly diagnosing ALD in females is much more difficult. The VLCFA test is accurate in the majority (85 percent) of cases. In most cases of women with ALD, though, results of adrenal tests and brain MRIs are usually normal.

Patients with ALD may be treated with adrenal hormones, which may be necessary to sustain the patient's life. As mentioned, some patients with ALD are treated with Lorenzo's oil. A bone marrow transplant is another treatment option, though it is experimental and very dangerous. A bone marrow transplant will decrease the amount of VLCFA in the tissue. Unfortunately, it does not seem to reverse any of the neurological deficits that the patient experiences, and thus, it is not usually recommended for patients with either adult-onset ALD or neonatal ALD.

For further information on ALD, contact the following organizations:

The Myelin Project
1747 Pennsylvania Avenue Northwest
Suite 950
Washington, DC 20006
(202) 452-8994
http://www.myelin.org

National Institute of Neurological Disorders
Building 31, Room 8A-96
31 Center Drive
MSC 2540
Bethesda, MD 20892
http://www.ninds.nih.gov

National Organization for Rare Disorders (NORD)
P.O. Box 1968
55 Kenosia Avenue
Danbury, CT 06813
(203) 744-0100
http://www.rarediseases.org

United Leukodystrophy Foundation
2304 Highland Drive
Sycamore, IL 60178
(815) 895-3211 or (800) 728-5483 (toll-free)
http://www.ulf.org

Laureti, S., et al. "Etiological Diagnosis of Primary Adrenal Insufficiency Using an Original Flowchart of Immune and Biochemical Markers." *Journal of Clinical Endocrinology & Metabolism* 83, no. 9 (1998): 3,163–3,168.

Moser, Hugo W., M.D., Ann B. Moser, and Steven J. Steinberg. "X-Linked Adrenoleukodystrophy." Available online. URL: http://www.geneclinics.org/ profiles/x-ald/details.html. Downloaded on February 15, 2004.

Moser, H. W., et al. "Adrenoleukodystropy: Survey of 303 Cases: Biochemistry, Diagnosis, and Therapy." *Annals of Neurology* 16, no. 6 (1984): 628–641.

AIDS (acquired immune deficiency syndrome) A severe and, as of this writing, incurable but highly treatable illness of the immune system. AIDS is caused by the human immunodeficiency virus (HIV). The time period from when the HIV virus is actually contracted to when a person is diagnosed with AIDS may be as long as 10 years or more, although some people are diagnosed with AIDS within two years of their initial infection with HIV. People with AIDS also have an increased risk for developing a wide variety of endocrine diseases and disorders, such as ADDISON'S DISEASE, thyroid disease, HYPOGLYCEMIA, lymphomas, and PANCREATITIS.

Thyroid Disease
The thyroid diseases that patients with AIDS may develop range from infections of the thyroid gland to HYPOTHYROIDISM or HYPERTHYROIDISM. They may also develop EUTHYROID SICK SYNDROME, in which their THYROID-STIMULATING HORMONE (TSH) level, the key test for diagnosing thyroid disease, may be only minimally abnormal.

Often patients with AIDS have abnormal levels of thyroid hormones, such as total T4 or free T4. Patients with AIDS also have abnormally high levels of thyroid-binding globulin (TBG), which increase as they become sicker. Because T4 is 99.7 percent bound (thus only a tiny amount is available to the cells for use), the increased TBG levels will lead to increased total T4 levels. This finding could lead the physician to believe that the patient has developed hyperthyroidism. However, in this case, this is a laboratory abnormality and is not indicative of true thyroid disease. The clinical significance of a rising TBG in AIDS patients is unknown, causes no symptoms, and is not treated.

Some medications used to treat patients with AIDS, such as rifampin (Rifampicin, Rifadin, Rimactane), can affect the thyroid laboratory results in patients with normal thyroid function. Some patients who are already taking levothyroxine as a thyroid supplement may need to take a higher dose of their thyroid medication when they are taking rifampin, as it will accelerate T4 metabolism.

Effects on the Adrenal Glands
Many AIDS patients have slightly increased adrenocorticotropic hormone (ACTH) and cortisol levels. As in many serious illnesses, the serum cortisol levels can increase, which is the body's reaction to stress. At autopsy, many AIDS patients have evidence of a cytomegalovirus (CMV) infiltration of the adrenal glands. Overall, about one in 20 patients with AIDS have ADRENAL INSUFFICIENCY. Most of this is secondary to CMV, tuberculosis, HIV itself, hemorrhage, and tumors.

Patients with AIDS also often have lower than normal levels of adrenal androgens, such as dehydroepiandrosterone (DHEA). Androgen replacement has not proven to be beneficial for these patients.

Some drugs that are given to patients with AIDS, such as ketoconazole (Nizoral) or megesterol acetate (Megace), can also affect the adrenal glands. For example, ketoconazole may cause adrenal insufficiency by decreasing the patient's synthesis of cortisol. Megestrol acetate is used to increase a patient's appetite, but it may on occasion also lead to the development of a secondary adrenal insufficiency.

The hormone itself has some glucocorticoid activity and thus can induce a Cushing's syndrome-type picture. If the drug is stopped suddenly, it can lead to a condition of a secondary adrenal insufficiency because the production of ACTH from the pituitary and corticotropin releasing factor (CRF) from the hypothalamus have been suppressed. On rare occasions, primary adrenal insufficiency has been diagnosed in patients on megestrol; the etiology is unknown.

Effects on the Pituitary Gland

Some studies have shown that the posterior pituitary function, where desmopressin acetate (DDAVP) is secreted after traveling from the hypothalamus, is impaired in many hospitalized patients with HIV. Additionally, as many as half of these hospitalized patients had HYPONATREMIA (below-normal levels of sodium in the blood due to the presence of excessive water). In some cases, hospitalized patients were treated with trimethoprim, an antibiotic that can cause or contribute to the development of hyponatremia.

Gonadal Function

As AIDS progresses, the testosterone levels of patients decrease, but FOLLICLE-STIMULATING HORMONE (FSH) and LUTEINIZING HORMONE (LH) do not decrease appropriately. As a result, patients can develop hypogonadotropic hypogonadism. In women with AIDS, the serum testosterone levels are usually slightly below those of their age-matched controls.

Effect on the Pancreas

Autopsies of patients with AIDS have revealed many pancreatic abnormalities that were not diagnosed prior to death. Studies have shown that infections and malignancies of the pancreas were much more common among deceased AIDS patients than among individuals who died of other causes.

Patients with AIDS may also have an increased risk for developing INSULIN RESISTANCE and HYPER-GLYCEMIA. Some patients initially experience hypoglycemia (low blood sugar) and later develop hyperglycemia.

Treatment with pentamidine (Nebupent or Pentaur) apparently increases the risk of the patient developing both hypoglycemia and diabetes. Treatment with megestrol acetate, a drug used to counteract anorexia (the loss of appetite, not to be confused with anorexia nervosa) and cachexia (a wasting away), both common characteristics among patients with AIDS, can sometimes cause diabetes mellitus.

Other Endocrine Effects

Other drugs that are given to many patients with AIDS may cause endocrine disorders that will need to be treated. For example, foscarnet (Foscavir) that is given to improve OSTEOPOROSIS may cause HYPOCALCEMIA and nephrogenic DIABETES INSIPIDUS. Megestrol acetate may cause lowered testosterone levels. Amphotericin B (Fungizone) that is given to patients to treat life-threatening fungal infections may result in renal (kidney) magnesium and potassium wasting. AIDS patients on antiretroviral therapy may develop lipodystrophy.

Growth Hormone as a Treatment

Some physicians have used growth hormone to treat their patients with AIDS. Growth hormone may help patients who suffer from cachexia. It has also been shown to be partially effective in treating HIV-induced lipodystrophy syndrome, perhaps by helping reduce fat content and by increasing lean (muscle) body mass.

See also CACHEXIA; GROWTH HORMONE; THYROID BLOOD TESTS.

Grinspoon, Steven, and Marie Gelato. "Editorial: The Rational Use of Growth Hormone in HIV-Infected Patients." Journal of Clinical Endocrinology & Metabolism 86, no. 8 (2001): 3,478–3,479.

Sellmeyer, Deborah E., and Carl Grunfeld. "Endocrine and Metabolic Disturbances in Human Immunodeficiency Virus Infection and the Acquired Immune Deficiency

Syndrome." *Endocrine Reviews* 17, no. 5 (1996): 518–532.

aldosterone A hormone synthesized by the adrenal glands (in the zona glomerulosa), that works to maintain normal electrolyte (mostly sodium and potassium) levels in the body as well as normal blood pressure. Aldosterone prevents the loss of salt and water when the patient is deficient in sodium or has low blood pressure. Aldosterone levels are regulated by the patient's potassium and sodium levels, blood pressure, angiotensin II, and renin as well as by the activity of the person's sympathetic nervous system.

A severe illness may cause the aldosterone levels to fall to very low levels. Either excessive levels of aldosterone (hyperaldosteronism) or insufficient levels of this hormone (hypoaldosteronism) will cause medical problems for the patient.

Aldosterone levels may be measured in both the blood and the urine. Patients who will be undergoing a test for their aldosterone levels may be asked to refrain from taking any diuretic medications, antihypertensive drugs, oral contraceptives, estrogens, and real licorice candy for about four hours to as long as one month before having the test to avoid invalid or confusing test results.

Patients with abnormally high aldosterone levels may have benign adrenal tumors, adrenal cancer, or liver disease, such as cirrhosis, or may have heart failure. Women in their third trimester of pregnancy may also have abnormally high levels of aldosterone.

Very low levels of aldosterone (hypoaldosteronism) may occur due to the surgical removal of the adrenal glands, ADDISON'S DISEASE, TYPE 2 DIABETES, renal tubular acidosis type 4 (TRA IV, also known as hyporeninemic hypoaldosteronism), or the toxemia that can occur in pregnancy.

See also ALDOSTERONISM; BLOOD PRESSURE; CONGENITAL ADRENAL HYPERPLASIA; HORMONES.

aldosteronism Refers to excessive levels of ALDOSTERONE within the bloodstream, a condition classified as primary aldosteronism, secondary aldosteronism, or idiopathic aldosteronism. Most cases of aldosteronism are associated with hypertension.

Primary aldosteronism, also known as primary hyperaldosteronism or Conn's syndrome, is usually caused and characterized by small benign adrenal tumors called aldosteronomas. Patients with primary aldosteronism have hypertension, hypokalemia (low potassium levels), and on occasion, muscle weakness and/or nonspecific malaise. Primary aldosteronism is also one of the few causes of hypertension that can be cured and is seen among only about 1–2 percent of all patients. Women are more likely to experience this condition than men.

Secondary hyperaldosteronism is a more common condition than primary hyperaldosteronism. Possible causes, in addition to hypertension, include heart failure, cirrhosis of the liver, or nephrotic syndrome. This ailment is caused by increased levels of aldosterone that have been induced by low blood pressure or other factors that may impair blood flow and/or the delivery of salt to the kidney. When this occurs, the kidney increases the production of aldosterone in an attempt to save salt and water and thus restore normal blood pressure and blood flow to the kidneys. Doctors can distinguish primary aldosteronism from secondary aldosteronism by measuring the patient's plasma renin levels.

Idiopathic aldosteronism is another form of the medical problem. It is found primarily among men. Patients with this condition are usually hypertensive.

Signs and Symptoms

Many patients with either primary or secondary aldosteronism have no signs or symptoms. If symptoms are present, they may include:

- Headaches
- Frequent urination
- Muscle cramps
- Muscle weakness and paresthesias (pins and needles); these symptoms are less frequently seen

Diagnosis and Treatment

Doctors who suspect aldosteronism will perform a physical examination and take a complete medical history. The patient's blood pressure is usually at least somewhat high. Routine laboratory tests for conditions such as hypokalemia or hypomagnesemia (low magnesium levels) may indicate the presence of aldosteronism. In fact, as many as 80 percent of patients with aldosteronism have hypokalemia.

Because low body potassium can impair the ability of the pancreas to produce insulin, patients with aldosteronism may also have abnormal glucose tolerance blood test results. Plasma renin levels are suppressed in patients with primary aldosteronism and are high in patients with secondary aldosteronism. The cortisol blood levels are usually normal.

After a biochemical diagnosis of primary hyperaldosteronism is made, and only then, imaging studies are obtained. COMPUTERIZED TOMOGRAPHY (CT) scans can reveal most aldosteronomas present in the adrenal glands. On some occasions, MAGNETIC RESONANCE IMAGING (MRI) and nuclear scans may be necessary to diagnose these lesions, which can be quite small.

If aldosteronomas are found, the preferred treatment is usually to remove the adrenal gland that contains them surgically (adrenalectomy). Existing hypertension improves shortly after the surgery is performed in about a third of patients. Some patients may also need spironolactone (Aldactone), an aldosterone agonist, for about three to four weeks before having the surgery. This therapy minimizes the risk of postoperative hypoaldosteronism as well as helps the body achieve normal potassium levels before surgery. Some patients have laparoscopic adrenalectomies. Although technically difficult for the surgeon, these procedures often give patients faster and easier recoveries.

When patients have idiopathic aldosteronism, they are usually not treated with surgery. Instead, they are treated with spironolactone therapy, with dosages ranging from 25–400 mg per day. Unfortunately, spirolactone is associated with many side effects, especially when patients take more than 100 mg per day. Side effects may include fatigue, ERECTILE DYSFUNCTION, GYNECOMASTIA (breast enlargement in males), hyperkalemia, irregular menstruation, and gastrointestinal problems. To minimize these side effects, men are usually prescribed 50 mg or less per day of spironolactone.

See also BLOOD PRESSURE/HYPERTENSION.

Ganguly, Arunabha, M.D. "Primary Aldosteronism." *New England Journal of Medicine* 339, no. 25 (December 17, 1998): 1,828–1,834.

Sawka, Anna M., M.D., et al. "Primary Aldosteronism: Factors Associated with Normalization of Blood Pressure After Surgery." *Annals of Internal Medicine* 135, no. 4 (August 21, 2001): 258–261.

alternative medicine   Refers to nontraditional or complementary medicine that relies on herbs, supplements, and other treatments such as acupuncture or massage therapy, rather than on traditional prescribed medications and over-the-counter treatments.

Dietary supplements, also known as nutraceuticals, are also popular with proponents of alternative medicine. In fact, alternative remedies are popular among many consumers. Some are seeking a quick fix for their often chronic medical problems. Others hope for improved general health or longevity by taking vitamins, minerals, and other substances. As a result, alternative medicine has become a multibillion dollar business in the United States.

Some individuals encourage people with endocrine diseases to use vitamins, herbal remedies, and supplements. For example, as of this writing, some purveyors of medications over the Internet encourage the use of coconut oil or sea kelp as a substitute for thyroid hormone or to increase the overall METABOLISM. This is dangerous advice. Individuals with HYPOTHYROIDISM need to take prescribed LEVOTHYROXINE to treat their hypothyroidism or they risk a serious worsening of their condition. In addition, people who have not been diagnosed with any thyroid disease should not seek to increase their metabolism with herbal remedies or other drugs.

Diseases such as DIABETES MELLITUS, hypertension, and many other serious chronic diseases cannot be cured with herbal remedies and may, in fact, be worsened by them. In addition, some patients may take an herbal remedy or supplement instead of a proven medication for their illnesses, which can lead to a worsening of their illness.

Vitamins, Herbs, and Supplements
According to an article published in a 2002 issue of the *Journal of the American Medical Association*, a survey of about 2,600 individuals ages 18 and older in the United States revealed that 40 percent of this

population took vitamins and minerals and 14 percent took at least one herbal or other supplemental drug. Among prescription drug users, an average of 16 percent took an herbal remedy or supplement. The greatest users of herbal remedies or supplements were patients taking fluoxetine (Prozac) or 22 percent of this group. Clearly, a large number of people in the United States use herbal remedies.

Multivitamins were the most popular vitamin used by the survey subjects, followed, in order of popularity, by vitamin E, vitamin C, calcium, magnesium, zinc, folic acid, vitamin B12, vitamin D, and vitamin A. The most popular herbal remedies and supplements were, in order, starting with the bestselling: ginseng, ginkgo biloba, *Allium sativum,* glucosamine, Saint-John's-wort, *Echinacea angustifolia,* lecithin, chondroitin, creatine, and *Serenoa repens.* Because of changes in advertising as well as trends among consumers, the most popular herbs and supplements among consumers will likely change from year to year. However, it is also likely that vitamins, herbs, and supplements as a group will continue to be popular among many consumers.

In 2003, the American Academy of Clinical Endocrinologists (AACE) published a comprehensive monograph providing information on dietary supplements and nutraceuticals. According to this report, nutraceuticals are "dietary supplements that contain a concentrated form of a presumed bioactive substance originally derived from a food, but now present in a nonfood matrix, and used to enhance health in dosages exceeding those obtainable from normal foods."

The report further explains that there are some disease-related claims, made by purveyors of nutraceuticals, that are actually approved by the Food and Drug Administration (FDA) and supported by strong evidence. Examples of such claims include calcium decreasing the risk of OSTEOPOROSIS, fiber decreasing the risk of CANCER and coronary artery disease, and soy protein decreasing the risk of coronary artery disease. In contrast, the FDA has particularly warned consumers against some specific nutraceuticals, such as hydroxybutyric acid, which can lead to seizure, coma, and death, and plantain, which may cause myocardial infarction (heart attack).

Ban of Ephedra

In late 2003, the FDA issued an announcement that the organization planned to ban all sales of any dietary supplements containing ephedra and *ma huang.* Because of the vagaries of the law surrounding dietary supplements, the ban did not become effective for 60 days from the date it was issued. However, the FDA actively and immediately solicited consumers to cease their use of any drugs such as ephedra and *ma huang* that contained ephedrine alkaloids.

According to the FDA press release, "Ephedra is an adrenaline-like stimulant that can have potentially dangerous effects on the heart. FDA's evaluation also reflects the available studies of the health effects of ephedra. This includes many studies reviewed by the RAND Corporation, which found little evidence for effectiveness other than short-term weight loss, as well as evidence suggesting safety risk. Other recent studies have also confirmed that ephedra use raises blood pressure and otherwise stresses the circulatory system, effects that have been conclusively linked to significant and substantial adverse health effects like heart problems and strokes."

Supplements Promoted for Endocrine Health, Questionably

Many manufacturers promote supplements and nutraceuticals for improving endocrine health although neither the AACE nor the FDA have evaluated the majority of these claims. For example, coenzyme Q10 is promoted to improve hypercholesterolemia, coronary artery disease, and congestive heart failure, while chromium, magnesium, vitamin E, zinc, and other supplements are claimed to be effective in improving glucose control. There is no evidence to date that such claims are valid.

Medication Interactions May Occur with Alternative Remedies

Some dietary supplements and nutraceuticals interact with medications that patients may already be taking and thus may consequently boost, weaken, or somehow change the effect of the prescribed drug. Saint-John's-wort has a potential interaction with many drugs, including amitriptyline (Elavil), simvastatin (Zocor), warfarin (Coumadin), and a variety of oral contraceptives. Ginkgo leaf is known to have potential drug interactions with aspirin, warfarin (Coumadin), and trazodone (Desyrel). Patients taking thyroid medication may experience a drug interaction when also taking bugleweed, red yeast, kelp, calcium, iron, or bonemeal.

Women who are taking estrogens may have a drug interaction if they also take androstenedione, chasteberry, grapefruit juice, fenugreek, licorice root, saw palmetto, or Siberian ginseng. Patients taking oral hypoglycemic medications may experience a drug interaction with many different supplements or nutraceuticals, such as devil's claw, fenugreek, feverfew, garlic, ginger, guar gum, psyllium, stinging nettle, and others. In one last example, patients taking insulin may experience a medication interaction if they also take chromium or ginseng.

Reasons for the Popularity of Alternative Remedies

Alternative medicine has a particular appeal for patients with chronic diseases that cannot be cured but can only be managed, especially illnesses or conditions that are very difficult for patients to deal with. Patients may become frustrated with their physicians and seek something more than what their doctors can provide. Unfortunately, patients also often fail to report the use of alternative medicines to their physicians and, consequently, risk dangerous medication interactions.

Sometimes doctors recommend alternative medicine to their patients. According to the National Center for Health Statistics in the "National Ambulatory Medical Care Survey: 2000 Summary," physicians ordered alternative therapies at 31 million visits in the United States in 2000. There were a total of 823.5 million visits to physicians in 2000, bringing the number of times that alternative remedies were recommended to about 4 percent of the total visits.

Benefits of Alternative Medicine

Supporters of alternative medicine and treatments say that herbal supplements, acupuncture, and other alternative options may provide relief to patients with chronic problems who have gained little or no

relief from following conventional medical treatment and therapies. For example, massage therapy or acupuncture may provide temporary relief for patients with aching muscles and stress-induced tension that have not responded to medications.

Occasionally, clinical studies back up the claims of alternative medicine proponents. For example, studies have indicated that patients with some chronic diseases, such as osteoarthritis, may benefit from taking regular dosages of supplements such as glucosamine. The problem is that many patients may generalize from these specific benefits, assuming that if glucosamine improves their arthritis, then another herb may improve their diabetes, thyroid disease, heart disease, or other serious chronic ailment. This is not a valid assumption.

Potential Problems with Alternative Remedies

Many people mistakenly believe that alternative remedies are inherently safe because they are natural. (Most prescribed medications are or were also plant based.) At the same time, some people believe that herbal remedies and supplements are somehow more powerful than medications prescribed to them by their physicians.

Despite this common belief in the inherent safety and efficacy of supplemental remedies, the reverse has been shown to be true. For example, when considering the safety issue, researchers have found that some drugs sold over the counter as herbal remedies actually contained prescribed drugs not listed on the container, such as testosterone. Other herbal remedies have been found to contain dangerously high levels of lead, mercury, and even arsenic.

Some forms of alternative medicine have caused disease or even death. A study in Japan reported that some Chinese dietary supplements were associated with causing HYPERTHYROIDISM and liver failure. In the United States in 2003, a baseball player died, reportedly from using a drug that contained ephedra. His was not the first death from using this supplement. Some herbal remedies are known to have toxicities. For example, licorice root and *ma huang* are cardiotoxic (dangerous to the heart), chapparal leaf, *ma huang* and pennyroyal oil are hepatotoxic (dangerous to the liver), and nux vomica and starfruit may cause convulsions.

This does not mean that all or even most herbal remedies are dangerous or toxic; however, it is very important for consumers to discuss their plan to take any such drug with their physicians beforehand.

Additionally, there is very little standardization from one manufacturer's herbal remedy or supplement to that produced by another manufacturer. Registered pharmacist Peter De Smet stated in his 2002 article in the *New England Journal of Medicine,* "Standardization of herbal remedies can be difficult, because herbs contain complex mixtures and because the constituents responsible for the claimed effects are often unknown. Since herbal remedies are exempt from rigorous regulation in the United States, there may be considerable variation in the composition of an herbal remedy among manufacturers and lots, as well as discrepancies between label information and actual content."

The Dietary Supplement and Health Education Act

The Dietary Supplement and Health Education Act in the United States has been a key force behind the explosive sales growth of herbs and supplements. Many people in the United States are unaware that herbs and supplements fall under the Dietary Supplement and Health Education Act, enacted by Congress in 1994.

This law upholds different standards and requirements for herbs and supplements compared with those held for both prescribed drugs and over-the-counter drugs in the United States. This law is also the reason why the FDA had such difficulty banning ephedra.

Many physicians believe this is a bad law. They feel it is far too lenient and believe that producers of herbs and other supplements should be subject to the same regulations that govern over-the-counter medications and prescribed drugs.

Those who produce herbal remedies and supplements have a broad freedom to sell their wares and do not have to perform extensive clinical testing beforehand, as must be done with prescribed and over-the-counter drugs. In addition, the FDA must prove that an herb or supplement is dangerous before removing it from the consumer market. As of this writing, politicians and drug companies contin-ue to battle over whether the Dietary Supplement and Health Education Act should be made stricter.

De Smet, Peter A. G. M. "Herbal Remedies." *New England Journal of Medicine* 347, no. 25 (December 19, 2002): 2,046–2,056.

Food and Drug Administration. "FDA Announces Plans to Prohibit Sales of Dietary Supplements Containing Ephedra." Available online. URL: http://www.fda.gov /oc/initiatives/ephedra.december2003/advisory.html. Posted December 30, 2003; downloaded January 16, 2004.

Kaufman, David W., et al. "Recent Patterns of Medication Use in the Ambulatory Adult Population of the United States: The Slone Study." *Journal of the American Medical Association* 287 (2002): 337–344.

Marcus, Donald M., M.D., and Arthur P. Grollman, M.D. "Botanical Medicines—The Need for New Regulations." *New England Journal of Medicine* 347, no. 25 (December 19, 2002): 2,073–2,075.

Mechanick, Jeffrey I., M.D., et al. "American Association of Clinical Endocrinologists Medical Guidelines for the Clinical Use of Dietary Supplements and Nutraceuticals." *Endocrine Practice* 9, no. 5 (September/October 2003): 417–470.

amenorrhea   Absence of the menstrual period in a woman or girl who would normally menstruate. Pregnancy is a normal cause of amenorrhea. In the absence of a pregnancy, most women of childbearing age should menstruate unless the uterus has been surgically removed, as with a hysterectomy. Amenorrhea may also be an indicator of an underlying illness or of INFERTILITY.

Primary Amenorrhea

Primary amenorrhea is a condition diagnosed in a woman who has failed to menstruate by the age of 18 years. Most females menstruate well before that age. However, if other pubertal changes have occurred, such as pubic and underarm hair and breast development, most doctors do not worry about the failure to menstruate until a female is 18 years old or older. They may, however, order clinical tests to reassure the patient about her health, including tests for estrogen levels and thyroid levels.

Doctors diagnose primary amenorrhea by taking a careful medical history, finding out the age of the patient's mother when she began to menstruate (in the event that late-age menstruation is common for the family), and asking about a present possible pregnancy as well as any recent weight changes and any gynecological surgery the woman has had. All of these factors can affect menstruation.

Some diseases that may cause primary amenorrhea are ACROMEGALY, ANOREXIA NERVOSA, Stein-Leventhal syndrome, TURNER SYNDROME, HERMAPHRODITISM, DIABETES, Crohn's disease, tuberculosis, thyroid disease, and heart disease. A tumor such as a prolactinoma may also cause amenorrhea.

If a patient is diagnosed with primary amenorrhea, doctors should check for cryptomenorrhea, a condition in which menstruation occurs but an imperforate hymen or other obstruction prevents the blood from leaving the body. The doctor may order X-rays of the patient's hands to determine the patient's bone age. If bones have fused, adult growth has been achieved, and menstruation should have commenced. If the bones have not yet fused, the first menstruation (menarche) may be anticipated to occur within a short period. Of course, a pelvic examination should also be performed by a gynecologist to check for the presence of any abnormalities.

When no medical problems are identified, doctors usually advise the female to come back in six months for a follow-up examination.

Secondary Amenorrhea

When a nonpregnant woman who has menstruated in the past has not menstruated for three or more consecutive months, she may be diagnosed with secondary amenorrhea. Doctors need to distinguish between amenorrhea and oligomenorrhea (which are scanty menstrual periods with fewer than 90 days between them).

As with primary amenorrhea, patients with secondary amenorrhea need a thorough physical examination and the taking of a complete medical history. They will also need a pelvic examination and appropriate laboratory tests.

Causes of secondary amenorrhea may include the following: ovarian cysts or tumors, POLYCYSTIC OVARY SYNDROME, pituitary damage caused by postpartum hemorrhage, and an endometrium that was destroyed in an overzealous curettage

(ASHERMAN'S SYNDROME). Some drugs, such as barbiturates, corticosteroids, ORAL CONTRACEPTIVES, and some tranquilizers, may also cause amenorrhea. In addition, arduous physical exercise, such as is seen with ballet dancers or professional athletes, may cause amenorrhea. Rarely, secondary amenorrhea is caused by ANDROGEN EXCESS or hyperandrogenism, which is an excessively high level of male hormones.

If the cause of the amenorrhea is resolved, then menstruation may either resume again or start for the first time in a female who has not menstruated before.

See also ANDROGEN RESISTANCE; ANDROGENS; EATING DISORDERS; MENSTRUATION, PAINFUL; POLYCYSTIC OVARY SYNDROME; THYROTOXICOSIS.

Ammer, Christine. *The New A to Z of Women's Health,* 4th ed. New York: Facts On File, Inc., 2000, pp. 23–25.
Lupo, Virginia R., M.D., and Catherine B. Niewoehner, M.D. "Endocrinology of Female Reproduction," in *Endocrine Pathophysiology.* Madison, Conn.: Fence Creek Publishing, 1998.

American Association of Clinical Endocrinologists (AACE) The leading professional organization of physicians who specialize in the clinical evaluation and care of patients with a variety of endocrine disorders, such as DIABETES MELLITUS, thyroid disease, OSTEOPOROSIS, and other illnesses. The AACE was founded in 1991 and has over 4,000 members from the United States and 63 other countries.

The AACE publishes a monthly peer-reviewed clinical journal, *Endocrine Practice.* It has also published numerous clinical guidelines on such topics as HYPERTHYROIDISM, HYPOTHYROIDISM, HYPOGONADISM, the Women's Health Initiative, and many other important topics.

The organization sponsors a yearly scientific clinical session where the latest advances in the diagnosis and treatment of endocrine disorders are reviewed and discussed.

The AACE offers annually updated, patient-oriented press releases to the public, including such releases as "Thyroid Awareness," "Stand Strong Against Osteoporosis," and "A Campaign for

Intensive Diabetes Self-Management." This information can be reviewed at the AACE Web site: www.aace.com. Patients can also go to this Web site to locate an endocrinologist near them who has an interest in their particular endocrine-related problem.

For further information, contact the AACE:

AACE
1000 Riverside Avenue, Suite 205
Jacksonville, FL 32304
(904) 353-7878
http://www.aace.com

American Diabetes Association (ADA)   A non-profit organization formed in 1940 by physicians concerned about diabetes treatment and research. Their mission is to prevent and cure diabetes as well as to improve the lives of everyone affected by the disease.

Along with major federal agencies, the ADA has cosponsored very large and significant clinical trials of patients with diabetes, such as the Diabetes Control and Complications Trial (DCCT), as well as many other important studies.

The American Diabetes Association provides information to both diabetes medical professionals and to consumers with diabetes. The organization produces the four most widely read, professional peer-reviewed journals published on diabetes, including *Diabetes, Clinical Diabetes, Diabetes Care,* and *Diabetes Spectrum.* In addition, the ADA publishes a weekly online newsletter, *DIABETES E-News Now!* available with other newsletters that individuals can sign up to receive at http://diabetes.org/site/PageServer?pagename=EM_signup.

The ADA also sponsors an online community forum, where patients and other interested individuals may discuss issues about diabetes of any type. The ADA Web site posts a tip of the day as well as information on opportunities to volunteer and donate to the ADA. In addition, the Web site also offers access to a vast array of diabetes-related resources. The ADA also has an advocacy center that allows people to advocate for their own diabetes-related causes in their local and state governments as well as the federal government.

For further information, contact the ADA:

American Diabetes Association (ADA)
1701 North Beauregard Street
Alexandria, VA 22311
(703) 549-1500 or (800) 342-2383 (toll-free)
http://www.diabetes.org

American Thyroid Association (ATA)   An organization of physicians and scientists interested in scientific research on the thyroid gland. The primary mission of the American Thyroid Association is to foster and support thyroid research, both on normal thyroid physiology and disease states. The organization also aims to disseminate new information on the thyroid gland to clinicians, researchers, and the general public. The Web site of the American Thyroid Association has a section, set aside for patients, that offers information on specific thyroid issues.

The American Thyroid Association publishes the journal *Thyroid,* which has clinical and basic science articles on the problems and physiology of the thyroid gland. It also publishes *Clinical Thyroidology,* a synopsis of research studies accompanied by expert commentary. The ATA advocates for the public in areas such as patient testing, public health issues, and insurance coverage. In addition, the ATA publishes updated laboratory guidelines for physicians, laboratories, hospitals, and teaching purposes.

For further information, contact:

American Thyroid Association
6066 Leesburg Pike, Suite 550
Falls Church, VA 22041
(703) 998-8890
http://www.thyroid.org

anabolic steroids   Refers to a group of synthetically created steroids that typically have glucocorticoid and androgen-like effects. These drugs are sometimes used illegally by body builders seeking to increase their muscle mass more quickly than weight lifting efforts can achieve. The term *anabolic* refers to the ability of these compounds to help build up the body, typically by increasing the incorporation of amino acids into proteins. The naturally occurring steroids, such as the male hormones (androgens such as TESTOSTERONE) produced by the testes, also have anabolic effects.

Anabolic steroids have systemic effects. Their use will also lead to oily skin, acne, increased hair growth in places other than the scalp, decreased hair growth on the scalp, and often cause users to have a more aggressive temperament.

As of this writing, grand jury hearings have been held about the use of illegal anabolic steroids by both amateur and professional athletes. In addition, a new anabolic steroid known as tetrahydrogestrinone (THG) was uncovered by authorities in 2003 and was subsequently banned by the Food and Drug Administration (FDA). This drug was formerly undetectable by even very sophisticated testing methods; however, the detection of this steroid is now possible.

Synthetic androgens are also available for medically indicated reasons, such as hypogonadism, or serious chronic conditions, such as the human immunodeficiency virus (HIV), severe burns, liver failure, pulmonary (lung) disease, kidney failure, wound healing, and postoperative recovery.

Androgens are also given to men with some forms of advanced CANCER, particularly prostate cancer. For men with prostate cancer, testosterone makes cancer grow. By suppressing testosterone, men's lives can be extended, sometimes for years. (Androgen therapy is not, however, a cure for prostate cancer or for any other form of cancer.)

For further information on the abuse of anabolic steroids, contact:

National Institute on Drug Abuse (NIDA)
6001 Executive Boulevard
Room 5213
Bethesda, MD 20892
(301) 443-1124
http://www.nida.nih.gov

See also ANDROGENS.

Basaria, Shehzad, Justin T. Wahlstrom, and Adrian S. Dobs. "Anabolic-Androgenic Steroid Therapy in the Treatment of Chronic Diseases." *Journal of Clinical Endocrinology & Metabolism* 86, no. 11 (2001): 5,108–5,117.

androgen excess The overproduction of male hormones; usually a problem experienced in women; also known as hyperandrogenism. Androgens are produced in the testes, ovaries, and the adrenal glands. Thus, an evaluation of this problem must sort out the degree of the excess and where the excess androgens are produced.

Androgen excess may result in HIRSUTISM in women (excessive body hairiness), acne, and AMENORRHEA (failure to menstruate) or oligomenorrhea (infrequent menstruation). Women with androgen excess may also have problems with hair loss (alopecia) rather than with hirsutism. Some women with severe androgen excess may also experience a deepening of their voice, clitoral enlargement, and increased muscle mass, symptoms known as virilization. When virilization is present, the physician must consider the possible diagnosis of an androgen-producing tumor, either benign or malignant.

Excessive levels of androgen may be a genetic problem. Androgen excess may also be caused by illnesses, such as ADRENAL CORTICAL CANCER, CONGENITAL ADRENAL HYPERPLASIA, or POLYCYSTIC OVARY SYNDROME.

androgen resistance Inability of the body to use some or all of the male hormones that are naturally produced. This problem is typically caused by a genetic defect. It may be due to a problem with the receptor for testosterone or due to an enzyme deficiency (as in a deficiency of the 5-alpha reductase enzyme that changes testosterone to dihydrotestosterone, the biologically active form of testosterone within the cells).

As a steroid hormone, testosterone must bind to the surface of the cell it is going to affect via a specific receptor. The receptor may be regarded as a loading dock, albeit a loading dock that is very specific to testosterone. Thus, most other steroid hormones are unable to bind (or dock) there as they have the wrong three-dimensional shape for binding. Once the testosterone is docked, it must then be internalized. Thus, the testosterone must be brought into the cell and moved to the nucleus of the cell. Once there, the testosterone will interact with the DNA within that particular cell to cause its effects.

When binding to the DNA, testosterone can stimulate the synthesis of new proteins or it may inhibit other processes. Thus, at any stage of the process, a defective protein or bonding can lead to androgen resistance because the androgen cannot bind and cause the appropriate effects.

Androgen resistance may range from severe to very mild forms. Three forms are described below.

Complete Androgen Resistance

At its most extreme, complete androgen resistance (previously called testicular feminization) prevents the development of normal male sexual characteristics. Consequently, the individual looks like a female but has no true uterus, ovaries, or vagina. During puberty, the individual develops secondary sexual characteristics, such as breasts; however, since there is no uterus, the individual cannot menstruate and is also infertile. These patients typically present during puberty, concerned because they have never menstruated. (Genetically, they are typically 46-X, Y and also have normal (for a male) or elevated testosterone levels and elevated luteinizing hormone (LH) levels.)

In some cases, the condition is actually unknown to the individual and the family, who have always assumed the person to be a female. The androgen resistance is not discovered until the time of expected puberty or even later, when the individual attempts to get pregnant. At that time, it is discovered that "she" is genetically a male, an obviously shocking revelation. The testicular remnants of the person are often found in the abdomen or inguinal area. Thus, in women with both primary amenorrhea and inguinal or labial masses, this diagnosis must be suspected.

Note that complete androgen resistance is *not* at all the same as transsexualism or gender dysphoria, which refers to a person who is born genetically and physically a male (or female) but who, at a very young age (as young as three or four years old), feels trapped in the wrong body. For example, a male feels he is truly female. These patients have normal hormone levels for their genetic makeup, and they do not have abnormalities of hormone resistance.

Incomplete/Partial Androgen Resistance

The two primary forms of incomplete or partial androgen resistance are categorized as incomplete androgen insensitivity and Reifenstein's syndrome.

With incomplete androgen insensitivity, the patient appears as a normal female with normal breasts and external genitalia, with the exception of an enlarged clitoris and/or fusion of the posterior labia. In contrast, the patients who have Reifenstein's syndrome appear to be males, but they present with GYNECOMASTIA (breast enlargement) and perineoscrotal hypospadias (an opening in the area behind the scrotum or directly in the scrotum).

In both of these syndromes, infants present with what is known as ambiguous genitalia. When evaluating these infants, the endocrinologist must also consider the diagnoses of 5-alpha reductase deficiency syndrome, mixed gonadal dysgenesis, and other defects in the synthesis of testosterone.

Among males, the size of the penis is usually the deciding factor for making the gender choice. Having a very tiny penis (MICROPENIS) may lead to the parents' decision to raise the child as a female; however, this is a controversial issue. (According to authors Erica A. Engster, M.D. and Antoinette M. Moran, M.D., in their chapter in *Endocrine Physiology,* a micropenis in an infant is a penis that is less than or equal to two centimeters in size.) In other cases of partial androgen resistance, the child is given large doses of testosterone to stimulate the growth of the penis. If a course of testosterone fails to induce growth, the parents may then be advised to raise the baby as a girl.

Mild Androgen Resistance

In its mildest form, androgen resistance may lead to symptoms such as infertility caused by insufficient sperm (oligospermia) or to minimal breast enlargement. However, despite these signs, the individual is clearly male in his physical appearance, orientation, and behavior.

Diagnosis and Treatment

The diagnosis of androgen resistance may be missed altogether in some cases of complete androgen resistance. This occurs when the family and doctors assume that the individual is actually a female rather than a male. However, if the child has both female and male characteristics (incomplete testicular feminization), the condition is usually diagnosed earlier.

Blood tests will reveal that for patients with androgen resistance, testosterone levels are in the range for males rather than females. In addition, levels of LUTEINIZING HORMONE (LH) will usually be high. FOLLICLE-STIMULATING HORMONE (FSH) levels will be in the normal range. An ultrasound test will reveal that no uterus is present, and it may also reveal the presence of intra-abdominal testes.

To differentiate androgen resistance from either an androgen deficiency or a deficiency of 5-alpha reductase enzyme, physicians may measure the concentrations of both testosterone and dihydrotestosterone (DHT). Individuals who have androgen resistance will have normal ratios of testosterone to dihydrotestosterone. However, with 5-alpha reductase deficiency syndrome, the DHT levels are decreased, and thus the testosterone to DHR ratio is then increased.

If doctors find the presence of intra-abdominal testes, these testes are usually removed after the individual is fully grown as they serve no purpose in an individual with a female gender identity and could later become malignant. After puberty, the individual with complete androgen resistance is given estrogen replacement therapy in order to maintain the female identity.

In rare cases, large doses of male hormone have been given to induce a normal development of the penis. For example, in an article in a 1989 issue of the *Journal of Clinical Endocrinology & Metabolism*, a baby had a very small penis and small testes that could be felt in the labialscrotal folds and had no vagina.

Laboratory tests revealed that the infant had normal 5-alpha reductase activity and androgen resistance. At the ages of $2^1/_2$ and $3^1/_2$ years, this child was given large doses of testosterone, which resulted in the further growth of the penis and also enabled the doctors to correct the child's hypospadias surgically. The doctors in this case hypothesized that the androgen receptor function causing the androgen resistance was successfully treated by the high doses of androgen. It is unknown if the boy later required any future doses of androgen.

When the androgen resistance is mild and the primary sign is infertility, treatment can be aimed at increasing testicular function with medications, such as human chorionic gonadotropin (HCG) and gonadotropin-releasing hormone (GnRH.)

See also AMENORRHEA; HERMAPHRODITISM; HYPOGONADISM; KLINEFELTER SYNDROME; OVARY; TESTES/TESTICLES; TURNER SYNDROME.

For further information on androgen resistance, contact the following organization:

Androgen Insensitivity Syndrome
  Support Group (AISSG)
P.O. Box 2148
Duncan, OK 73534-2148
http://www.medhelp.org/ais

Engster, Erica A., M.D. and Antoinette M. Moran, M.D. "Sexual Determination, Sexual Differentiation, and Puberty," in *Endocrine Physiology.* Madison, Conn.: Fence Creek Publishing, 1998, 1,237–1,255.

Grino, P. B., et al. "Androgen Resistance Associated with a Qualitative Abnormality of the Androgen Receptor and Responsive to High Dose Androgen Therapy." *Journal of Clinical Endocrinology & Metabolism* 68, no. 3 (1989): 578–584.

androgens   Male hormones that play a key role in sexual development, sexual interest and ability, muscle mass, weight, body hair, energy levels, bone density, and other functions. The most prominent male hormone is TESTOSTERONE, a hormone that affects sexual desire and potency, muscle mass, and the presence of body hair. Women also have some testosterone, although the testosterone levels in females are normally lower than those found in most men. Most androgens in men are produced in the TESTES. Some androgens are also produced by the ADRENAL GLANDS.

When men become androgen deficient for any reason, they will have less muscle mass, decreased bone density (which may lead to OSTEOPOROSIS), sparser body hair, and significantly decreased libido. They may develop ERECTILE DYSFUNCTION, although most men with very low androgen levels may retain a normal ability to have erections but find they have very little sex drive (as well as other medical problems). The voice will remain deep in the adult male because he has already undergone puberty. However, hypogonadal men may develop GYNECOMASTIA, or enlargements of the breast tissue.

Androgen Therapies

Low androgen levels seen with hypogonadism are treated with supplemental androgens, typically in the form of testosterone. Rarely, very small amounts are used in boys who have delayed puberty and then for only a short time. Androgen replacement is available as an intramuscular injection or a topical gel or skin patch. It is also available in pill form. However, pills are not used for long-term replacement therapy as such use can lead to serious problems, including tumors.

The topical approach is best, as it allows for physiological concentrations of androgens in the bloodstream. In contrast, when injections are used, initially the testosterone level normalizes, but then it goes too high for several days, after which it returns to normal. In addition, prior to the next injection, the testosterone level may fall below normal. As a result, injections are best given every 10–14 days, although many men prefer to receive them only every three to four weeks.

Some patients receive androgens to help control Fanconi's anemia or aplastic anemia. Androgens are also used to treat sickle cell anemia or other forms of blood diseases, such as the anemia caused by kidney failure.

Women and Androgen Therapy

The main use of androgens in women is in the treatment of decreased libido. In this situation, the androgen is often combined with an estrogen, as in the combination trade medications Estratest and Estratest HS. On other occasions, an androgen is used in the treatment of endometriosis, a condition in which the cells from the endometrial lining implant in a variety of places around the pelvis and abdomen, causing the woman to develop pain, menstrual derangements, and infertility. Women taking such drugs may experience temporary masculinizing side effects, such as HIRSUTISM, smaller breast size, and INFERTILITY.

Abuse of Androgen Drugs

Some individuals, especially some athletes and body builders, take artificially synthesized androgens, not for a medical purpose but to increase their muscle mass. The Drug and Enforcement Administration (DEA) in the United States classifies these anabolic steroids as controlled or scheduled drugs, just as drugs such as narcotics are scheduled drugs.

Apparently, anabolic steroids can improve athletic performance for some individuals. However, their use may also cause severe side effects such as liver damage, tumor growth in the liver and brain, and wild personality swings, with fits of rage and uncontrolled behavior. Other side effects include acne, oily skin, increased blood pressure, infertility, sleep apnea, and gynecomastia.

Women who abuse androgens may experience acne, hirsutism, amenorrhea, and virilization.

Although men and women may both develop psychological and physical dependencies on anabolic steroids, most abusers are males. In some cases, users become not only more aggressive but may also exhibit symptoms of mental illness.

See also ANABOLIC STEROIDS; DELAYED PUBERTY; HYPOGONADISM; HYPOGONADOTROPISM.

Bagatell, Carrie J., M.D., and William J. Bremner, M.D. "Androgens in Men—Uses and Abuses." *New England Journal of Medicine* 334, no. 11 (March 14, 1996): 707–714.

anorexia nervosa A severe eating disorder and psychiatric problem that is primarily characterized by purposeful self-starvation. About 5 million Americans suffer from anorexia nervosa. Some experts define anorexia nervosa quantitatively as a BODY MASS INDEX (BMI) of equal to or less than 17.5 kg/m^2. (The average healthy person has a BMI within the range of about 19–24.)

The term *anorexia nervosa* should not be confused with the single word *anorexia*, which indicates a usually temporary lack of appetite in people who are ill. Individuals with anorexia nervosa are usually hungry but purposely avoid food, often because of a delusional belief that they are fat, despite the fact that they are significantly below normal in body weight. The condition can be life threatening and may require the treatment of a variety of specialists, including an ENDOCRINOLOGIST, a psychiatrist, and other physicians.

Occasionally, experts misdiagnose patients as having anorexia nervosa because of a significant weight loss due to a different condition. This can occur when the patient has ADDISON'S DISEASE, TYPE 1 DIABETES, GRAVES' DISEASE, and other illnesses that cause extreme weight loss. As a result, any individual suspected of having anorexia nervosa should receive a thorough medical screening before a definitive diagnosis is given.

Patients with anorexia nervosa also have a significantly greater risk of abusing substances such as alcohol, cocaine, and other drugs. According to *Food for Thought: Substance Abuse and Eating Disorders,* a 2003 report by the National Center on Addiction and Substance Abuse at Columbia University, researchers have found that teenage girls with eating disorders have a five times greater risk of abusing alcohol or illegal drugs than girls of the same age who do not have an eating disorder; a 50 percent risk versus a 9 percent risk.

Risk Factors

Anorexia nervosa occurs in about 1–2 percent of the population. It is much more prominent among females, who have a 20 times greater risk of developing the condition than males. Caucasian females are more likely to develop anorexia nervosa than women of other races, although females of other races also exhibit this behavior. Women who are active in modeling, ballet dancing, or athletic pursuits are more likely to develop anorexia nervosa than others, as are females who are perfectionists. Some studies indicate that overprotective parenting may be a factor leading to the development of anorexia nervosa.

When males exhibit anorexia nervosa, they are more likely to be athletes or dancers, for whom attaining and maintaining a specific weight is considered important by their peers.

A Genetic Problem

Some studies have indicated a genetic influence on anorexia nervosa, with a seven to 12 times greater risk among the relatives of individuals with anorexia nervosa. A study of 672 female twins, ages 16–18 years, performed by K. L. Klump and colleagues and reported in a 2001 issue of *Psychological Medicine,* identified 26 individuals with anorexia nervosa who had a strong genetic component.

Sometimes adolescent girls with Type 1 diabetes develop eating disorders such as anorexia nervosa. Generally, the scenario is that a girl, once very slender due to undiagnosed diabetes, is diagnosed with the illness and properly placed on insulin therapy. She gains weight with better blood glucose levels. In addition, her appetite usually improves when she is less ill, leading to a larger caloric intake.

The increased weight may greatly distress the female adolescent. In an attempt to revert to her former lower weight, an adolescent may radically reduce the amount of food that she eats or may manipulate her insulin dosages to induce a weight loss. Some adolescents with diabetes will binge on food and then purge (bulimia nervosa), although such behavior does not appear to be characteristic for the adolescent with diabetes.

Signs and Symptoms of Anorexia Nervosa

In addition to a significant weight loss, other indicators of anorexia nervosa include:

- Menstrual problems or the lack of menstruation (AMENORRHEA) for three or more months
- Very fine hair on the side of the faces and arms
- Thinning hair
- Brittle nails
- Unexplained fatigue
- Sensitivity to cold
- Light-headedness

Diagnosis and Treatment of Anorexia Nervosa

Doctors primarily diagnose anorexia nervosa based on the signs and symptoms exhibited by a patient as well as the presence of a significant weight loss and a below-normal body weight. Laboratory tests for patients with anorexia nervosa are often in the normal range, although some patients are anemic or hypoglycemic. Some tests of thyroid function may be abnormal, such as abnormal levels of reverse triiodothyronine (rT3). In most cases, if the anorexia nervosa is resolved, any negative laboratory results will normalize as well.

Electrolytes will often be out of balance if the patient has abused diuretic drugs or laxatives.

Cortisol blood levels may be elevated. Scans of bone loss indicate bone density abnormalities in as many as 50 percent of patients with anorexia nervosa. Experts report that bone loss can occur in young anorexic women as early as six months from the onset of the anorexic behavior.

Treatment for anorexia nervosa may include taking antidepressants or other psychiatric medications as well as receiving psychological counseling. Individuals who are severely ill will need hospital care or long-term residential treatment. Generally, hospitalized patients are those who are 25–30 percent below the ideal body weight for their height. In contrast, patients who are 85–90 percent of their normal weight may often be treated successfully on an outpatient basis.

Physicians treating patients with anorexia nervosa need to be careful with what is known as refeeding syndrome, a problem that may occur when a severely anorexic patient is given meals that are high in calories. This problem is most likely to occur in the first two to three weeks of refeeding. It may cause cardiovascular collapse and even heart failure because the severely malnourished person cannot cope with higher-than-normal (for her) calories. To avoid this problem, the hospitalized patient should have the electrolyte levels, especially of phosphorus, monitored at least every other day. After several weeks of gaining weight, such monitoring is usually no longer needed.

See also AIDS; DIABETES MELLITUS; EATING DISORDERS; GHRELIN; PRADER-WILLI SYNDROME.

For further information on anorexia nervosa, contact the following organizations:

National Association of Anorexia Nervosa and
    Associated Disorders
P.O. Box 7
Highland Park, IL 60035
(847) 831-3438
http://www.anad.org

Becker, Anne E., M.D., et al. "Eating Disorders." *New England Journal of Medicine* 340, no. 14 (April 8, 1999): 1,092–1,098.

Colton, Patricia A., et al. "Eating Disturbances in Young Women with Type 1 Diabetes Mellitus: Mechanisms and Consequences." *Psychiatric Annals* 29, no. 4 (April 1, 1999): 213–218.

Klump, K. L., et al. "Genetic and Environmental Influences on Anorexia Nervosa in a Population-Based Twin Sample," *Psychological Medicine* 31, (2001): 737–740.

Mehler, Philip S., M.D. "Diagnosis and Care of Patients with Anorexia Nervosa in Primary Care Settings." *Annals of Internal Medicine* 134, no. 11 (2001): 1,048–1,059.

National Center on Addiction and Substance Abuse at Columbia University. *Food for Thought: Substance Abuse and Eating Disorders.* New York: National Center on Addiction and Substance Abuse at Columbia University, 2003.

anovulation   The failure to release an egg in the ovulation process, which then leads to INFERTILITY. Women with regular menstrual cycles typically have predictable times of ovulation. Those women with AMENORRHEA (failure to menstruate) usually have complete anovulation and, thus, do not ovulate at all. Women with irregular cycles (oligomenorrhea) have an erratic pattern of ovulation.

Anovulation has many different etiologies (causes). POLYCYSTIC OVARY SYNDROME (PCOS) is often a cause of anovulation. Patients with PCOS often have insulin resistance syndrome (IRS). In addition to IRS, LUTEINIZING HORMONE secretions are often abnormal. The combination leads to hyperandrogenism, the likely underlying cause of the anovulation. Other causes of anovulation are HYPOTHYROIDISM and MENOPAUSE. The physician should screen the patient for thyroid dysfunction before attempting any direct treatment for anovulation.

Said Brinda N. Kalro, M.D., in a 2003 article in *Endocrinology and Metabolism Clinics*, "With the availability of ovulation-inducing agents, there is a possibility that thyroid disorders may be overlooked in women presenting with menstrual irregularities and anovulation. Pregnancy in women with overt thyroid disease is uncommon, but when it does occur, it can be fraught with complications and have grave consequences. Therefore, evaluation of the thyroid axis in women presenting with thyroid problems is imperative."

Successful diagnosis and treatment of the underlying disease may resolve a woman's anovulation. If the cause cannot be determined, sometimes ovulation can be stimulated with fertility drugs. These drugs should be administered and monitored by a physician who is experienced in treating women with infertility.

Diagnosis of Anovulation

Before diagnosing a patient with anovulation, the physician takes a thorough medical history and gives the patient a physical examination, including a pelvic examination. In addition, the physician orders tests of the woman's hormone levels, such as luteinizing hormone (LH), FOLLICLE-STIMULATING HORMONE (FSH), ESTRADIOL, progesterone, PROLACTIN, and thyroid hormones.

The woman's basal body temperature (her temperature immediately upon arising in the morning) may also be measured to determine if ovulation is occurring, as there is an increase of 0.5–1.0 degree Fahrenheit in body temperature during ovulation. However, most physicians consider it more accurate and simpler to measure hormonal changes in the woman's blood and/or urine than to rely upon the woman's basal temperature. An ultrasound scan may also show the presence or lack of a developing follicle that precedes ovulation.

PCOS and Anovulation

According to experts, although PCOS is the most common cause of anovulation, why anovulation occurs with this endocrine disorder is unknown. What is known is that women with PCOS and anovulation present with normal serum FSH levels and elevated LH levels. Usually there is also evidence of hyperandrogenism leading to HIRSUTISM (excess body hair within areas where women typically do not have hair but men do, such as on the face and chest). In addition, the patient usually does not menstruate (amenorrhea) or has infrequent menstrual periods (oligomenorrhea). The woman's ovaries may be found to be polycystic (with multiple cysts) on an ultrasound.

In vitro fertilization, a procedure to create an embryo outside the womb, is generally not the first line of treatment for women with PCOS who wish to become pregnant. Instead, the antidiabetes drug metformin is generally the first therapy used for infertility/anovulation if PCOS is suspected. Note

that metformin is not approved by the Food and Drug Administration (FDA) for treating PCOS as of this writing. Many times the changes that occur with insulin resistance after taking this drug will cause ovulation to occur in the first month of treatment. As added benefits, metformin can also lead to weight loss, decrease the risk of diabetes, decrease the woman's triglyceride levels, and also diminish the androgen levels and help ameliorate any hirsutism that is present.

If metformin fails to resolve infertility, an estrogen therapy, such as clomiphene citrate, can be utilized. This medication stimulates FSH secretion and leads to ovulation in about 75 percent of patients, according to Stephen Franks in his 2003 article for *Endocrinology and Metabolism Clinics of North America.* If this treatment does not work, ovulation may be successfully induced with gonadatropin medications.

Patients may also be given injections of human menopausal gonadotropin (HMG). Ultrasound scans and measurements of estradiol will then reveal if a follicle is produced. If not, the dosage of the HMG is often increased and the doctor will continue to monitor the patient.

When a dominant follicle is identified, the HMG is stopped and the patient is given one intramuscular injection of human chorionic gonadatropin (HCG) in order to trigger her ovulation. If this treatment is not effective at causing ovulation to occur, HMG is given again in order to create follicles.

Sometimes surgery is used to treat infertile women with PCOS, particularly women who are resistant to clomiphene. Such women receive a laparoscopic ovarian diathermy. Patients may find this procedure preferable to multiple injections.

See also FEMALE REPRODUCTION; THYROID BLOOD TESTS.

Barbieri, R. L. "Metformin for the Treatment of Polycystic Ovary Syndrome." *Obstetrics & Gynecology* 101, no. 4 (2003): 785–793.

Franks, Stephen, M.D. "Assessment and Management of Anovulatory Infertility in Polycystic Ovary Syndrome." *Endocrinology and Metabolism Clinics of North America* 32, no. 3 (2003): 639–651.

Kalro, Brinda N., M.D. "Impaired Fertility Caused by Endocrine Dysfunction in Women." *Endocrinology and Metabolism Clinics of North America* 32, no. 3 (2003): 573–592.

antibodies Proteins that are synthesized mainly by B lymphocytes. Antibodies are also known as immunoglobulins. There are five different classes of antibodies, including IgG, IgA, IgD, IgE, and IgM. The immune system creates immunoglobulins to fight off foreign invaders, such as bacteria and viruses. Many of the known autoimmune conditions seen in endocrinology are caused by an immunoglobulin-mediated attack, which then leads to the damage and destruction of an organ.

HASHIMOTO'S THYROIDITIS is an example of an autoimmune disease. With Hashimoto's thyroiditis, antibodies to thyroid protein, which are known as peroxidase, are created. They gradually destroy the thyroid gland, leading to HYPOTHYROIDISM. Often T lymphocytes also participate in the destructive autoimmune process, exacerbating it even further.

apolipoproteins Particles that circulate throughout the body carrying blood, fats, or lipids. Cholesterol and triglycerides are insoluble in plasma and thus must be transported. They circulate as lipoproteins, which are combinations of phospholipids and apoproteins. The aproteins support the structure of these particles, making them soluble in the blood. They also activate enzymes critical for normal lipid metabolism and act as targets for receptors. They are recognized by the receptors on cells and thus can dock and be taken up into those cells for specific purposes.

There are five classes of lipoproteins. These include chylomicra, high-density lipoproteins (HDL), intermediate-density lipoproteins (IDL), low-density lipoproteins (LDL), and very low-density lipoproteins (VLDL).

As of this writing, researchers have identified at least nine types of apolipoproteins. These apolipoproteins can be measured and may represent surrogate measurements for lipid levels. If apolipoprotein (apo) B levels are elevated, typically LDL levels are elevated. If apo A-I levels are high, usually the HDL is high. At this time, they are mainly used as research tools to study how the body metabolizes these lipids and to help in designing medical therapies to improve lipid levels and decrease the risk of ATHEROSCLEROSIS.

Individuals with high levels of apolipoprotein B may face a greater risk of suffering from coronary heart disease since apo B is the primary protein within LDL cholesterol. In contrast, apolipoprotein E is associated with LDL cholesterol.

See also CHOLESTEROL; HYPERLIPIDEMIA.

Asherman's syndrome Secondary amenorrhea (cessation of menstruation) caused by damage to and scarring of the endometrium. It is not a reversible condition. Typically, Asherman's syndrome is caused by a postpartum hemorrhage (heavy bleeding) and an overzealous dilation and curettage (D and C) procedure. Asherman's syndrome can also occur after an instrumentation of the uterus that leads to infection or inflammation.

The diagnosis of Asherman's syndrome is confirmed by an ULTRASOUND that fails to reveal any uterine lining stripe as well as by a failure of the patient to have a withdrawal bleed after the administration of progesterone hormone. The lack of lining and the scarring of the uterus can also be visualized and the diagnosis confirmed by a hysteroscopy, which is an instrument scan into the uterus.

Klein, S. M., and C. R. Carcia. "Asherman Syndrome: A Critique and Current Review." *Fertility and Sterility* 24, no. 9 (1973): 722–735.

atherosclerosis/arteriosclerosis A complex pathological condition in which the body reshapes and also damages the surface of the blood vessels as a direct consequence of various interactive metabolic processes that involve lipids (fats), white blood cells, antibodies, platelets, and other hormones and proteins. The current theory about what causes atherosclerosis is that most atherosclerosis is a product of an inflammation of the endothelium (the lining of blood vessels that comes into direct contact with circulating blood). This inflammatory process is ongoing and may progress and regress, depending upon the local conditions to which the endothelium is exposed.

If the damaging process to the vessel continues, the blood vessel may become occluded (blocked). However, more frequently, plaque accumulates from within the endothelium and finally ruptures into the lumen of the blood vessel, exposing lipids and other proteins directly into the bloodstream. This sets off a massive cascade of events that perpetuates the problem locally. The body harnesses the white blood cells, proteins, hormones, interleukins (hormones made by the white blood cells), and the platelets, ultimately creating an occlusive blood clot (thrombus).

This clot results in even more blocking of blood flow and also prevents sufficient oxygen from reaching the affected organ. Depending on the severity of the blood flow blockage, atherosclerosis may lead to a heart attack, stroke, or other serious medical problems.

Experts now know that most myocardial infarctions (heart attacks) occur in blood vessels that are only initially less than 50 percent blocked but, because of less stable caps on the vessel's lining, are much more likely to rupture. In contrast, vessels that have not yet ruptured but have progressed to 80–99 percent occlusion have thick, fibrous coverings which, although they limit blood flow, are much less likely to rupture and lead to a complete occlusion. In addition, as the condition has typically progressed slowly, the tissue that is endangered has often had sufficient time to develop collateral blood vessels upon which to rely. These are vessels that have bypassed the diseased area and, thus, help the organ—and the patient—to survive.

Risk Factors

Risk factors for atherosclerosis, include the following:

- High levels of "bad" cholesterol (low-density lipoproteins)
- Low levels of "good" cholesterol (high-density lipoproteins)
- Obesity
- DIABETES MELLITUS
- Hypertension
- An age of 65 and older (the risk for atherosclerosis increases with age)
- Lack of exercise
- Insulin resistance syndrome
- A family history of atherosclerosis

Diagnosis and Treatment

Atherosclerosis is diagnosed by a physician taking a complete medical history and doing a physical exam. The physician will note any history of prior heart attack, stroke, positive family history of atherosclerosis, symptoms suggesting angina, transient ischemic attack (TIA) (a ministroke), or claudication. During the physical examination, the doctor will check for the absence of pulses, presence of bruises, and tobacco-stained fingers and teeth. These may suggest the presence of atherosclerosis.

The doctor will also order laboratory tests to measure factors that contribute to the development of atherosclerosis, such as lipids, glucose, kidney function, C-reactive protein (CRP), homocysteine, and lipoprotein a (Lp a). Individuals who already have atherosclerosis need treatment, usually in the form of medications that improve their lipid profiles, lower their blood pressure, normalize their glucose, and make their platelets less sticky. Some individuals may respond well to taking very low doses (81 mg) of aspirin, such as a baby aspirin, each day.

Most physicians treating patients with atherosclerosis also recommend lifestyle changes. These include stopping smoking, increasing the daily intake of fiber, obtaining at least minimal exercise every day, such as walking (30 minutes, five times per week), and following a heart-healthy nutritional plan.

See also CHOLESTEROL.

basal-bolus therapy   The concept of treating DIA-BETES MELLITUS with INSULIN by using a combination of a long-acting (NPH/Lente/Ultra Lente) or very long-acting (glargine) insulin with rapid-acting (aspart, lyspo) insulin in order to mimic the normal mode of insulin secretion in the pancreas. The basal insulin is given once or twice a day to shut off production of excess glucose from the liver, while the bolus insulin is given to help metabolize the calories (mainly carbohydrates) that are consumed with each meal or snack. This technique allows for very tight control of blood glucose levels and enables patients to vary the times and types of their meals.

This therapy is also done with insulin pump therapy, where one or more basal rates are preprogrammed, to allow the pump to deliver small amounts of insulin continuously for 24 hours. The patient "plugs in" boluses for each meal or snack, depending upon the glucose level, anticipated carbohydrate intake and activity levels. For pump patients, only short-acting insulin is used.

bisphosphonates   Drugs used to treat patients with OSTEOPOROSIS, PAGET'S DISEASE, humoral hypercalcemia of malignancy, and disorders of dystrophic bone deposition. Bisphosphonates are particularly effective at inhibiting the action of OSTEOCLASTS, the cells that break down bone. They have also been used to treat patients with cancer that has metastasized (spread) to the bones leading to bone pain and/or hypercalcemia. Some examples of bisphosphonate medications are etidronate (Didronel), alendronate (Fosamax), risedronate (Actonel), zoledronate (Zometa), tiludronate (Skelid), and pamidronate (Aredia).

Many patients are now able to receive their bisphosphonate doses weekly due to the long half-lives of the newer medications. (The medications remain in the bone for a long time.) Typically, bisphosphonates are all poorly absorbed and must be taken on an empty stomach with water only (not coffee, tea, juice, or any fluids other than water). Patients must then remain upright for at least one hour, because these compounds can irritate the esophagus and cause inflammation (esophagitis) or ulceration if they reflux from the stomach into the esophagus.

Newer bisphosphonates can also be given intravenously. The only indication for this treatment currently approved by the Food and Drug Administration is for humoral hypercalcemia of malignancy and bone pain due to metastases.

As of this writing, researchers are trying to develop bisphosphonates that can be given only once per year for the treatment of osteoporosis.

See also HYPERCALCEMIA; OSTEOBLASTS.

Fleisch, Herbert. "Bisphosphonates: Mechanisms of Action." *Endocrine Reviews* 19, no. 1 (1998): 80–100.

blood pressure/hypertension   Blood pressure is a measure of diastolic and systolic pressure as exerted upon the walls of the blood vessels and arteries. Blood pressure may be temporarily elevated during sickness or times of stress, or it may be temporarily lowered. Hypertension refers to chronically high levels of blood pressure. It is defined as a systolic pressure (the upper number in the measurement of blood pressure) of 140 mm Hg or higher and a diastolic pressure (the lower number) of 90 mm Hg or greater. About 50 million people in the United States are hypertensive. Hypertension is most common among African Americans and individuals age 65 years and older. The Pima Indians of Arizona have the highest rates of hypertension in the world.

New Category of Prehypertension

In 2003, the National Heart, Lung, and Blood Institute released new hypertension guidelines that included a new prehypertension category of patients. It includes individuals with systolic blood pressures between 120 and 139 and diastolic blood pressures between 80 and 89. Although prehypertension is not a disease state, patients whose blood pressure falls within this range should be carefully watched by their physicians. In addition, if they have specific additional medical problems, such as DIABETES MELLITUS, chronic kidney disease, or a previous history of heart attack, or if they are at high risk for coronary heart disease or recurrent stroke, these particular prehypertensive patients should also be given antihypertensive medications.

Causes of Hypertension

Hypertension is a medical problem accompanying many endocrine diseases, such as HYPERPARATHYROIDISM, ACROMEGALY, CUSHING'S SYNDROME, diabetes mellitus, HYPERTHYROIDISM, PHEOCHROMOCYTOMA, DIABETIC NEPHROPATHY, and ALDOSTERONISM. Other causes of high blood pressure include obstructive sleep apnea, kidney disease, and heart disease. In most cases, hypertension is treated with recommendations for therapeutic lifestyle changes, such as appropriate nutrition, weight loss, exercise, and stress management as well as medications. Rarely, hypertension can be cured, such as when the cause is aldosteronism or pheochromocytoma, conditions that can be resolved with surgery known as an ADRENALECTOMY.

Sometimes medication causes hypertension. For example, ORAL CONTRACEPTIVES may raise an individual's blood pressure to hypertensive levels. They often do so by increasing the synthesis of angiotensinogen in the liver, which is converted to angiotensin, a potent vasoconstrictor on its own, and which will also stimulate the adrenal glands to synthesize excess aldosterone, leading to further vasoconstriction and salt and water retention. Smoking also exacerbates the risk for hypertension.

CLASSIFICATION AND MANAGEMENT OF BLOOD PRESSURE FOR ADULTS

Category	Systolic (mm Hg)		Diastolic (mm Hg)
Normal	Less than 120	and	Less than 80
Prehypertension	120–139	or	80–89
Stage 1 hypertension	140–159	or	90–99
Stage 2 hypertension	More than 160	or	More than 100

Source: National Heart, Lung, and Blood Institute. "JNC 7 Express: The Seventh Report of the Joint National Committee on Prevention, Detection, Evaluation, and Treatment of High Blood Pressure." National Institutes of Health, National Heart, Lung, and Blood Institute, National High Blood Pressure Education Program, NIH Publication No. 03-5233, May 2003.

Diagnosis of Hypertension

Blood pressure is measured with a cuff device after the patient has been sitting quietly for at least five minutes in a chair. Hypertension is best diagnosed by medical staff, such as the nurse or the doctor, rather than by patients themselves using home devices. At least two measurements of a patient's blood pressure should be taken to ensure accuracy. Individuals who are smaller or larger than most adults should be tested with a pressure device that is suitable to their size and that can cover at least 80 percent of the patient's arm. Once hypertension has been established, home monitoring of blood pressure may help patients to track their own blood pressure levels and enable them to report any dramatic increases to their physicians.

Laboratory tests can provide further information about hypertension. Doctors generally order a urinalysis as well as blood tests that measure complete blood count, serum electrolytes (especially sodium and potassium), blood urea nitrogen (BUN) levels, calcium blood levels, creatinine, glucose levels, and plasma lipid levels. The patient's urine may also be checked for albumin excretion, and an electrocardiogram may be ordered as well.

Treatment of Hypertension

Most physicians treat hypertension by helping bring down the patient's systolic pressure. For most patients, once their systolic pressure has dropped, their diastolic pressure will fall as well. If hypertension is caused by or related to a medical problem, successful treatment of that medical problem should improve the patient's hypertension.

Weight loss among obese individuals should improve or even normalize high blood pressure. Hypertension can also be treated with improvements in diet; increasing the intake of fruits and vegetables can lower blood pressure in many individuals. Highly salted foods should be avoided. Foods rich in potassium, such as bananas, should generally be consumed. Some medications reduce potassium levels, making it even more important that patients eat a diet that is rich in potassium. Some patients will also need to take supplemental potassium.

Patients who smoke should be advised to stop smoking immediately to improve their blood pressure levels. Patients who drink alcohol should sharply curtail drinking or avoid alcohol altogether. Male hypertensive patients should consume no more than two drinks per day and females and other individuals of lighter weight should limit their consumption to a maximum of one drink per day.

Regular exercise is another important lifestyle component of keeping hypertension within control. Even taking a brisk walk for 30 minutes on most days of the week can be sufficient to improve health for many hypertensive patients. Some exercises, however, should be avoided, such as heavy weight lifting or exercises that would tend to raise the patient's blood pressure.

Many people with high blood pressure need two or more medications to keep their blood pressure at an acceptable level. Many studies have shown that the average patient with hypertension requires 3.5 drugs per day to normalize blood pressure. Many different types of medications may be prescribed to patients with hypertension, including thiazide-based diuretics, beta-blockers, angiotensin-converting enzyme (ACE) inhibitors, calcium channel antagonists, alpha-blockers, and angiotensin-receptor antagonists. Each type of drug has its own indications, contraindications, and side effects.

Follow-ups on Patients with Hypertension

Once hypertension has been diagnosed, regular follow-ups with a physician are essential. The timing of the medical follow-ups (weekly, biweekly, monthly, or on some other schedule) is up to the individual doctor. It usually depends on how severe the hypertension is, how effective treatment has been, as well as other factors, such as whether the patient has another serious coexisting illness such as diabetes. The patient's serum creatinine and potassium levels should be checked at least once or twice each year.

In general, if blood pressure goals have been reached, patients may be followed up at three- to six-month intervals. However, patients with diabetes or heart disease may need more frequent visits with their physicians.

See also ATHEROSCLEROSIS/ARTERIOSCLEROSIS; CHOLESTEROL; HYPOTENSION; ORTHOSTATIC HYPOTENSION; TYPE 1 DIABETES; TYPE 2 DIABETES.

August, Phyllis, M.D. "Initial Treatment of Hypertension." *New England Journal of Medicine* 348, no. 7 (2003): 610–617.

blood sugar Refers to glucose, although other forms of sugar can be found in the bloodstream. Blood sugar can be measured by drawing a sample of blood from a patient's vein. It is now often measured immediately in the doctor's office, using a glucose monitor and a small sample (one to 10 microliters) that is taken from a fingertip or the forearm. The presence of unusually high levels of blood sugar is referred to as HYPERGLYCEMIA, while unusually low levels indicate HYPOGLYCEMIA.

People with sustained levels of hyperglycemia (a fasting glucose that is greater than 126 mg/dl on two occasions, or a random glucose level that is greater than 200 mg/d, or an abnormal glucose tolerance test) are diagnosed with DIABETES MELLITUS, typically either TYPE 1 DIABETES or TYPE 2 DIABETES. If the patient's levels of blood sugar are above normal but not high enough for a diagnosis of diabetes, he or she may be diagnosed with PREDIABETES.

Individuals both with and without diabetes can have hypoglycemia. This condition is typically defined as a glucose level less than 55 mg/dl along with the appropriate signs and symptoms of hypoglycemia.

Patients with prediabetes must work to get this high blood sugar problem under control with a proper nutrition plan and exercise. They are at risk for developing diabetes. This is especially true if there is a family history of diabetes.

People with diabetes must maintain a glucose level that is as close to normal as possible. Numerous major studies have proven that keeping blood sugar close to normal will greatly reduce the risk for many complications of diabetes, such as DIABETIC NEPHROPATHY, DIABETIC NEUROPATHY, and DIABETIC RETINOPATHY.

See also IMPAIRED GLUCOSE TOLERANCE.

body mass index (BMI)   A specific formula based on an individual's height and weight that helps to determine whether a person is underweight, of optimal weight, overweight, obese, or severely obese. BMI is derived from a person's weight in kilograms divided by the height in meters squared. For patients with very small frames or with significant muscle mass, the calculation does not give a very accurate assessment.

Since the mathematical formula is difficult for most people to calculate easily, tables have been created that enable patients to use their height in inches and their weight in pounds to determine whether they fit into the below-normal normal weight, overweight, obese, or severely obese category.

According to the National Heart, Lung, and Blood Institute (NHLBI) of the National Institutes of Health, weight categories of BMI are as follows:

Optimal weight: 21–24.9
Overweight: 25.0–29.9
Obese: 30–39.9
Severely obese: 40.0 and greater

According to the Centers for Disease Control and Prevention (CDC), individuals with a BMI of less than 18.5 are underweight.

Individuals with a BMI of 40 or greater are considered to be potential candidates for surgical intervention with a gastric bypass procedure. Other considerations for this procedure include the regional distribution of the fat. For example, people whose fat lies primarily around the waist area are at greater risk for serious health problems than are people whose fat is primarily located in their hip area. Patients with a BMI of 35.0 who also have other serious illnesses (comorbidities), such as dia-betes and/or hypertension, may also be candidates for weight loss surgery.

See also ANOREXIA NERVOSA; CUSHING'S SYNDROME/CUSHING'S DISEASE; EATING DISORDERS; GASTRIC SURGERY FOR WEIGHT LOSS; OBESITY; PRADER-WILLI SYNDROME.

National Institutes of Health. "The Practical Guide: Identification, Evaluation, and Treatment of Overweight and Obesity in Adults." National Heart, Lung and Blood Institute, NIH Publication No. 00–4084, October 2000.

bone age   The age of a person based on the individual's skeletal maturity. Bone age is also known as skeletal age. It is determined by taking X-rays of the hand and the wrist (usually the left hand/wrist of a child) and considering the size of the growth plates at the ends of the bones (the epiphyses). These bone shapes are then compared with standards to determine bone age. Usually the Greulich and Pyle atlas of radiographic standards are used for a comparison basis. X-rays taken to determine an individual's bone age can be easily misinterpreted, however, and an experienced radiologist is crucial to provide the correct interpretation.

The bone age represents a percentage of the adult age, and it can also be used to calculate a child's growth potential. Delayed bone age can be caused by HYPOTHYROIDISM, a growth hormone deficiency, chronic illnesses, as well as other causes.

Sometimes physicians check the bone age in children whose actual age and birth date are known, such as in the case of adolescents who have a DELAYED PUBERTY or an EARLY PUBERTY or who have experienced growth failure or delay. Sometimes the child's age is not known, such as with some children adopted from foreign orphanages. The bone age information will help the physician determine whether further growth can be anticipated in a child.

If the child's long bones (at the epiphyses) have not yet fused, this is an indication that some potential for growth remains. Thus, if a child is age 12 or older, is significantly shorter than normal for the child's age, and has a bone age of 9.5 years, the child still has significant growth potential. Conversely, if a child is age 17 and has a bone age of 18 years, the epiphyses are closed and the child has no further potential for growth in height.

If a child has short stature and has growth hormone deficiency, physicians may decide that growth hormone can be prescribed as long as the epiphyses are not yet fused.

See also GROWTH HORMONE.

bone diseases Illnesses that cause an underproduction of bone mass, such as osteoporosis, an overproduction of bone, such as PAGET'S DISEASE and ACROMEGALY, or abnormal bone, seen to varying extents in OSTEOPOROSIS, fibrous dysplasia, and Paget's disease. Disorders of bone may be induced by nonendocrine causes, such as cancer, infection, vitamin deficiency, disorders of cartilage production, and genetic defects.

Bone density can be measured using a variety of techniques, most commonly with the dual-energy X-ray absorptiometry scan (DEXA SCAN). Bone biopsies are helpful in some cases. Blood and urine tests can help to determine the activities of the major cells within the bone, namely, the osteoclasts, which help to break down the bone, and the osteoblasts, which help to create the new bone.

See also CALCIUM BALANCE; OSTEOBLASTS; OSTEO-CLASTS; OSTEOMALACIA; OSTEOPENIA; OSTEOPOROSIS; RICKETS.

bone mass measurement A test to determine the density of bone mass. In most cases, bone mass is measured with a dual-energy X-ray absorptiometry (DEXA) scan. Typically, bone measurements are made in the spine and the hip, but they can also be taken in other areas of the body. With primary hyperparathyroidism, cortical bone is lost prior to trabecular bone. Thus bone density is also measured at the wrist, where there is a greater preponderance of cortical bone.

An experienced clinician is needed to interpret these X-rays, because osteoarthritis can falsely elevate readings, especially in the spine. Positioning the patient for the scan is critical, especially if serial data are being compared, as there can be significant differences in bone mineral density if even slightly different areas of a bone are being measured.

Bone mass density can also be tested using what is called quantitative computerized tomography (QCT) scanning and can be estimated with forms of ultrasound. However, this technique is primarily used for screening as opposed to making serial measurements.

Low bone mass density is computed at 2.5 standard deviations versus the peak bone mass seen in a person of the same sex between the ages of 20–30 years old. This is known as the T-score. Another measure, the Z-score, compares a patient's bone density with an age-matched control.

Low bone density is known as OSTEOPOROSIS. Individuals with osteoporosis are at risk for developing serious fractures, particularly fractures of the hip. Sometimes patients have a bone mass density that is not sufficiently low to merit a diagnosis of osteoporosis but that may be low enough to fit the criteria for OSTEOPENIA. Patients with osteopenia also need to work to improve their bone density so that their condition does not further deteriorate to the level of osteoporosis.

See also BONE AGE; CALCIUM BALANCE.

breast-feeding Providing nutrition to newborns, older infants, and sometimes toddlers through milk produced by a woman's breasts. Breast-feeding is also known as lactation. Breast-feeding is strongly encouraged in the United States and other countries as a positive and nutritious way to feed a baby.

Some studies have indicated that women with HYPOCALCEMIA (below-normal levels of calcium in their blood) may actually show improvement in this condition during pregnancy and lactation, largely because of the production of PROLACTIN, a hormone linked to pregnancy, childbirth, and breast-feeding. Some women who were hypocalcemic may even become temporarily hypercalcemic while breast-feeding, as may some women with previously normal calcium blood levels.

A very small number of women, however, such as women with DIABETES MELLITUS who have proliferative retinopathy (an eye disease that may cause blindness), should consider refraining from breast-feeding their babies. The act of breast-feeding can worsen their retinopathy. Physicians have also discouraged breast-feeding among women being treated for hyperthyroidism, although this view is moderating. A recent report in the *Journal of Clinical Endocrinology & Metabolism,* which studied 51 infants who were nursed by mothers taking methimazole (Tapazole), an antithyroid drug, revealed that the babies had normal THYROID-STIMULATING HORMONE (TSH) levels as well as other normal thyroid levels. The children's intellectual development, at 48 and 74 months, was normal as well.

See also HYPERCALCEMIA; INFANTS; POSTPARTUM THYROID DISEASE; PREGNANCY.

For further information on breast-feeding, contact:

La Leche League International
1400 North Meacham Road
Schaumburg, IL 60173–4840
(847) 519-7730
http://www.lalecheleague.org

Azizi, F., et al. "Thyroid Function and Intellectual Development of Infants Nursed by Mothers Taking Methimazole." *Journal of Clinical Endocrinology & Metabolism* 85 (2000) no. 9: 3,233–3,238.

bromocriptine (Parlodel) A medication that increases dopamine secretion in the brain and can be used to treat patients with hyperprolactinemia (whether it is associated with a pituitary tumor or not) and ACROMEGALY. Bromocriptine is a dopamine agonist. This means that it is a medication that increases the amount of dopamine in the brain and thus inhibits prolactin secretion from the pituitary gland. It can cause some patients to experience significant nausea. Therefore the medication must be started at very low doses and slowly increased in order to obtain the appropriate clinical and biochemical response in the patient. Bromocriptine is usually given once per day.

CABERGOLINE (Dostinex) is usually used as the second-line drug in the treatment of hyperprolactinemia. It causes less nausea than bromocriptine, and it can often be dosed only one or two times per week. Pergolide (Permax) is another medication used to treat patients with hyperprolactinemia.

cabergoline (Dostinex)   A medication used to treat patients with hyperprolactinema and, on occasion, those with ACROMEGALY. In the treatment of hyperprolactinemia, which is mainly caused by microadenomas of the pituitary gland, cabergoline causes less nausea than BROMOCRIPTINE (Parlodel) and needs to be dosed only one or two times per week.

Cabergoline works by increasing the amount of dopamine in the brain and thus decreasing the secretion of PROLACTIN. Similar drugs, such as pergolide (Permax) and bromocriptine have been successful in improving the quality of life of many patients with hyperprolactinemia and acromegaly.

cachexia   A state of abnormal metabolism causing a wasting away of the body's muscle mass as well as body weight. It generally occurs due to an inadequate intake of nutrition to meet the body's metabolic needs. It may also be caused by the increased stress on the body from an illness, which then results in increased metabolic needs that the body is unable to meet. Some elderly patients fail to eat enough food to meet their nutritional needs.

Cachexia is found in severely ill patients with such diseases as cancer, acquired immune deficiency syndrome (AIDS), rheumatoid arthritis, and other very serious illnesses and medical conditions. Some untreated endocrine disorders can lead to cachexia. These include HYPERTHYROIDISM (of any cause), ADDISON'S DISEASE, and CUSHING'S SYNDROME caused by the ectopic secretion of excess adrenocorticotropic hormone (ACTH), typically caused by a malignant tumor.

It is important for physicians to treat cachexia because for some patients, treatment may mean the difference between life and death. Said authors Daniel L. Marks and Roger D. Cone, in their 2001 article in *Recent Progress in Hormone Research*, "The severity of cachexia in these illnesses is often the primary determining factor in both quality of life and eventual mortality."

Signs and Symptoms

The primary indicators of cachexia include:

- Severe fatigue
- Lack of appetite (anorexia, not to be confused with anorexia nervosa)
- A weight loss of as much as 10 percent of body weight or more
- Severe weakness

Diagnosis and Treatment

The diagnosis is made based on the patient's current weight compared with the recent past weight. Patients in a state of cachexia are often treated with small, frequent, high-fat meals; nutritional supplements; and drugs, such as megestrol acetate or cyproheptadine, to stimulate the appetite. In a study reported in a 2003 issue of *Gut*, the researchers studied 200 patients with pancreatic cancer who had cachexia. They found that omega-3 fatty acid supplements increased lean body mass and appetite in these patients. The researchers also noted that the subjects' weight gain also improved their quality of life.

Elderly patients are often afflicted with cachexia. According to an article in a 1999 issue of *The American Journal of Clinical Nutrition*, cachexia is associated with above-normal levels of proinflammatory cytokines, such as tumor necrosis factor-alpha, interleukin, serotonin, and interferon. Said the authors, "Reduction in the concentrations of these cytokines is associated with weight gain." They stated that drugs that stimulate appetite and weight gain in geriatric patients, such as progestational agents, pentoxifylline, cyproheptadine, and thalidomide, may decrease cytokine levels and thus increase appetite and weight.

Fearon, K. C. H., et al. "Effect of a Protein and Energy Dense N-3 Fatty Acid Enriched Oral Supplement on Loss of Weight and Lean Tissue in Cancer Cachexia: A Randomised Double Blind Trial." *Gut* 52, no. 10 (2003): 1,479–1,486.

Marks, Daniel L., and Roger D. Cone. "Central Melanocortins and the Regulation of Weight During Acute and Chronic Disease." *Recent Progress in Hormone Research* 56, (2001): 359–376.

Yeh, Shing-Shing, and Michael W. Schuster. "Geriatric Cachexia: The Role of Cytokines." *American Journal for Clinical Nutrition* 70, no. 2 (August 1999): 183–197.

calcitonin A hormone produced by the parafollicular c cells of the thyroid gland. The exact physiological reasons for the existence of calcitonin are unclear. However, it is known that calcitonin is involved with calcium and bone metabolism as well as in breast milk letdown and lactation. Calcitonin may be secreted in large quantities in patients who have a rare form of THYROID CANCER: medullary carcinoma of the thyroid (MCT). As a result, the measurement of calcitonin in the bloodstream can be used to help diagnose and monitor this form of thyroid cancer.

Injectable, synthetically derived calcitonin may be used to treat already diagnosed OSTEOPOROSIS. It was first approved for this purpose by the Food and Drug Administration (FDA) in 1984. (Calcitonin is not, however, approved for the prevention of osteoporosis.) Both nasal calcitonin (Miacalcin) and injectable calcitonin (Calcimar) are FDA-approved to treat postmenopausal osteoporosis.

Calcitonin may also be used to treat PAGET' DISEASE and the HYPERCALCEMIA caused by malignant tumors (humoral hypercalcemia of malignancy, or HHM). With Paget's disease, due to the need for long-term usage, the calcitonin may lose its efficacy because of the formation of antibodies that bind to it.

Most patients use calcitonin in the form of a nasal spray and find using the nasal calcitonin (Miacalcin) to be more attractive than using the other forms. However, it is absorbed more slowly and less efficiently, and thus larger amounts are required. Some patients are given calcitonin in combination with HORMONE REPLACEMENT THERAPY, which has been found to increase the bone density in some patients significantly. Calcitonin may also be injected subcutaneously or intramuscularly.

Some patients may be allergic to the salmon-derived form of calcitonin, although this reaction can also be seen with recombinant human calcitonin. Calcitonin may also cause such side effects as flushing, nausea, and diarrhea, although these effects are not common, and when they appear, are often short-lived. In contrast, due to the large amounts of endogenous calcitonin secreted by patients with medullary carcinoma of the thyroid (MCT), these symptoms may be severe.

Some studies have shown that calcitonin also has an analgesic (pain-killing) effect on patients who have acute bone fractures. Most of this data has been accumulated by studying the injectable form of calcitonin. However, the inhaled nasal spray has also been utilized. In one study, the nasal spray was found to be more effective than the injectable calcitonin.

Controversy remains about whether either the nasal spray or the injected calcitonin is effective in treating the pain of fractures and, if so, which is superior. Neither preparation is approved by the Food and Drug Administration (FDA) for the treatment of bone pain caused by FRACTURE, but endocrinologists have found it to be useful.

See also BISPHOSPHONATES; CALCIUM BALANCE.

Lyritis, G. P., et al. "Analgesic Effects of Salmon Calcitonin in Osteoporotic Vertebral Fractures: A Double-Blind Placebo Controlled Case Study." *Calcification Tissue International* 49, no. 6 (December 1991): 369–372.

Overgaard, K., et. al. "Effect of Salcatonin Given Intranasally on Bone Loss and Fracture Rates in Established Osteoporosis." *British Medical Journal* 305, no. 6,853 (September 5, 1992): 556–561.

Overgaard, K., et. al. "Effect of Salcatonin Given Intranasally on Early Postmenopausal Bone Loss." *British Medical Journal* 299, no. 6,697 (August 19, 1989): 477–479.

Silverman, Stuart L., M.D. "Calcitonin." *Endocrinology and Metabolism Clinics of North America* 32 (2003): 273–284.

calcitriol Synthetic vitamin D that is prescribed for people with a calcium deficiency/HYPOCALCEMIA. Most commonly, these are patients who have either kidney failure or HYPOPARATHYROIDISM. Calcitriol increases the absorption of calcium from the gut into the blood. It is commercially available as Rocaltrol in 25- and 50-microgram capsules. Generic formulations of calcitriol are also available to patients.

Because it is the most potent and longest-acting vitamin D metabolite available, calcitriol can also easily lead to HYPERCALCEMIA (excessively high levels of calcium in the blood) and to hypercalciuria (excessive levels of calcium in the urine) among patients who take the medication. Thus, calcitriol should be used judiciously by physicians, with regular monitoring of a patient's blood calcium levels.

See also CALCIUM ABSORPTION; CALCIUM BALANCE; VITAMIN D; VITAMIN D RESISTANCE.

calcium absorption The continuing process by which calcium is absorbed, usually in the intestines. Calcium absorption is monitored by physicians by measuring the amount of calcium found in the urine over a period of 24 hours. A normal level that indicates good absorption and generally adequate vitamin D levels is between 2 and 4 mg/kg/day.

Calcium absorption in the intestines is primarily driven by VITAMIN D. Thus, deficiencies of vitamin D lead to poor calcium absorption, a decreased serum calcium (calcium in the blood), and a rise in parathyroid hormone (PTH) levels. This increased PTH helps to decrease the loss of calcium from the kidneys, and it also helps to move some calcium from the bone back into the bloodstream. Typically, 40–50 percent of ingested calcium is absorbed, but a large portion of absorbed calcium is lost via intestinal secretion.

Medications may also affect calcium absorption. Some antibiotics, such as penicillin and chloramphenicol, may increase calcium absorption. Factors that decrease calcium absorption include high fiber in the diet, foods high in oxalic acid or phytic acid, an existing lactase deficiency, and some medications. These medications include GLUCOCORTICOIDS, anticonvulsants, tetracycline, and estrogens, such as those found in ORAL CONTRACEPTIVES or in ESTROGEN REPLACEMENT THERAPY.

If patients who take calcium supplements need a short-term increase in their calcium absorption, they may wish to spread out their intake of calcium supplements throughout the day. They should take the calcium supplement with their meals and avoid taking it along with foods that are high in oxalate, such as spinach or nuts, or that are high in phytates, such as wheat bran or soybeans.

The most commonly used forms of calcium supplements are oyster shell calcium or calcium carbonate. Other forms of calcium, such as calcium citrate, maltase, and glaciate, can be used, although they are usually more expensive. Calcium lactate is another form of calcium, but it is often difficult to obtain.

See also CALCIUM BALANCE; HYPERCALCEMIA; HYPOCALCEMIA; HYPOPARATHYROIDISM; PARATHYROID GLANDS.

Levenson, David I., M.D., and Kevin Al Ohayon. "A Practical Analysis of Calcium Supplements." *Alternative Therapies in Women's Health Archives* 2 (April 1, 2000): 28–31.

calcium balance Refers to the processes involving the gut (absorption), kidneys (filtering and reabsorption as well as vitamin D metabolism), parathyroid glands (the four glands in the neck, by the thyroid gland), and bone (where calcium is stored and used for structural integrity). Among other functions, calcium is needed for muscle contractions, to activate nerves, and to cause blood to clot. Some experts believe that insufficient calcium in childhood and adolescence may contribute to the development of OSTEOPOROSIS in later adulthood.

Although many people are mildly or moderately deficient in calcium, elderly adults (age 65 and older) and adolescents are the most likely to have below-normal levels of calcium (hypocalcemia) in their bloodstreams, primarily because of diets that are low in calcium and/or vitamin D. Others have excessive levels of calcium in the bloodstream. The most common cause of excess calcium in the blood is primary hyperparathyroidism.

Individuals who cannot gain sufficient calcium from their diets may take calcium supplements, usually in tablet form. In addition, prescribed vitamin D (CALCITRIOL) is usually given to such individuals to boost their blood levels of calcium. According to a 2000 article in *Alternative Therapies in Women's Health Archives,* calcium carbonate is the most popular calcium supplement, followed by calcium citrate. Some patients take bonemeal to boost their calcium levels, while others take dolomite, which is a combination of calcium carbonate and magnesium carbonate.

Less popular means of increasing calcium intake include taking supplements of calcium lactate, calcium gluconate, and calcium citrate malate. If intravenous calcium is needed, in the event of a medical emergency, calcium gluconate is usually used.

See also CALCIUM ABSORPTION; HYPERCALCEMIA; HYPOCALCEMIA; HYPOPARATHYROIDISM.

Bove, Lisa Anne. "Restoring Electrolyte Balance: Calcium & Phosphorus" 59, no. 3 *RN* (March 1996): 47–5l.

Levenson, David I., M.D., and Kevin Al Ohayon. "A Practical Analysis of Calcium Supplements." *Alternative Therapies in Women's Health Archives* 2 (April 1, 2000): 28–31.

Tordoff, Michael G. "Calcium: Taste, Intake, and Appetite." *Physiological Reviews* 81, no. 4 (October 1, 2001): 1,567–1,597.

Canadian Diabetes Association (Association Canadienne du Diabète)   Formed in 1953, the Canadian Diabetes Association is a nongovernmental advocacy organization for research and education that helps an estimated 2 million Canadians who have diabetes. It has 150 branches throughout the country. The organization also funds research through the Charles H. Best Research Fund. The Canadian Diabetes Association estimates that by 2010, the number of Canadians with diabetes will increase to 3 million.

National Office:

National Life Building
1400-522 University Avenue
Toronto, Ontario M56 2R5
(416) 363-0177 or (800) BANTING (toll-free in
   Canada)
www.diabetes.ca

Provincial Offices:

British Columbia–Yukon Division
360-1385 West 8th Avenue
Vancouver, BC V6H 3V9
(604) 732-1331 or (800) 665-6526 (toll-free)

Alberta/Northwest Territories Division
1010-10117 Jasper Avenue NW
Edmonton, AB T5J 1W8
(780) 423-1232 or (800) 563-0032 (toll-free)

Saskatchewan Division
104-2301 Avenue C North
Saskatoon, SK S7L 5Z5
(306) 933-1238 or (800) 996-4446 (toll-free)

Manitoba Division
102-310 Broadway Avenue
Winnepeg, MB R3C 0S6
(204) 925-3800 or (800) 226-8464 (toll-free)

Ontario Division
15 Toronto Street
Suite 800
Toronto, ON M5C 2E3
(416) 363-3373 or (800) 226-8464 (toll-free)

New Brunswick Division
165 Regent Street
Suite 3
Fredericton, NB E3B 7B4
(506) 452-9009 or (800) 884-4232 (toll-free)

Nova Scotia Division
6080 Young Street
#101
Halifax, NS B3K 5L2
(902) 453-4232 or (800) 326-7712 (toll-free)

Prince Edward Island Division
Charlottetown Area Health Centre
1 Rochford Street
Charlottetown, PEI C1A 9L2
(902) 894-3005

Newfoundland and Labrador Division
354 Water Street
Suite 217
St. John's, NF A1C 1C4
(709) 754-0953

Affiliate:

Association Diabète Québec (Quebec Diabetes
   Association)
5635, Rue Sherbrooke Est
Montreal, PQ H1N 1A2
(514) 259-3422 or (800) 361-3504 (toll-free number)

cancer A malignant tumor. Any organ within
the endocrine system (or within the entire body)
can develop a malignant tumor. Physicians who
suspect a cancerous tumor will almost always perform a biopsy, which is the removal of tissue from
the area that may be cancerous. A pathologist eval-
uates whether the tissue is actually cancerous.

The cancer is then staged by the physician,
which means that the severity of the cancer is evaluated. Whether the cancer has spread to other
parts of the body or to other organs is also determined. Most physicians assess the stage of cancer
using the TNM (tumor/node/metastasis) system,
which varies somewhat depending on the form of
the cancer.

When possible and if identified early enough,
cancer is often surgically excised. If the tumor is
not operable because it is too difficult to reach, is at
an advanced stage of tumor, or for other reasons
(such as the ill health of the patient), the patient
may be treated with radiation therapy, chemotherapy, and other forms of treatment. Patients who
have advanced cancers may seek to join clinical trials, in which they may be selected to test medications or therapies that are not available to the general public.

Hormone therapy (also called endocrine therapy
by the physicians who use it) is sometimes used to
treat advanced cancer. For example, with prostate
cancer, oncologists may give men hormone medications to block the production of TESTOSTERONE.
The reason is that testosterone enhances cancer
growth, and thus, lower levels of testosterone will
mean less aggressive tumor growth.

Hormone therapy usually includes luteinizing
hormone-releasing hormone (LH-RH) agonists and
sometimes other drugs, such as antiandrogens, to
treat prostate cancer. These drugs frequently cause
men to experience a wide variety of side effects,
including reduced sex drive, impotence, hot flashes, mood swings, breast swelling, weight gain, and
loss of muscle mass. Though hormone therapy
eventually fails and men become hormone resistant, the therapy may be effective in extending their
lives for years.

See also OVARIAN CANCER; PANCREATIC CANCER;
PARATHYROID CANCER; PHEOCHROMOCYTOMAS; TESTIC-
ULAR CANCER; THYROID CANCER.

For further information on cancer, contact:

American Cancer Society
1599 Clifton Road NE
Atlanta, GA 30329
(404) 320-2408 or (800) 227-2345 (toll-free)
http://www.cancer.org

National Cancer Institute
Division of Cancer Epidemiology and Genetics
6120 Executive Boulevard, MSC-7242
Executive Plaza South
7th Floor
Bethesda, MD 20892
(301) 496-1611

Lange, Paul H., M.D., and Christine Adamec. *Prostate
   Cancer for Dummies.* New York, N.Y.: Wiley Publishing,
   2003.

Carney complex A rare condition, originally
described by J. A. Carney in 1985. Carney complex
is caused by a genetic mutation and is usually considered a form of a multiple endocrine neoplasia
(MEN) syndrome. Symptoms of Carney complex
include skin lesions, such as pigmented lentigines
and blue nevi on the eyes, face, lips, neck, and
trunk, as well as endocrine tumors (adrenal, pituitary, testicular, and thyroid) and nonendocrine
tumors (atrial, breast, and skin).

Carney complex is considered a developmental
disorder, although it may not be diagnosed until
early adulthood. Men and women are about equally affected by this disorder, and half the cases are
diagnosed after the age of 20 years. In many cases,
the characteristic skin changes occur during puberty and may fade by the time the patient is in his or
her 40s. All patients are found to have some adrenal gland abnormalities at the time of surgery and
biopsy or at autopsy.

Carney complex causes a form of Cushing's syndrome, due to bilateral adrenal micronodular hyperplasia, in about one of every four patients. The pituitary tumors are typically adenomas. About 15 percent of the pituitary tumors cause gigantism. The atrial tumors are typically myxomas and may cause obstruction of the mitral valve of the heart, embolism, and constitutional symptoms such as weight loss, fever, and fatigue (with anemia and thrombocytopenia). Some patients have thyroid tumors and some may also have acromegaly. The disease decreases the normal expected life span in most patients.

Patients with Carney complex should receive regular medical attention, and any tumors should be treated. Physicians should vigilantly check for the development of further tumors.

See also ACROMEGALY; CUSHING'S SYNDROME/ CUSHING'S DISEASE; GIGANTISM; MULTIPLE ENDOCRINE NEOPLASIA.

Carney, J. A., et al. "The Complex of Myxomas, Spotty Pigmentation, and Endocrine Overactivity." *Medicine* 64, no. 4 (July 1985): 270–283.

Stratakis, Constantine A., Lawrence S. Kirschner, and J. Aidan Carney. "Clinical and Molecular Features of the Carney Complex: Diagnostic Criteria and Recommendations for Patient Evaluation." *Journal of Clinical Endocrinology & Metabolism* 87, no. 9 (2001): 4,041–4,046.

Centers for Disease Control and Prevention (CDC)

The primary federal agency in the United States that oversees the government agencies that provide research and information on diabetes and other major diseases. For example, the National Center for Health Statistics compiles data and statistics on incidence of diseases, deaths, hospitalizations, and many other topics.

The National Institute of Diabetes and Digestive and Kidney Diseases (NIDDK) is an important branch of the CDC. Contact the NIDDK at:

Building 31
Room 9A04
Center Drive
MSC 2560

Bethesda, MD 20892-2560
(800) 860-8747 or (301) 654-3327
http://www.niddk.nih.gov

For further information on the CDC, contact the organization at:

1600 Clifton Road NE
Atlanta, GA 30333
(404) 639-3534 or (800) 311-3435 (toll-free)
http://www.cdc.gov

cerebral vascular diseases   Diseases that cause damage to the blood vessels in the brain and neck and that can lead to stroke or heart disease. People with some endocrine diseases, such as DIABETES MELLITUS or hypertension, have a higher risk of developing cerebrovascular diseases than do nondiabetics. Elderly individuals (age 65 and older) are at particular risk for developing cerebral vascular diseases.

cholesterol   One of several fats (lipids) that circulate in the body as lipoproteins, including low-density lipoproteins (LDL) and high-density lipoproteins (HDL). HDL is considered to be good cholesterol because it works to keep blood vessels healthy via a process known as reverse cholesterol transport. Conversely, LDL is considered to be bad cholesterol because it damages the blood vessels and can lead to ATHEROSCLEROSIS and then heart attack, stroke, peripheral vascular disease, and finally, death.

Patients with some diseases, such as Type 2 DIABETES MELLITUS, typically have lower-than-normal HDL levels. Even when they have normal or only slightly elevated LDL levels, they are at greater risk of developing complications. This is because their LDL cholesterol tends to be more atherogenic as it has been glycosylated—that is, glucose molecules have attached atop the proteins in the LDL, rendering the LDL more likely to attach to blood vessel walls and cause problems. In addition, the HDL of patients with Type 2 diabetes does not work as well as it should either. It is less efficient than among nondiabetics in transporting cholesterol from the blood vessel to the liver.

Thus, the target LDL cholesterol level is lower for those with diabetes. Patients with diabetes should contact their physicians for information on the LDL cholesterol levels that are appropriate in their case.

Risk Factors

Other individuals in addition to those with diabetes have a greater-than-normal risk for developing health problems associated with their cholesterol levels. These at-risk individuals tend to be those who:

- Have hypertension
- Are obese
- Have a very inactive lifestyle
- Are either African American or Native American
- Eat a very high-fat diet

Recommended Levels of Cholesterol

The National Heart, Lung, and Blood Institute released their new guidelines for cholesterol control in 2002, provided in the chart that follows.

CLASSIFICATION OF LDL, TOTAL AND HDL CHOLESTEROL (MG/DL)

LDL Cholesterol: Primary Target of Therapy

Less than 100	Optimal
100–129	Near optimal/above optimal
130–159	Borderline high
160–189	High
190+	Very high

Total Cholesterol

Less than 200	Desirable
200–239	Borderline high
240+	High

HDL Cholesterol

Less than 40	Low
60+	High

Source: National Cholesterol Education Program. "Third Report of the National Cholesterol Education Program (NCEP) Expert Panel on Detection, Evaluation, and Treatment of High Blood Cholesterol in Adults (Adult Treatment Panel III)." NIH Publication No. 02-5215, September 2002.

Diagnosis and Treatment

Cholesterol problems are diagnosed based on the patient's blood levels of HDL and LDL. Thus, LDL levels of 160 and above are considered high, and 190 and above is very high. A level of HDL cholesterol below 40 is considered problematic.

Patients diagnosed with cholesterol disorders are first asked to work on therapeutic lifestyle changes, including changes in nutrition (lower fat and cholesterol intake and increased fiber intake) and attention to weight and exercise. If these measures fail to bring a patient's lipid levels to the goal, medications are frequently needed.

Patients with diabetes as well as cholesterol disorders are urged to get their glucose levels as close to normal as possible. Patients with hypertension will be advised to bring their blood pressure levels down as well. Regular exercise is also usually recommended. It need not be strenuous or difficult; even a daily walk is a good exercise that can help to improve health.

If a patient has high LDL levels and dietary modifications do not bring about sufficient changes, doctors may then decide to prescribe cholesterol-lowering drugs in the statin series of medications. (Statins were formerly known as HMG CoA reductase inhibitors.) Aspirin therapy may also be considered, especially if the patient is at risk for a heart attack or stroke, has diabetes, or has ever had either a heart attack or stroke in the past.

For further information on cholesterol levels, contact:

The National Heart, Lung, and Blood Institute
Building 31, Room 5A52
31 Center Drive MSC 2486
Bethesda, MD 20892
(301) 592-8573
http://www.nhlbi.nih.gov

National Cholesterol Education Program. "Third Report of the National Cholesterol Education Program (NCEP) Expert Panel on Detection, Evaluation, and Treatment of High Blood Cholesterol in Adults (Adult Treatment Panel III)." NIH Publication No. 02-5215, September 2002.

Pearlman, Brian L., M.D. "The New Cholesterol Guidelines: Applying Them in Clinical Practice." *Postgraduate Medicine* 11, no. 2 (August 2002): 13–26.

chromogranin A   A peptide hormone cosecreted with catecholamines. It is elevated in patients who have neuroendocrine tumors, such as a PHEOCHRO-MOCYTOMA, GASTRINOMA, or carcinoid and medullary carcinoma of the thyroid. However, chromogranin A is not specific nor is it sensitive enough to be used as a diagnostic test. It is mainly used as a tumor marker, if no better markers are available, to help physicians follow the progress of a patient's therapy for a specific tumor.

See also THYROID CANCER.

Chvostek's sign   A simple test used during a physical examination to check for severely low levels of calcium in the blood, originally noted by 19th-century Austrian surgeon Frantisek Chvostek. Chvostek's sign is considered a classic sign of hypocalcemia.

With this test, the physician taps the midcheekbone near the area where the facial nerve is located (where the seventh cranial nerve exits the salivary/parotid gland). If the person is hypocalcemic, this action will usually elicit a sneering-like contraction in the patient's cheek, nose, and corner of the mouth.

Patients who exhibit Chvostek's sign will need supplemental doses of calcium and will often also need vitamin D supplements to stimulate the further absorption of calcium from their gut. Unfortunately, about 20–25 percent of patients who do not have hypocalcemia will also demonstrate some facial twitching with this test. In addition, some patients who actually do have hypocalcemia will not produce the Chvostek's sign.

Chvostek's sign is also sometimes positive in the absence of hypocalcemia when patients have other illnesses, such as myxedema, rickets, measles, and diphtheria. In addition, some healthy patients may show a positive Chvostek's sign, while some patients who actually have hypocalcemia will show a negative Chvostek's sign. At best, Chvostek's sign is merely a good basic indicator of possible hypocalcemia and should be followed up by a blood test of the patient's calcium level.

Another diagnostic test for hypocalcemia, TROUSSEAU'S SIGN, was noted by 19th-century French physician Armand Trousseau. Most experts believe that this sign, which uses a blood pressure cuff to elicit the characteristic flexing of the wrist and finger joints, is more reliable (sensitive and specific) than is Chvostek's sign.

See also CALCIUM BALANCE; HYPOCALCEMIA; HYPOPARATHYROIDISM; TETANY.

Hofmann, E. "Chvostek Sign." *American Journal of Surgery* 96, no. 1 (1958): 33–38.
Urbano, Frank L., M.D. "Signs of Hypocalcemia: Chvostek's and Trousseau's Signs." *Hospital Physician* 36, no. 3 (March 2000): 43–45.

clonidine suppression test   A diagnostic/confirmatory medical test given when there is a very high suspicion of the presence of a PHEOCHROMOCYTOMA, an adrenal gland tumor that causes paroxysmal hypertension, flushing, headaches, and orthostatic hypertension. This test is only done for a patient whom the endocrinologist strongly suspects of having a pheochromocytoma, and whose total blood plasma levels are borderline, typically between 1,000 and 2,000 pg/ml (or 5.9–11.8 nmol/l). For patients whose levels are even lower than this range, other stimulatory tests may need to be done to ascertain a diagnosis.

The clonidine suppression test should only be conducted in patients who are well hydrated to avoid the onset of severe hypotension (low blood pressure). The patients are instructed to avoid eating for at least four hours before the test. Some types of medications must be completely avoided before the test, such as beta-blockers, diuretics, and tricyclic antidepressants. Other medications for the treatment of hypertension should be withheld for about 12 hours prior to this test to minimize any effect on the test results.

Clonidine is a commercially available oral antihypertensive drug that works to lower blood pressure by stimulating alpha-2 adrenoreceptors in the brain, thus leading to a decrease in sympathetic nervous system outflow from the brain. This typically causes there to be lower levels of catecholamine in the system, which, in turn, allows blood vessels to relax and thus blood pressure to drop. Patients with a pheochromocytoma have less of a decrease in their plasma catecholamines.

The drug can cause drowsiness and dry mouth in 30–40 percent of patients who receive it. It also has a potent first-dose effect, whereby a patient's blood pressure may drop precipitously with the first dose.

Baseline plasma catecholamine levels are measured from an indwelling intravenous catheter in the patient. (The simple act of inserting a needle or intravenous drip will cause the release of some catecholamines and thus "falsely" elevate the catecholamine levels. Physicians realize this.)

After baseline catecholamine levels are taken, 0.3 mgs of clonidine is orally ingested by the patient. Three hours later, the patient's plasma catecholamine levels are remeasured.

If the patient's total plasma catecholamine levels fall to less than 500 pg/ml (or 2.96 nmol/l) or to less than a 50 percent decline from the patient's baseline levels, the diagnosis of a pheochromocytoma is excluded with a 92 percent certainty. Overall, the clonidine suppression test has a 97 percent sensitivity, which means that 97 percent of patients with a pheochromocytoma will have an abnormal test. It also has a 67 percent specificity, which means that two-thirds of patients without a pheochromocytoma will have a normal response and one-third will have a false positive test.

Abnormal blood levels are as follows:

Epinephrine: over 90 pg/ml
Norepinephrine: over 550 pg/ml
Dopamine: over 150 pg/ml

In looking at the combination of the epinephrine, norephinephrine, and dopamine levels (the total plasma catecholamines), abnormal blood levels are those that are greater than 500 pg/ml.

Segen, Joseph C. and Joseph Stauffer. *The Patient's Guide to Medical Tests*. New York, N.Y.: Facts On File, Inc., 1998.
Sjoberg, R. J., K. J. Simcic, and G. S. Kidd. "The Clonidine Suppression Test for Pheochromocytoma: A Review of Its Utility and Pitfalls." *Archives of Internal Medicine* 152, no. 6 (1992): 1,193–1,197.

coma A state of unconsciousness that may last for days, weeks, or even years. Often physicians cannot predict if and when the person will regain consciousness. DIABETIC KETOACIDOSIS, a severe imbalance of glucose and acids in the bloodstream, may cause a coma. There are also other endocrine causes of coma, such as severe HYPOTHYROIDISM, from which the patient may suffer from a myxedema coma. In some cases, a blow to the head may cause a coma, as may an overdose of medications or a severe medication interaction. Sometimes a patient enters a coma state and the cause cannot be determined.

The comatose individual needs emergency treatment and usually also requires hospitalization. Rarely, a patient will recover from coma after many years. Some patients have recovered after 20 years or more in a comatose state.

See also DIABETES MELLITUS; MYXEDEMA COMA; TYPE 1 DIABETES; TYPE 2 DIABETES.

computerized tomography (CT) A specific type of X-ray imaging study that is frequently used to diagnose and monitor a wide variety of medical diseases and conditions. The CT scan is also known as a computerized axial tomography or CAT scan. Sometimes physicians will order contrast dye to be injected into the patient's veins to highlight particular organs or areas of the body.

For endocrine disorders, the CT scan is particularly helpful in assessing problems with the ADRENAL GLANDS as well as in evaluating any of the cancers associated with the endocrine system. The CT scan can also be used to image the HYPOTHALAMUS and PITUITARY GLAND, but most of this imaging, as of this writing, is done with MAGNETIC RESONANCE IMAGING (MRI).

See also ULTRASOUND.

congenital adrenal hyperplasia (CAH) Refers to a set of inherited disorders that cause an increased size in the adrenal glands and that are nearly always (about 95 percent of the time) caused by mutations in genetic coding. These disorders cause an insufficient synthesis of CORTISOL.

The most common genetic defect within the category of congenital adrenal hyperplasia is a 21-hydroxylase 21-OH deficiency, which represents over 90 percent of all the cases of congenital adrenal hyperplasia. This defect is found in an estimated one in 12,000 to one in 15,000 births in the United States. It is transmitted as an autosomal recessive condition.

Signs and Symptoms

Newborns and children with congenital adrenal hyperplasia present with either the salt-wasting form (with HYPOTENSION, low sodium levels and high potassium levels) or the simple virilizing form (with ambiguous genitalia). These are the classical forms of 21-hydroxylase 21-OH congenital hyperplasia. Six to seven out of 10 newborns with congenital hyperplasia have the salt-wasting form. HIRSUTISM is not typically evident until later in life.

These patients cannot synthesize adequate cortisol and ALDOSTERONE (and lose excess sodium but retain excess potassium). Thus they will also secrete greater-than-normal amounts of adrenocorticotropic hormone (ACTH). Because of this increased androgen production, women may also become virilized.

Patients with CAH may also suffer from catecholamine deficiency, which can worsen shock.

The nonclassical or late form of CAH presents in puberty or after puberty. Females with this form have menstrual irregularities and hirsutism/virilization that is clinically impossible to distinguish from POLYCYSTIC OVARY SYNDROME (PCOS). Many females have adrenal incidentalomas (adenomas). Boys may have testicular tumors that are actually comprised of adrenal tissue that grows in the scrotum.

Diagnosis and Treatment

The diagnosis of congenital adrenal hyperplasia is based on signs and symptoms as well as medical history. If physicians suspect CAH, the gold standard test for this disorder is used: the corticotrophin (Cortrosyn) stimulation test. With this test, cosyntropin (synthetic ACTH) is injected after measuring the basal levels of 17-(OH) progesterone, and the patient's blood levels of 17-hydroyprosterone are measured 60 minutes later. Salt wasting is measured through testing the blood for serum electrolytes, plasma renin, and aldosterone.

Patients with congenital adrenal hyperplasia are treated with glucocorticoids such as prednisone (Deltasone) or cortisone acetate (Cortef). If this therapy fails, the removal of the adrenal glands (ADRENALECTOMY) may be needed. If performed, this surgery is usually done on adults. Surgery will induce the symptoms of full-blown ADDISON'S DISEASE, but many physicians argue that Addison's disease is easily more manageable than CAH with bilaterally enlarging adrenal glands.

Children with CAH also need annual X-rays to determine their BONE AGE and their growth.

In the less common cases of congenital adrenal hyperplasia that is due to deficiency of 3 beta-hydroxysteroid dehydrogenase, levels of 17 OH progesterone and 17-hydroxypregnenolone accumulate. In congenital adrenal hyperplasia that is due to 17 OH deficiency, androgens and cortisol cannot be produced. With the 11 beta-hydroxylase deficiency form of CAH, aldosterone and cortisol are not produced in adequate amounts. In the 17-ketosteroid reductase deficiency form of congenital adrenal hyperplasia, TESTOSTERONE cannot be synthesized from androstenedione.

See also ADRENAL GLANDS.

Gmyrek, Glenn A., M.D., et al. "Bilateral Laparoscopic Adrenalectomy as a Treatment for Classic Congenital Adrenal Hyperplasia Attributable to 21-Hydroxylase Deficiency." *Pediatrics* 109, no. 2 (February 2002). Available online. URL: http://pediatrics.aapublications.org/cgi/content/full/109/2/e28. Downloaded January 15, 2004.

Speiser, Phyllis W., M.D. and Perrin C. White, M.D. "Congenital Adrenal Hyperplasia." *New England Journal of Medicine* 349, no. 8 (August 21, 2003): 776–788.

congenital hypothyroidism   A rare condition in which low levels of thyroid hormone are found in newborn infants. An estimated one in every 4,000 infants has congenital hypothyroidism, according to the American Academy of Clinical Endocrinologists. Of these cases, 85 percent are sporadic and 15 percent are inherited. Most of these cases are caused by a genesis of thyroid tissues or ectopic tissue. For unknown reasons, congenital hypothyroidism occurs twice as frequently in girls as boys. Interestingly, the incidence is more common in

Hispanic children (one in 2,000) and much rarer in African-American children (one in 32,000). Some of the cases have a central etiology and are often associated with other midline defects, such as cleft palate and eye abnormalities.

Infants who have Down syndrome have an increased risk for the diagnosis of congenital hypothyroidism. In one large population study of newborn infants that identified 97 infants with congenital hypothyroidism, reported in a 1997 issue of the *American Journal of Medical Genetics*, the researchers found that newborn babies with Down syndrome had a 35 times greater risk of having congenital hypothyroidism compared with babies without Down syndrome. In addition, babies with Down syndrome are at a greater risk for developing hypothyroidism later in infancy. As a result, the American Academy of Pediatrics recommends that babies with Down syndrome be screened for acquired hypothyroidism at birth, at the four- to six-month stage, at the 12-month stage, and once a year afterward.

An early diagnosis is important. If infants with hypothyroidism are not diagnosed and treated, they will develop cretinism, which is manifested by mental retardation, slowed growth, intolerance to cold, constipation, dry skin, as well as other symptoms typical of hypothyroidism. Untreated children will often also be deaf and mute. At birth, these children may have few signs and symptoms because their bodies still have some thyroid (T4) hormone from their mothers. They may have slightly increased birth weight, enlarged fontanels (soft spots), hoarse cries, poor movement, constipation, enlarged tongue, jaundice, and low body temperature.

All states in the United States require neonatal screening for congenital hypothyroidism. Infants afflicted with congenital hypothyroidism are treated with supplemental thyroid hormone (levothyroxine), and their pediatricians and pediatric endocrinologists also carefully monitor them. Even with treatment, some infants born with severe congenital hypothyroidism may experience mild cognitive defects later in life according to a study reported in a 2001 issue of *Acta Paediatrics*.

Transient congenital hypothyroidism can occur due to excess iodine, caused by the mother taking amiodarone (Cordarone), a heart medication, or by iodine-containing contrast agents ingested by the mother, thus inducing the production of antibodies by the mother while pregnant.

See also HYPOTHYROIDISM.

Leger, J., et al. "Severity of Hypothyroidism and Inadequate Treatment Limit School Achievement in Children with Congenital Hypothyroidism." *Acta Paediatrics* 90 (2001): 1,249–1,256.

Roberts, Helen E., et al. "Population Study of Congenital Hypothyroidism and Associated Birth Defects, Atlanta, 1979–1992." *American Journal of Medical Genetics* 71, no. 1 (July 11, 1997): 29–32.

Vogiatzi, Maria G., M.D. and John L. Kirkland, M.D. "Frequency and Necessity of Thyroid Function Tests in Neonates and Infants with Congenital Hypothyroidism." *Pediatrics* 100, no. 3 (September 1997). Available online. URL: http://pediatrics.aapublications.org/cgi/content/full/100/3/e6. Downloaded January 20, 2004.

Conn's syndrome   See ALDOSTERONISM.

cortisol   An important hormone synthesized and released by the adrenal glands to help activate many critical body processes, including alertness, vigilance, blood pressure, blood glucose level, and the ability to respond to physical and social stressors.

Cortisol is synthesized in the adrenal cortex in the layer known as the zona fasciculata, under the control of hypothalamic corticotropin releasing factor (CRF) and pituitary adrenocorticotropic hormone (ACTH). It has a circadian rhythm; cortisol levels usually drop when an individual sleeps and begin to rise again shortly before awakening occurs. If very low levels of cortisol are produced, this is called Addison's disease or hypocortisolism, a condition that can become life threatening, requiring emergency doses of hydrocortisone. Very high levels of cortisol cause Cushing's disease. Cortisol is one of the COUNTERREGULATORY HORMONES, a hormone that is released in response to an action elsewhere in the body.

See also ADDISON'S DISEASE; CUSHING'S SYNDROME/CUSHING'S DISEASE; HORMONES.

cortisone Synthetically produced cortisol. Cortisone is used in replacement for the glucocorticoid hormone, meaning it helps to maintain blood glucose levels among its many actions. Some individuals have below-normal levels of cortisol, such as patients with ADDISON'S DISEASE. These patients can be treated with daily doses of cortisone acetate, allowing them to live long and full lives. Without cortisone or other glucocorticoids, however, these patients would die.

In an acute crisis, such as a patient with previously undiagnosed or inadequately treated Addison's disease or among patients who have developed a secondary adrenal insufficiency (typically due to being tapered off their glucocorticoid therapy too quickly), intravenous forms of cortisone as well as normal saline are administered. These treatments are lifesaving.

Cortisone is also used to treat patients with a variety of medical problems, such as various forms of arthritis.

See also CORTISOL; HORMONES.

counterregulatory hormones Hormones released in response to an action elsewhere within the body. For example, if a person develops HYPOGLYCEMIA (low blood sugar), glucagon is released to stimulate the breakdown of glycogen from the liver to counteract the hypoglycemia. Counterregulatory hormones include CORTISOL (the body's natural cortisone), GLUCAGON, epinephrine (ADRENALINE), and GROWTH HORMONE. Cortisol and epinephrine are released by the adrenal glands. Epinephrine and norepinephrine are also synthesized by the sympathetic nervous system. The pituitary releases growth hormone, and the pancreas releases glucagon.

Another example of a counterregulatory hormone at work occurs when a person undergoes severe stress. Epinephrine is released to help the individual deal with that stress by maintaining blood pressure and pulse as well as by increasing blood flow to muscles, part of the fight-or-flight response.

Some people with DIABETES MELLITUS develop reduced rates of response from their counterregulatory hormones. This may be caused by either tight glycemic control or by autonomic neuropathy. When patients have had excellent blood sugar control plus episodes of hypoglycemia, the brain, which can use only glucose for fuel, adapts by improving its ability to extract glucose from the bloodstream. It does this by increasing the synthesis of glucose transporters (GLUT).

This increase means that although patients should begin to feel the symptoms of hypoglycemia at a blood glucose level of about 65 mg/dl (with symptoms such as an increased pulse, sweating, nervousness, tremulousness, nausea, and hunger), such symptoms will not occur as the brain has been able to extract enough glucose to keep functioning in a normal fashion. However, as the blood glucose continues to fall, the brain then begins to malfunction, which is the neuroglycopenic phase of hypoglycemia. At this time, patients are typically unable to make the correct decisions to obtain food or drink to correct the hypoglycemia, and will need help from someone else or they may develop a seizure or fall into a coma.

Fortunately this process can be ameliorated. It is one of the few times in diabetes management when the endocrinologist will instruct patients to allow their glucose blood levels to run higher than normal. Over a three- to six-week period, this will help to reset the alarm system in the brain and will most likely return the patient to a normal counterregulatory response.

In patients who develop hypoglycemic unawareness due to the complication of autonomic neuropathy, this problem is not reversible. These patients must be treated cautiously to avoid hypoglycemia. Interestingly, after five years of Type 1 diabetes, most patients will not be able to release glucagons in response to hypoglycemia although it is, in fact, present in their pancreases.

See also HORMONES.

Creutzfeldt-Jakob disease (CJD) A brain disorder that affects memory, behavior, coordination, and vision. Creutzfeld-Jakob disease was named after two German neurologists, Dr. Hans Gerhard Creutzfeld and Dr. Alfons Maria Jakob, who identified the disease in the 1920s. CJD is a very rare disease, occurring in only about one per million patients. In the most severe form of the illness, the individual becomes blind and mentally unstable, with rapidly progressing dementia, and loses all voluntary control of movements. The patient may lapse into a COMA. The disease is always fatal: death occurs within a year of the onset for most (90 percent) of patients.

When CJD is present, it is usually found among patients ages 60 and older. However, some patients have developed CJD as young as age 26. Patients with an early onset present with emotional symptoms, such as anxiety, insomnia, and social withdrawal. However, they are not usually diagnosed until they present with neurological symptoms, such as abnormal gait, paresthesias (pins and needles), and pain.

The diagnosis of CJD has been enhanced by the establishment of the National Prion Disease Pathology Surveillance Center, located at Case Western University. The Center performs free tests for patients suspected of having CJD, including analysis of DNA extracted from the blood or brain tissue, analysis of the cerebrospinal fluid, and other tests.

CJD is categorized as a transmissible spongiform encephalopathy (TSE), a medical condition common to humans and animals. The most prominent form of animal TSE is bovine spongiform encephalopathy, popularly known as mad cow disease, although it also affects sheep and goats.

Types of CJD

There are three primary forms of CJD. Sporadic CJD is the most common form, accounting for about 85 percent of all cases. Hereditary CJD occurs in about 5–10 percent of all cases. The third type, acquired CJD, results from damage to the brain or nervous system.

Causes of CJD

What causes CJD is unknown, although theories do exist. Some researchers believe that a slow-acting virus can cause CJD, although no one has been able to isolate such a virus.

With hereditary CJD, the disorder results from a genetic mutation. However, not everyone with the mutated gene actually develops CJD. Therefore there may be other yet-undiscovered factors, such as something that triggers the action of the mutated gene to lead to the disease's onset.

Prior to the development and availability of recombinant growth hormone, a synthetic substance, this hormone was obtained from cadavers. There were several cases of CJD that resulted from transfers of these growth hormone extracts to pediatric patients who were using them to remedy short stature. This horrible complication ended the cadaver growth hormone program.

For further information, contact the following organizations:

Creutzfeldt-Jakob Disease Foundation
P.O. Box 5312
Akron, OH 44334
(800) 659-1991 (toll-free)
http://www.cjdfoundation.org

National Organization for Rare Disorders (NORD)
55 Kenosia Avenue
P.O. Box 1968
Danbury, CT 06812
(203) 744-0100
http://www.rarediseases.org

Tyler, Kenneth L., M.D. "Creutzfeldt-Jakob Disease." *New England Journal of Medicine* 348, no. 8 (February 20, 2003): 681–682.

Crow-Fukase syndrome/POEMS syndrome   First described by Dr. R. S. Crow in 1956 and then by Dr. M. Fukase in 1968, this condition was once known as Crow-Fukase syndrome. Most experts now use the acronym POEMS for this medical condition, which stands for polyneuropathy, organomegaly, endocrinopathy, monoclonal gammaopathy, and skin changes. Patients with POEMS have disorders in at least three of the areas described by the acronym. Only several hundred cases of this medical condition have been identified worldwide.

The polyneuropathy involves dysfunction of many sensory and motor nerves and becomes progressively worse. The organomegaly refers primarily to the enlarged spleen, lymph nodes, and liver. The endocrine disorders experienced by men with this syndrome include GYNECOMASTIA and ERECTILE DYSFUNCTION, while many women with this syndrome have AMENORRHEA. Patients of both genders may have glucose intolerance and DIABETES MELLI-

TUS as well as HYPOTHYROIDISM, HYPOPARATHY-ROIDISM, and hyperprolactinemia.

POEMS is somewhat more commonly seen among men than women, and the onset of the syndrome usually occurs when patients are in their 50s or early 60s. Patients present with severe diarrhea, shortness of breath, peripheral edema, weakness, and paresthesias (numbness and tingling). Skin changes, such as flushing, may occur as well as alopecia (loss of some or all of the hair). The syndrome appears to be caused by a disorder of plasma blood cells, although what drives this change is unknown. Treatment is usually corticosteroids, such as prednisone, given at high doses.

Rehmus, Wingrield, M.D. "POEM Syndrome." Available online. URL: http://www.emedicine.com/derm/topic771.htm. Downloaded on February 1, 2004.

Cushing's syndrome/Cushing's disease   Rare endocrine disorders that occur in about 10–15 patients per million people each year. These disorders are named after Dr. Harvey Williams Cushing, who first identified the symptoms in 1932.

Both disorders are due to excessive levels of cortisol in the bloodstream. However, Cushing's disease refers specifically to the condition in which the excess secretion of cortisol is due to a problem in the central nervous system. Cushing's disease includes either an overproduction of adrenocorticotropic hormone (ACTH) by the pituitary or an overproduction of corticotropin releasing factor (CRF) by the hypothalamus. In some cases, both ACTH and CRF are overproduced.

Cushing's syndrome refers to any clinical syndrome where the effects of excessive glucocorticoids are present, as with the administration of exogenous steroids (such as the use of prednisone in the treatment of asthma, lupus, and or rheumatoid arthritis), or in the cases of the ectopic production of ACTH and adrenal tumors.

In 90 percent of the cases of Cushing's syndrome, the patient is an adult. In 10 percent, the patient is a child or adolescent. Most patients are adult females between the ages of 20 and 50 years old.

In patients with rapidly progressive Cushing's syndrome caused by the ectopic production of ACTH, as in a small cell tumor of the lung, the patient may present with only weight loss, hypokalemia (low potassium blood levels), and hyperglycemia. The patient may show none of the typical physical features associated with excess glucocorticoid activity.

Symptoms of Cushing's Syndrome in an Adult

- HYPERGLYCEMIA
- Menstrual disturbances such as AMENORRHEA or oligomenorrhea (periods become irregular or stop altogether)
- OSTEOPOROSIS
- Muscle weakness (more prominent in the shoulder and hip girdle muscles, also called proximal muscle weakness or myopathy)
- Depression
- Extreme fatigue
- Thin skin that is easily bruised and heals slowly
- HIRSUTISM (excess hair growth and in atypical areas) in women, especially on the face, neck, chest, thighs, and abdominal area
- Decreased fertility among men and/or lack of interest in sex and diminished libido
- Moon-shaped face
- Stretch marks on the skin, especially on the abdomen, typically greater than one centimeter in diameter and violet colored
- Large deposition of fat at the base of the neck, sometimes called buffalo hump
- Sleep disorders

Symptoms of Cushing's Syndrome in a Child or Adolescent

- Delayed growth
- Hyperglycemia (a high glucose/high blood sugar level) and diabetes
- Excessive weight gain, particularly in the face, neck, and abdomen (also called central, truncal, or centripetal OBESITY)
- Hypertension

- DELAYED PUBERTY or a very EARLY PUBERTY in a child
- Amenorrhea (missed periods in females) or oligomenorrhea (irregular menses)
- Extreme fatigue

Diagnosis

Cushing's syndrome/disease is diagnosed with laboratory tests, including a 24-hour measurement of urinary free cortisol, measurement of cortisol in the blood at different times throughout the day, and a dexamethasone suppression test. In addition, CRF testing and direct measurements of ACTH and dehydroepiandrosterone (DHEAS) in the blood can be used. Sometimes physicians will order a measurement of 17-hydroxycorticosteroids, which are the metabolites of cortisol in the urine. Cortisol levels that are greater than 50–100 mcg per day in the 24-hour urine collection test may indicate that the patient has Cushing's disease/syndrome.

With the dexamethasone test, the patient is given dexamethasone, which is a glucocorticoid drug. Cortisol levels are then measured at specific times in both the blood and urine. If a person has a normal hypothalamic-pituitary-adrenal (HPA) axis, the ingestion of excessive dexamethasone should suppress the production of CRF and ACTH, thus leading to decreased amounts of cortisol in the blood and the urine. If a patient has Cushing's disease or syndrome, production of cortisol will not respond normally, and the cortisol levels will remain inappropriately high in the blood and urine.

As with all laboratory tests, some false positives and false negatives will occur. For example, the patient who has used excessive alcohol or taken estrogen can affect the test results. Drugs such as phenobarbital and phenytoin (Dilantin) can also affect results. Alcoholic patients may develop a form of pseudo-Cushing's syndrome.

As with other endocrine disorders, imaging tests are done only after a biological diagnosis is made. This order of events helps the doctor avoid focusing on any false-positive results, as adrenal incidentalomas are quite common. Typically, COMPUTERIZED TOMOGRAPHY (CT) scans of the adrenal glands are used, as are MAGNETIC RESONANCE IMAGING (MRI) scans of the pituitary, depending on the case. Because Cushing's disease or syndrome is often difficult to diagnose, angiographic studies of the arteries, and sometimes the veins, are done to make absolutely certain where the pathology lies.

Treatment

Once diagnosed, treatment of Cushing's disease or syndrome depends on the underlying cause. It can be treated with medication, chemotherapy, radiation treatments, surgery, or a combination of these treatments. Surgery can provide a cure if the cause is an adrenal tumor. For ectopic syndromes, treatment is aimed at the underlying cancer and medications are given to decrease the production of cortisol.

If the syndrome is secondary to exogenous steroid use, the glucocorticoid medication being used is tapered to the lowest possible dosage for the particular patient.

See also CORTISOL.

For further information, contact:

Cushing's Support and Research Foundation, Inc.
65 East India Row 22B
Boston, MA 02110
(617) 723-3824

Pituitary Network Association
223 East Thousand Oaks Boulevard
Suite 320
Thousand Oaks, CA 91360
(805) 496-4932

Amos, Aaron, and J. William Roberts. "Cushing's Syndrome Associated with a Pheochromocytoma." *Urology* 52, no. 2 (1998): 331–335.

Lindholm, J., et al. "Incidence and Late Prognosis of Cushing's Syndrome: A Population-Based Study." *Journal of Clinical Endocrinology & Metabolism* 86, no. 1 (2001): 117–123.

Moro, Mirella, et al. "The Desmopressin Test in the Differential Diagnosis between Cushing's Disease and Pseudo-Cushing States." *Journal of Clinical Endocrinology & Metabolism* 85, no. 10 (2000): 3,569–3,574.

Newell-Price, John, et al. "The Diagnosis and Differential Diagnosis of Cushing's Syndrome and Pseudo-Cushing's States." *Endocrine Reviews* 19, no. 5 (1998): 647–672.

dehydration   Severely low levels of fluid in the body that are insufficient to meet the individual's needs. Symptoms of dehydration include thirst, dry skin and mucous membranes, light-headedness, and nausea.

Risk Factors

Children who are ill and feverish may be at risk for dehydration if they do not receive appropriate medical treatment. Sometimes elderly people (ages 65 and over) become dehydrated because they are not given sufficient fluids by staff members in a nursing home or by their own family members. This may constitute poor care, particularly if the patient becomes unconscious. The elderly may also fail to drink sufficient fluids because of forgetfulness associated with problems such as Alzheimer's disease or depression.

People with some diseases, particularly DIABETES MELLITUS, are at risk for developing dehydration. Dehydration can occur in patients with poorly controlled diabetes mellitus as they have very high levels of glucose that can lead to osmotic diuresis. In this circumstance, the high levels of sugar that are filtered and lost in the kidney pull along extra water and lead to increased urination. This will lead to dehydration if there is inadequate fluid replacement. This situation is more likely to occur in the very young and the elderly, who may not be able to obtain fluids on their own or who may have disordered senses of thirst.

Individuals with DIABETES INSIPIDUS are clearly at risk for rapid and severe dehydration, leading to death, if they are not properly treated. They need adequate replacement of desmopressin acetate (DDAVP), their antidiuretic hormone, to avoid huge losses of fluid in the urine.

Individuals taking certain medications are also at risk, especially patients who are taking diuretic drugs. Individuals who are wounded and are bleeding severely are at risk of dehydration and need intravenous fluids as soon as possible.

The primary causes of dehydration are as follows:

- Inadequate fluid intake
- Hyperglycema (high blood sugar levels)
- Excessive vomiting
- Severe diarrhea
- Diuretic medications
- Excessive bleeding
- Diabetes insipidus

Diagnosis and Treatment

Dehydration is diagnosed by assessing the medical history, conducting a physical examination, and taking laboratory tests of the patient. In a person with vomiting or diarrhea, a history of poor fluid intake may be all that is needed to make the diagnosis of dehydration. In the elderly and the young, however, sometimes the history is not accurate or is not obtained at all. Thus physical signs, such as poor skin turgor (when the skin is pulled, it does not quickly resume to normal) may indicate dehydration. Another indicator of dehydration is decreased blood pressure, especially when the patient is standing, or a clinically significant decrease in blood pressure when the patient changes position from lying to sitting or standing.

Laboratory tests such as the blood urea nitrogen (BUN) level, creatinine, complete blood count (CBC), and electrolytes will often reinforce the diagnosis.

The doctor treats dehydration by first determining the cause of the problem and then replacing fluids to an adequate level. Sometimes merely encouraging the individual to drink fluids may solve the problem. At other times, medical intervention is required. A severely dehydrated person may need fluid replacement intravenously until he or she is able to take fluids in the usual manner, by drinking.

Dehydration may become a serious problem if left untreated. Dehydration may contribute to or exacerbate such medical problems as DIABETIC KETOACIDOSIS and even COMA.

delayed puberty A later-than-average onset of the normal physical maturation that occurs in males and females during adolescence, or later than age 13 in girls and age 14 in boys. Delayed puberty is more common among boys than girls. Often it is an inherited trait and is not due to any underlying endocrine disease or other illness. Delayed puberty that is not caused by disease is also known as constitutional delay of growth and maturation or simply CD.

In one study of 158 boys and 74 girls with delayed puberty, published in a 2002 issue of the *Journal of Clinical Endocrinology & Metabolism,* researchers found that the majority of children studied (53 percent) had CD. In the other children, many different medical problems were identified, including a growth hormone deficiency, HYPOTHYROIDISM, poor nutrition, seizure disorders, KALLMANN'S SYNDROME, KLINEFELTER SYNDROME, PRADER-WILLI SYNDROME, TURNER SYNDROME, sickle cell anemia, ANOREXIA NERVOSA, and other causes. As a result, even though most children with delayed puberty are merely late bloomers, physicians should rule out other potential causes for the delay in physical maturation.

In a study reported in a 2003 issue of the *New England Journal of Medicine,* the researchers studied 600 Caucasian girls, 805 African-American girls, and 781 Mexican-American girls and considered their onset (or lack of onset) of puberty. The researchers found there was a significant relationship between high blood lead concentration and delayed puberty in the African-American and Mexican-American girls but not in the Caucasian

girls, although the reason for this finding was unclear. The greatest delays in breast development were seen in African-American girls with high blood lead concentrations.

Signs and Symptoms of Delayed Puberty
Delayed puberty is indicated more by a lack of signs than the presence of signs. For example, the child lacks hair in the underarm or genital area. The female has not menstruated or developed breasts. The male genitals have not developed beyond childhood. However, both males and females with delayed puberty are usually smaller in size than their peers.

Diagnosis and Treatment
A key determinant of delayed puberty is the child's BONE AGE. In a bone age study, physicians take X-rays of certain bones, such as those of the wrist. Physicians look at whether the bones have fused (the epiphyseal plates or growth plates at the ends of the bones), which occurs during adolescence.

If the child has a younger bone age than his or her chronological age, physicians should also note the child's hormonal levels to check for a deficiency. In boys, testosterone levels should be checked, and in girls the estradiol level should be taken. The thyroid levels of both boys and girls with delayed puberty should also be checked since the underlying problem may be hypothyroidism.

The treatment for delayed puberty depends on the underlying cause. If an illness is identified, that medical problem is treated and the delayed puberty may then resolve. If no cause is found, physicians must decide whether to treat the child.

Some physicians may treat patients with delayed puberty with growth hormone, although pediatricians disagree on whether growth hormone should be administered at all as well at what age it should be considered. Others may treat males with delayed puberty with intramuscular injections of testosterone, given every four weeks for a period of about four to six months. Hormonal treatment for females with delayed puberty is considered controversial. However, some physicians treat girls with low doses of oral estrogen or estradiol daily for three to four months.

If treatment does occur, it should be started or at least monitored by an endocrinologist rather than by an internist or family practitioner.

Effects of Delayed Puberty on the Child

Delayed puberty can cause emotional problems such as DEPRESSION in some children and adolescents, who may feel shunned and ridiculed by their peers. Especially during their early adolescent years, children are likely to be verbally abused and sometimes physically abused by others, particularly if they are males. Said Sharon Travers and Robert Slover in their discussion of the disorders of puberty, "Both boys and girls may be distressed because of their small size and sexually immature appearance. They are often treated as if they were younger, teased by peers, and denied participation in certain athletic activities."

It can also be very difficult for parents to see their children feel humiliated and maligned due to their small size and lack of pubertal development.

See also EARLY PUBERTY; GROWTH HORMONE; TANNER STAGES.

Seldmeyer, Ines L., and Mark R. Palmert. "Delayed Puberty: Analysis of a Large Case Series from an Academic Center." *Journal of Clinical Endocrinology & Metabolism* 87, no. 4 (2002): 1,613–1,620.

Selevan, Sherry G., et al. "Blood Lead Concentration and Delayed Puberty in Girls." *New England Journal of Medicine* 348, no. 16 (April 17, 2003): 1,527–1,536.

Travers, Sharon H., M.D., and Robert H. Slover, M.D. "Disorders of Puberty." *Endocrine Secrets*, 3d ed. Philadelphia, Pa.: Hanley & Belfus, Inc., 2002, 334–347.

depression   Clinically abnormal condition of low mood state with the inability to enjoy life and function at optimal levels. Depression may be caused by events in a person's life, or it may be triggered by an endocrine disorder or other illness. In some cases, depression is misdiagnosed when the underlying problem is actually an endocrine disease, such as HYPOTHYROIDISM or CUSHING'S SYNDROME, and the patient is not truly clinically depressed. It is also true that patients may have an endocrine disorder as well as depression.

Most physicians consider depression highly treatable, and many patients respond very well to antidepressant medications. Most of the modern selective serotonin reuptake inhibitors (SSRIs) have response rates in the 80 percent range. Many different types of antidepressants are available. Consequently, even if the first medication does not work, another medication may be efficacious. Patients may also need to receive short-term therapy, such as cognitive-behavioral therapy (CBT), in which the therapist teaches the patient how to identify and challenge irrational beliefs that are self-defeating and destructive.

For further information, contact the following organizations:

American Psychiatric Association
1400 K Street NW
Washington, DC 20005
(202) 682-6000
http://www.psych.org

American Psychological Association
750 First Street NE
Washington, DC 20002
(202) 336-5500
http://www.apa.org

desiccated thyroid   Thyroid hormones obtained from animal thyroids, such as pork thyroid. These extracts contain thyroid hormones and thyroglobulin. They are inexpensive, but their potency is harder to standardize than that of other thyroid medications.

Desiccated thyroid hormone is available in 15, 30, 60, 90, 120, 180, 240, and 300 mg tablets. The 60 mg tablets contain about 30 mg of T4 (THYROXINE) and 9 mg of T3 (TRIIODOTHYRONINE) and are equivalent to about 75 mg (or 0.075 mg) of LEVOTHYROXINE.

DEXA scan (dual-energy X-ray absorptiometry)   A special type of X-ray used to determine the level of bone density. Assessment of a DEXA scan can help a physician make the diagnosis of OSTEOPOROSIS or the less severe condition known as OSTEOPENIA. The DEXA scan is considered by many experts as the gold standard, not only in making the diagnosis of osteoporosis but also in following the patient's response to therapy for the treatment of osteoporosis.

diabetes insipidus (DI) A rare metabolic/endocrine disorder characterized by massive losses of body fluids through urination. The antidiuretic hormone (ADH), also known as vasopressin, which is made by the hypothalamus and stored in the pituitary gland, is at a reduced level among patients with DI. In a healthy person, ADH works to decrease urine flow by increasing the reabsorption of salt and water in the kidney tubules.

Diabetes insipidus has no relationship to DIABETES MELLITUS, although the twin symptoms of frequent urination and extreme thirst are common to both diseases. Diabetes insipidus may occur abruptly in individuals of any age, although it is more common among adults.

Types and Causes of Diabetes Insipidus

DI is caused by damage to the pituitary gland, which may result from a head injury, an infection, a tumor, or a variety of other causes. Some experts believe DI may be a form of autoimmune disorder. Diabetes insipidus may also be an inherited disease. Hereditary forms of DI are called familial diabetes insipidus or familial neurohypophysial diabetes insipidus.

Central DI is the most common form of diabetes insipidus. Unless otherwise stated, researchers who are discussing diabetes insipidus are referring to central DI. Another form of DI is nephrogenic DI, caused by a disorder of the kidneys in which they are unable to respond to the ADH that is produced. Nephrogenic DI may sometimes be caused by medications such as lithium.

Dipsogenic DI, a rare form of diabetes insipidus, is caused by a disorder in the hypothalamus that affects the mechanism causing thirst. In rare cases, pregnant women may develop gestational diabetes insipidus, which is caused by an enzyme in the placenta.

Signs and Symptoms of Diabetes Insipidus

Whether the illness is inherited or acquired, the symptoms of diabetes insipidus include frequent urination (typically, greater than four liters per day, with very dilute urine), fatigue, and excessive thirst. Unless the person with diabetes insipidus drinks copious quantities of fluid, he or she will become severely dehydrated and constipated. However, the patient will not have hyperglycemia (high levels of blood glucose), which is the hallmark feature of both Type 1 and Type 2 diabetes. Some patients with DI also have severe night sweats.

Infants and Children with DI

If infants with the disease are not treated quickly, they may suffer from irreversible brain damage or developmental problems, such as mental retardation and physical delays. Symptoms of diabetes insipidus in a baby are fever, vomiting, and convulsions, with high levels of sodium found in the blood upon laboratory examination. Infants and children with diabetes insipidus may also have FAILURE TO THRIVE and experience growth deficits.

Researchers studied 79 children with diabetes insipidus and reported on their findings in the *New England Journal of Medicine*. The children had a median age of seven years. The researchers performed MAGNETIC RESONANCE IMAGING (MRI) scans on the children, and they found that most of the children had certain abnormalities. For example, 18 of the patients had an intracranial tumor, two had skull fractures, and 12 of the children had Langerhans' cells histiocytosis.

Many of the children (61 percent) showed anterior pituitary deficiencies, particularly of growth hormone, within about a year from the onset of their diabetes insipidus.

In about 25 percent of the children, there appeared to be a link between contracting a virus and the subsequent onset of diabetes insipidus. In about 30–50 percent of the cases, the cause for the diabetes insipidus was unknown.

Adults and DI

Among adults, diabetes insipidus is commonly caused by pituitary tumors of many types as well as by the surgery and/or radiation used to treat them. Typically these tumors are benign. However, they damage the pituitary gland by their mass effect, as there is very little extra room in the sella turcica where the pituitary gland sits. Malignant tumors may also metastasize to the pituitary gland and cause DI.

A significant head trauma, such as that which can be caused by motor vehicle accidents or by gunshot wounds, can also cause DI to occur. Granulomatous diseases may also cause DI. These diseases cause the body to respond by creating granulomas, which are large cells derived from white blood cell monocytes and used as part of the body's immune system defense.

Anything that damages the hypothalamus, which sits directly adjacent to the pituitary gland, may also lead to DI. This occurs because the hypothalamus is where ADH is made prior to its transit to the pituitary gland.

Diagnosis and Treatment

The diagnosis of diabetes insipidus is based on the patient's symptoms and on blood tests of glucose levels that rule out a diagnosis of either Type 1 or Type 2 diabetes. In order to diagnose DI, the endocrinologist must document that the patient is producing a large flow of urine that is quite dilute and that fails to concentrate to the appropriate stimuli. In healthy people, if they do not drink water over a period of time, appropriate hormonal changes will ensue that cause the urine to become more concentrated and thus they will lose less water in their urine and their lives will be sustained. However, in contrast, when individuals with DI fail to drink water, the hormonal changes do not occur and instead, the body continues to pour out diluted urine. As a result, the water deprivation test is used to diagnose DI.

To determine the presence of diabetes insipidus, a fluid deprivation test is needed on occasion, especially if the ADH deficiency is only partial. Sometimes a test known as a dehydration test is used. This test is used especially if the ADH deficiency is partial or if there is a suspicion of the presence of psychogenic polydipsia, which is an extreme intake of water that may stem from an emotional or psychotic disorder such as untreated schizophrenia.

Diabetes insipidus is usually treated with desmopressin acetate (DDAVP), a hormone that is available in several forms: an intravenous or subcutaneous preparation, a nasal spray, a liquid, or a tablet. Physicians must be careful to prescribe the correct dose of this medication. If excessive amounts of DDAVP are administered, patients may become water intoxicated. Patients taking this drug must also be reassessed several times per year.

Other drugs besides DDAVP that increase ADH secretion are generally not very effective and, consequently, are rarely used. However, in a study reported in a 1999 issue of the *Archives of Internal Medicine*, researchers treated 20 patients with central diabetes insipidus with indapamide (Lozol), an antihypertensive diuretic. The drug worked well on most patients.

In the case of nephrogenic diabetes insipidus, recommendations of low-salt diets, thiazide diuretics, and nonsteroidal anti-inflammatory drugs (NSAIDs) are often used for patients. Gestational DI usually resolves when the pregnancy ends.

For further information, contact the following organizations:

Diabetes Insipidus Foundation, Inc.
4533 Ridge Drive
Baltimore, MD 21229
(410) 247-3953

National Kidney and Urologic Diseases
    Information Clearinghouse
3 Information Way
Bethesda, MD 20892
(800) 891-5390 (toll-free)

Nephrogenic Diabetes Insipidus Foundation
P.O. Box 1390
Eastsound, WA 98245
(888) 376-6343 (toll-free)
http://www.ndif.org

Maghnie, Mohamad, M.D., et al. "Central Diabetes Insipidus in Children and Young Adults." *New England Journal of Medicine* 343, no. 14 (October 5, 2000): 998–1,007.

Petit, William A. Jr., M.D., and Christine Adamec. *The Encyclopedia of Diabetes.* New York: Facts On File, Inc., 2002.

Tetiker, Tamer, M.D., Murat Sert, M.D., and Mustafa Kocak, M.D. "Efficacy of Indapamide in Central Diabetes Insipidus." *Archives of Internal Medicine* 159, no. 17 (1999): 2,085–2,087.

diabetes mellitus (DM) Common name for both Type 1 and Type 2 diabetes. Diabetes mellitus is a complex disorder of carbohydrates, proteins, and fats that leads to premature death, usually due to heart attack and stroke. Many experts think that although diabetes is commonly considered a disease of sugar, it is more accurately a vascular disease that severely affects blood vessels throughout the body.

Type 1 diabetes is an autoimmune disorder in which all the insulin-producing beta cells in the pancreas are destroyed, with patients dependent upon taking insulin to live. With Type 2 diabetes, patients' bodies do make insulin but have resistance to its effects. They are unable to make adequate insulin to control their glucose levels and the resulting metabolic disarray. Most patients with Type 2 diabetes can be treated with nutrition, exercise, and oral medications. About 7 percent of patients with Type 2 diabetes lose the ability to make insulin and, consequently, require insulin therapy.

Risk Factors

According to the Centers for Disease Control and Prevention (CDC), as of this writing about 18 million people in the United States, or 6.3 percent of the population, have diabetes. This number includes about 6 million people who have the disease but do not realize it. From 90–95 percent of all patients with diabetes mellitus have Type 2 diabetes, while 5–10 percent have Type 1 diabetes, requiring insulin injections. These figures do not include women with gestational diabetes, which refers to an estimated 135,000 pregnant women in the United States who did not have diabetes prior to their pregnancies.

About one in every five adults over age 65 has diabetes. The National Diabetes Information Clearinghouse estimated that the direct medical costs of diabetes mellitus were $92 billion in 2002.

There are racial differences among patients with diabetes. African Americans and Native Americans/Alaska Natives have a greater risk for developing Type 2 diabetes than Caucasians. In contrast, Caucasians are more likely to be diagnosed with Type 1 diabetes.

Most people with diabetes are diagnosed in adulthood. According to the CDC, only 7.2 percent of adults with diabetes were diagnosed between birth and age 19 years (see Table I).

The percentages of people in the United States who have been diagnosed with diabetes also varies greatly from state to state according to surveillance data for 2001 from the CDC. The greatest percentages were found in Puerto Rico (9.8 percent), Alabama (9.6 percent), and Guam (9.5 percent). The lowest percentages were found in Alaska (4.0 percent), Utah (4.2 percent), and Minnesota (4.4 percent) (see Table II).

TABLE I: DISTRIBUTION OF AGE AT DIAGNOSIS OF DIABETES AMONG ADULTS AGED 18–79 YEARS, UNITED STATES, 2000

Age in Years	Percent
0–9	2.4
10–19	4.8
20–29	6.6
30–39	14.4
40–49	24.2
50–59	24.8
60–69	17.0
70–79	5.7

Source: Diabetes Surveillance System, National Center for Chronic Disease Prevention and Health Promotion, Centers for Disease Control and Prevention.

Risks Are Increasing for Developing Diabetes

The risk of developing diabetes mellitus is rising. For example, according to an article in a 2003 issue of the *Journal of the American Medical Association,* researchers estimated the lifetime risk of developing diabetes among children born in 2000. They estimated that the risk was 32.8 percent for males and 38.5 percent for females.

Hispanics had the highest potential risks for developing diabetes, or 45.4 percent for males and 52.5 percent for females. Said the researchers, "The lifetime risk of diabetes is comparable with or higher than that for many diseases and conditions that are perceived as common. For example, the lifetime risk of diabetes is considerably higher than the

TABLE II: PREVALENCE OF ADULTS WHO REPORTED EVER HAVING BEEN TOLD BY A
HEALTH PROFESSIONAL THAT THEY HAD DIABETES, 1991, 2000, AND 2001, AND BY SEX, 2001—
UNITED STATES, BEHAVIORAL RISK FACTOR SURVEILLANCE SYSTEM

State or Territory	Both sexes						(%) Difference 1991–2001	Men (2001)		Women (2001)	
	2001		2000		1991						
	%	95% CI* (±)	%	95% CI (±)	%	95% CI (±)		%	95% CI (±)	%	95% CI (±)
Alabama	9.6	1.2	7.4	1.2	5.1	1.0	89.3	10.5	2.0	8.8	1.4
Alaska	4.0	1.0	3.8	1.4	4.3	1.3	−7.8	4.0	1.4	4.0	1.4
Arizona	6.1	1.0	5.9	2.2	3.8	1.0	60.1	7.3	1.8	4.9	1.2
Arkansas	7.8	1.2	6.2	1.0	4.8	1.2	63.9	8.4	1.8	7.2	1.4
California	6.5	1.0	6.8	1.2	4.8	0.9	36.8	5.8	1.2	7.1	1.4
Colorado	4.6	1.0	5.1	1.2	2.9	0.8	56.5	5.6	1.8	3.7	1.2
Connecticut	6.3	0.6	5.5	0.8	4.6	1.1	37.6	6.5	1.0	6.0	0.8
Delaware	7.1	1.0	6.4	1.2	4.9	1.2	43.7	7.5	1.8	6.7	1.4
District of Columbia	8.3	1.6	7.2	1.4	6.7	1.7	24.3	9.6	2.5	7.2	1.8
Florida	8.2	1.0	6.9	0.8	5.1	1.0	60.5	9.1	1.6	7.3	1.2
Georgia	6.9	0.8	6.8	1.0	5.6	1.2	23.2	6.5	1.4	7.2	1.2
Hawaii	6.2	1.2	5.2	0.8	6.5	1.2	−4.0	6.8	2.0	5.6	1.2
Idaho	5.4	0.8	4.9	0.8	3.7	0.9	45.2	5.2	1.0	5.7	1.0
Illinois	6.6	0.8	6.2	1.0	5.1	1.0	30.2	6.7	1.4	6.6	1.2
Indiana	6.5	0.8	6.0	1.0	5.4	1.0	20.8	6.3	1.2	6.8	1.0
Iowa	5.7	0.8	6.1	1.0	3.8	1.0	51.6	5.8	1.2	5.6	1.0
Kansas	5.8	0.8	5.9	0.8	-†	—	—	5.5	1.0	6.1	1.0
Kentucky	6.7	0.8	6.5	0.8	4.8	1.0	40.8	6.9	1.2	6.4	0.8
Louisiana	7.6	0.8	6.6	0.8	6.3	1.3	20.3	6.9	1.2	8.2	1.0
Maine	6.7	1.2	6.0	1.2	4.2	1.2	60.3	7.0	2.0	6.5	1.4
Maryland	6.9	1.0	6.4	1.0	5.2	1.2	32.7	7.1	1.6	6.6	1.4
Massachusetts	5.6	0.6	5.8	0.6	4.4	1.3	26.7	6.0	1.0	5.2	0.8
Michigan	7.2	1.0	7.0	1.0	5.4	0.9	34.3	6.8	1.4	7.6	1.2
Minnesota	4.4	0.6	4.9	1.0	3.7	0.7	18.3	4.4	1.0	4.3	1.0
Mississippi	9.3	1.2	7.6	1.2	7.0	1.4	32.1	8.8	2.0	9.7	1.4
Missouri	6.6	1.0	6.7	1.0	4.1	1.0	63.0	7.0	1.6	6.2	1.2
Montana	5.6	1.0	4.9	1.0	4.9	1.3	13.4	4.9	1.2	6.2	1.6
Nebraska	5.2	0.8	4.9	1.0	4.8	1.2	8.3	4.9	1.2	5.5	1.0
Nevada	5.7	1.4	6.8	2.0	—	—	—	5.2	1.4	6.2	2.2
New Hampshire	5.4	0.8	4.4	1.0	4.7	1.2	14.2	5.8	1.2	5.0	1.0
New Jersey	7.1	1.0	5.8	0.8	4.3	1.1	64.0	7.3	1.4	7.0	1.2
New Mexico	6.2	1.0	6.5	1.0	3.4	1.1	80.2	5.9	1.4	6.5	1.2
New York	6.6	1.0	6.3	1.0	5.2	1.1	27.7	6.4	1.4	6.8	1.4
North Carolina	6.7	1.0	6.4	1.0	6.3	1.2	6.2	6.8	1.4	6.7	1.0
North Dakota	5.1	1.0	5.2	1.2	4.4	1.0	16.4	4.7	1.4	5.6	1.2
Ohio	7.2	1.0	6.4	1.2	4.5	1.4	61.8	7.5	1.6	6.9	1.2
Oklahoma	7.7	1.0	5.5	0.8	4.0	1.0	91.1	8.3	1.6	7.2	1.2
Oregon	5.7	1.0	6.0	1.0	4.8	0.8	19.0	5.5	1.4	5.8	1.4
Pennsylvania	6.7	0.8	7.1	1.0	6.5	1.1	3.4	6.6	1.4	6.7	1.2
Rhode Island	6.4	1.0	6.0	0.8	5.6	1.1	14.9	7.4	1.4	5.6	1.2
South Carolina	8.1	1.0	7.1	1.0	6.5	1.2	24.8	8.4	1.8	7.7	1.4
South Dakota	6.1	0.8	5.7	0.8	3.4	0.9	79.4	6.6	1.2	5.6	0.8
Tennessee	7.7	1.2	7.2	1.2	7.2	1.1	6.4	7.6	2.0	7.9	1.4
Texas	7.1	0.8	6.2	0.8	4.7	1.1	50.7	7.0	1.2	7.2	1.0
Utah	4.3	0.8	5.4	1.2	3.9	1.0	10.3	4.3	1.4	4.2	1.2
Vermont	5.1	0.8	4.4	0.8	4.5	1.2	13.1	4.6	1.0	5.5	1.0

(continues)

**TABLE II: PREVALENCE OF ADULTS WHO REPORTED EVER HAVING BEEN TOLD BY A
HEALTH PROFESSIONAL THAT THEY HAD DIABETES, 1991, 2000, AND 2001, AND BY SEX, 2001—
UNITED STATES, BEHAVIORAL RISK FACTOR SURVEILLANCE SYSTEM** *(continued)*

| | Both sexes | | | | | | (%) | Men | | Women | |
| | 2001 | | 2000 | | 1991 | | Difference | (2001) | | (2001) | |
State or Territory	%	95% CI* (±)	%	95% CI (±)	%	95% CI (±)	1991–2001	%	95% CI (±)	%	95% CI (±)
Virginia	6.0	1.0	6.2	1.4	4.2	1.1	43.9	6.2	1.4	5.8	1.4
Washington	5.7	0.8	5.5	0.8	5.0	1.0	13.3	6.2	1.2	5.2	1.0
West Virginia	8.8	1.2	7.6	1.2	6.0	1.0	47.7	8.9	1.6	8.8	1.6
Wisconsin	5.6	0.8	6.1	1.0	4.9	1.2	15.0	5.9	1.4	5.3	1.2
Wyoming	4.5	0.8	5.0	1.0	–	–	–	4.1	1.2	4.8	1.0
Guam	9.5	2.5	–	–	–	–	–	9.9	3.9	9.1	3.1
Puerto Rico	9.8	1.2	8.5	1.0	–	–	–	9.1	1.8	10.5	1.6
Virgin Islands	7.2	1.2	–	–	–	–	–	4.3	1.6	9.5	2.0

Summary

| | Both sexes | | | Men | Women |
	2001	2000	1991	(2001)	(2001)
No. of states/territories	54	52	48	54	54
Median	6.6	6.2	4.8	6.6	6.5
Range	4.0–9.8	3.8–8.5	2.9–7.2	4.0–10.5	3.7–10.5
Mean	6.6	6.1	4.9	6.6	6.5

* Confidence interval.
†Not available or sample size <50 .
Source: Centers for Disease Control and Prevention, "State-Specific Prevalence of Selected Chronic Disease Related Characteristics—Behavioral
Risk Factor Surveillance System, 2001," *Morbidity and Mortality Weekly Report* 52, no. 55–8 (August 22, 2003): 39.

widely publicized 1 in 8 risk for breast cancer among US women."

Communication Is Critical Between Patients with Diabetes and Their Doctors

It is very important that people who have diabetes understand the basics about their illness as well as what they need to do in order to manage it successfully. In one study, reported in a 2003 issue of the *Archives of Internal Medicine,* interactions were observed between 38 doctors and 74 of their English-speaking patients when the physicians were explaining new concepts to their patients. The researchers found that when patients understood what their doctors were telling them, they were more likely to have good glycemic control. This is particularly important among patients who may have a poor grasp of their illness and what they need to do to control it. Of particular help is when doctors assess the patients' understanding level. According to the researchers, doing so can

"can uncover health beliefs, reinforce and tailor health messages, and activate patients by opening a dialogue."

Poor Compliance with Treatment

The National Institute of Diabetes and Digestive and Kidney Diseases (NIDDK) stated that study results released in 2004 showed that less than 12 percent of people with diagnosed diabetes meet their recommended treatment goals for blood glucose, blood pressure, and cholesterol. This occurs even though research has clearly shown that controlling these conditions dramatically delays or prevents diabetes complications.

Further, the percentage of people complying with treatment recommendations has improved little in the last decade. This is discouraging because failure to control diabetes leads to an increased risk for many complications, such as heart attack, stroke, amputations, DIABETIC RETINOPATHY, DIABETIC NEUROPATHY, DIABETIC NEPHROPATHY, and death.

Complications from Diabetes

Although many people can control their diabetes with diet, medication, exercise, and weight control, an estimated 200,000 Americans die each year from complications due to diabetes, making diabetes the sixth leading cause of death in the United States. The key cause of diabetes-related complications is heart disease. Patients with diabetes have a two to four times greater risk of dying from heart disease than patients who do not have diabetes. In addition, patients with diabetes have a two to four times greater risk of suffering from a stroke than nondiabetic patients. In addition, 73 percent of adults with diabetes have high blood pressure or are taking medications for hypertension.

Diabetes is also the leading cause of adult-onset blindness. Between 12,000–24,000 people in the United States become blind each year as a result of complications from diabetes. Others develop kidney diseases; an estimated 38,000 people with diabetes die from kidney failure each year in the United States.

Diabetes is the leading cause of nontraumatic amputation in the United States. Many patients with diabetes suffer amputations of the toes, feet, and legs. An estimated 82,000 Americans have body parts amputated each year as a result of diabetic complications. People with diabetes are also more likely to die from complications of flu or pneumonia, and from 10,000–30,000 people with diabetes die of flu or pneumonia each year. Only slightly more than half of them (55 percent) get an annual flu shot although nearly all are eligible for such injections.

Increasing numbers of people with diabetes are being hospitalized. For example, according to the National Center for Health Statistics, in the years 1990–91, there were 121.0 hospital discharges per 10,000 people among those individuals ages 45–54 years old. This rate has steadily increased. Over the period 2000–01, it was 156.6 per 10,000 people. The rates of hospitalization also increased for individuals in the age brackets of 55–64 years, 65–74 years, and 75 years and older (see Table III). Clearly, diabetes is becoming a greater problem for middle-aged and senior adults than in past years, possibly because so many more individuals in these age groups are either overweight or obese in comparison to past years.

TABLE III: HOSPITAL DISCHARGE RATES FOR DIABETES AMONG ADULTS 45 YEARS OF AGE AND OLDER BY AGE, DISCHARGES PER 10,000 POPULATION: UNITED STATES: 1990–2001

Year	45–54	55–64	65–74	75 years+
1990–1991	121.0	270.3	487.3	648.0
1992–1993	139.4	302.9	536.9	699.5
1994–1995	140.3	307.3	561.6	746.6
1996–1997	148.5	322.1	576.1	791.1
1998–1999	151.1	347.8	628.0	831.3
2000–2001	156.6	344.0	632.4	830.6

Source: Centers for Disease Control and Prevention. *Chartbook on Trends in the Health of Americans*. Health, United States, 2003.

Costs of Diabetes

The federal government in the United States estimates that the direct and indirect costs of diabetes are about $130 billion per year and the average health care cost for a person with diabetes is about five times greater than that of an age-matched person without diabetes. Some experts believe that these figures are underestimated.

Medications for Diabetes

The medications used to treat diabetes mellitus depend on whether the patient has Type 1 diabetes, which invariably requires some form of insulin delivery, or Type 2 diabetes, which can often be treated with oral medications. The Diabetes Prevention Program studied more than 3,000 people at risk for developing Type 2 diabetes (they had impaired glucose tolerance/prediabetes). Researchers compared the effects of diet and exercise to treatment with medication. One group was given medication (metformin), and individuals in a second group (the lifestyle group) were given information and the goal of dropping their body weight by 7 percent by exercising. A third group was a placebo group.

The study was ended about a year earlier than planned because the benefits of weight loss and medication were so clear. The lifestyle group had a 58 percent lower incidence rate of diabetes than the placebo group. The medication group had a 31 percent reduced occurrence of developing Type 2 diabetes compared with the placebo group. Clearly, exercise and medication can prevent or delay Type 2 diabetes in many people.

Among those who are already diagnosed with diabetes, studies have shown that improving glycemic control to reduce hemoglobin A1c blood tests by even 1 percent will reduce the risk of diabetic complications by 40 percent.

Prevention of Diabetes and Diabetic Complications

To date, Type 1 diabetes is a disease that is difficult or even impossible to prevent, although it can be well controlled with a careful diet, exercise, and insulin therapy. Ongoing clinical studies are looking at various means to delay or prevent the onset of Type 1 diabetes in susceptible individuals, such as those with impaired glucose tolerance.

Studies have indicated that Type 2 diabetes can be prevented or delayed in patients at high risk. These high-risk individuals are obese, have impaired glucose tolerance and are considered to have prediabetes, and are people with first-degree relatives (such as a parent or sibling) with Type 2 diabetes.

See also DIABETIC KETOACIDOSIS; GESTATIONAL DIABETES; HYPERGLYCEMIA; HYPOGLYCEMIA; IMPAIRED GLUCOSE TOLERANCE; TYPE 1 DIABETES; TYPE 2 DIABETES.

For further information, contact the following organizations:

American Diabetes Association (ADA)
1701 North Beauregard Street
Alexandria, VA 22311
(703) 549-1500 or (800) 342-2383 (toll-free)
http://www.diabetes.org

National Diabetes Information Clearinghouse
1 Information Way
Bethesda, MD 20892
(800) 860-8747 (toll-free)
http://diabetes.niddk.nih.gov

American Diabetes Association. "Economic Costs of Diabetes in the U.S. in 2002." *Diabetes Care* 26, no. 3 (March 2003): 917–932.

Bardsley, Joan K., and Maureen Passaro, M.D. "ABCs of Diabetes Research." *Clinical Diabetes* 20, no. 1 (2002): 5–8.

Centers for Disease Control and Prevention, Chronic Disease Prevention. "The Promise of Prevention: Reducing the Health and Economic Burden of Chronic Disease." Department of Health and Human Services, 2003.

Cherry, Daniel K., Catharine W. Burt, and David A. Woodwell. "National Ambulatory Medical Care Survey: 2001 Summary." Division of Health Care Statistics, Centers for Disease Control and Prevention, no. 337, August 11, 2003.

Narayan, K. M., M.D., et al., "Lifetime Risk for Diabetes Mellitus in the United States," *Journal of the American Medical Association* 290, no. 14 (October 8, 2003): 1884–1890.

National Institute of Diabetes and Digestive and Kidney Diseases. "Most People with Diabetes Do Not Meet Treatment Goals." Press Release, National Institutes of Health, January 20, 2004.

Petit, William A. Jr., M.D., and Christine Adamec. *The Encyclopedia of Diabetes.* New York: Facts On File, Inc., 2002.

Schillinger, Dean, M.D., et al. "Closing the Loop: Physicians Communication with Diabetic Patients Who Have Low Health Literacy." *Archives of Internal Medicine* 163, no. 1 (January 13, 2004): 83–90.

Tuomilehto, Jaako, M.D., et al. "Prevention of Type 2 Diabetes Mellitus by Changes in Lifestyle Among Subjects with Impaired Glucose Tolerance." *New England Journal of Medicine* 344, no. 18 (May 3, 2001): 1,343–1,350.

diabetic ketoacidosis (DKA)   An acute and often severe metabolic complication that occurs to some patients with diabetes (both TYPE 1 DIABETES and TYPE 2 DIABETES). DKA involves a combination of HYPERGLYCEMIA (excess acid in the blood) and DEHYDRATION.

DKA is so serious that it requires patients to be hospitalized (usually in the intensive care unit) until they are stabilized. In the worst cases, DKA may lead to coma and death. Experts report a death rate of 5–10 percent among patients who lapse into diabetic ketoacidosis. DKA may also cause cerebral (brain) edema, which greatly heightens the risk of death, especially among children with Type 1 diabetes.

Risk Factors for Developing DKA

The presence of diabetes is the major risk factor for the development of DKA. Poor glycemic control (patients' inadequate monitoring of blood glucose levels, poor nutrition, and inadequate therapy) is another risk factor. However, sometimes blood levels can change precipitously no matter how conscientious patients are about checking their blood.

One major problem is that not everyone who has diabetes mellitus is actually aware that they have the disease. In fact, they may first discover their illness when they are hospitalized and diagnosed with DKA. Ethnicity is another key factor in DKA. African Americans are twice as likely to be admitted to the hospital for DKA as Caucasians. Age is another risk factor, as DKA risks increase with age.

Symptoms of DKA

Blurred vision, nausea, abdominal pains, and lack of appetite are all common symptoms of DKA. The individual may also experience increased urination and great thirst. Dehydration may be both a symptom and a cause of DKA.

Diagnosis and Treatment

The diagnosis of DKA is based on the patient's clinical presentation as well as on the results of tests, such as blood glucose levels and urine and/or serum acetone levels, all typically high in patients with DKA. In addition, often an arterial blood gas is drawn to measure the pH level in the blood, which shows the level of acidity or alkalinity. Normal pH is 7.4, while in patients with DKA, it is less than 7.3.

Once DKA is diagnosed, the patient is given aggressive fluid resuscitation as well as insulin. Typically, short-acting insulin is administered intravenously and is followed by a continuous intravenous drip of the same insulin at a lower level. The fluid that is usually given initially is normal saline. Once the patient is producing urine, potassium generally needs to be administered as the vast majority of patients with DKA have a total body deficit of potassium. Once the emergency issues are treated, the physician must determine the underlying cause of the DKA and treat that cause aggressively.

Once the patient has sufficiently recovered, the physician will emphasize the importance of maintaining blood glucose levels that are as close to normal as possible with the hope that there will be no

further relapses into DKA. Patients who have been hospitalized for DKA should wear a medical identification bracelet that shows they have diabetes so that if the condition recurs, they will be likely to obtain proper medical care in a timely manner. For patients with diabetes, speed in treatment may mean the difference between life and death.

See also COMA.

Glaser, Nicole, M.D., et al. "Risk Factors for Cerebral Edema in Children with Diabetic Ketoacidosis." *New England Journal of Medicine* 344, no. 4 (January 25, 2001): 264–269.

Rewers, Arleta, M.D. "Predictors of Acute Complications in Children with Type 1 Diabetes." *Journal of the American Medical Association* 287, no. 19 (May 15, 2002): 2,511–2,518.

diabetic nephropathy Kidney disease that stems directly from DIABETES MELLITUS and that may ultimately result in kidney failure. According to the National Diabetes Information Clearinghouse, in 2001 nearly 43,000 patients with diabetes began treatment for end-stage renal disease (another name for kidney failure).

Patients who have diabetic nephropathy represent nearly half (42 percent) of all the kidney failure patients in the United States. Diabetic nephropathy is also the cause for either kidney dialysis or a kidney transplant among an estimated 100,000 people each year. Most patients with diabetic nephropathy also suffer from DIABETIC RETINOPATHY, a disease of the eye.

Unfortunately, patients with kidney disease usually do not have any symptoms until less than 25 percent of their kidney function remains. However, diligent testing by physicians, such as testing for very small amounts of protein in the patient's urine, can often detect an early onset of kidney dysfunction. Blood tests to measure creatinine and blood urea nitrogen (BUN) can also be monitored by physicians every three to six months, but these tests are less sensitive than monitoring the urine for protein. Increases in creatinine and BUN levels are also indicators of kidney disease.

The current standard of care is to monitor the patient first with a simple dipstick urine test. If protein is present in the urine, the patient has overt proteinuria. The patient will need strict attention to glycemic control, blood pressure, and lipids as well as treatment with angiotensin-converting enzyme (ACE) inhibitor mediations or angiotensin receptor blockers (ARBs).

If no protein is seen in the urine dipstick test, a second, more sensitive test for urine microalbuminuria can be obtained. Typically, this is a radioimmunoassay that detects tiny amounts of protein in the urine. If patients have less than 30 mcg of albumin per mg of creatinine, their levels are considered normal. If the level is 30–300 mcg albumin per mg of creatinine, patients have microalbuminuria. These patients are treated with ACE and/or ARB drugs, and strict attention is paid to their glucose and lipid levels.

When the level is greater than 300 mcg of albumin per mg of creatinine, patients have macroalbuminuria or overt proteinuria. Once a patient has a serum creatinine level greater than 1.8 mg/dl or has had greater than 1,000 mg of protein in their urine over 24 hours, he or she should be referred to a nephrologist for further consultation and therapy.

Causes of Nephropathy

The cause of diabetic nephropathy is often a combination of both hypertension and diabetes. Patients with these two medical problems have a mortality risk that is increased by 37 times over that of patients with one of these ailments. Patients with diabetes who do not have hypertension can also develop diabetic nephropathy, although their risk is reduced compared with patients who have both medical problems.

Because of the links connecting diabetes and hypertension with kidney disease, patients with both hypertension and diabetes must comply closely with the medical regimens prescribed by their physicians for decreasing high blood pressure. These regimens include taking medication, losing weight (if weight loss is recommended), and following other medical advice.

Patients with diabetes should work hard to keep their glucose levels as close to normal as possible by testing their blood on a regular basis and, if necessary, acting on the information provided by the blood tests. In a major study of people with dia-

betes, the federally funded Diabetes Control and Complications Trial Research Group, 1,441 subjects with Type 1 diabetes were studied from 1983–93. The study definitively proved that the group that successfully and tightly controlled their diabetes had a 50 percent reduced risk for kidney disease (and also a 60 percent reduced risk for nerve disease).

Signs and Symptoms

In the early stages of the disease, there may be few or no symptoms, although there may be microscopic levels of albumin and increased creatinine levels. As the illness progresses the albumin and creatinine levels increase, and the proteinuria becomes apparent. If the patient's kidneys further deteriorate, symptoms such as malaise and itchy skin may develop. Patients may show fatigue and decreased endurance. They may also retain fluid in the ankles and elsewhere in the body.

Physicians should check the urine of their patients with diabetes on a regular basis to detect any early signs of diabetic nephropathy. That way, it can be treated before the condition becomes too advanced and the patient requires kidney dialysis and a kidney transplant.

Genetic Risks

Researchers have found that the siblings of patients who have both diabetes and kidney disease have five times the risk of developing diabetic nephropathy themselves. In the future, doctors may be able to estimate a patient's risk by the detection of various forms of the *ACE* gene.

Diagnosis and Treatment

The diagnosis of diabetic nephropathy is based on the patient's symptoms and laboratory tests. Physicians may order a 24-hour urine collection, a test that provides a good estimate of kidney function and also measures excess amounts of protein being lost in the urine. If detected early, diabetic nephropathy can be treated with medications. In most cases, ACE inhibitors and/or ARB blockers are used to slow down the progression of kidney disease.

Blood pressure is also a consideration. The goal blood pressure may be as low as 120/70 if clinically indicated in patients with kidney disease.

See also BLOOD PRESSURE/HYPERTENSION; TYPE 1 DIABETES; TYPE 2 DIABETES.

Petit, William A. Jr., M.D., and Christine Adamec. *The Encyclopedia of Diabetes.* New York: Facts On File, Inc., 2002.

diabetic neuropathy Nerve damage directly caused by diabetes. Diabetic neuropathy may result in a variety of ailments, including a loss of feeling in the feet or hands, the delayed digestion of food, ERECTILE DYSFUNCTION, and many other medical problems. About 60–70 percent of all patients with diabetes will eventually suffer from some neuropathy, ranging from a mild to a severe form. Maintaining excellent glucose control may delay or prevent the development of neuropathy.

When the nerves of the face are affected, diabetic neuropathy can mimic symptoms of a stroke and may also cause a facial droop similar to that found in Bell's palsy. Diabetic neuropathy may also cause an eyelid droop. These types of neuropathies are caused by nerve attacks, a sudden blockage of blood flow to the nerve. This problem is similar to that of a heart attack or a stroke. Syndromes affecting the cranial nerves are called cranial mononeuropathies.

A radiculopathy is a painful neuropathy in which a nerve root is directly affected. If the nerve root supplying the area is located just below the right lower ribs of the patient, it can mimic a gallbladder attack. If the radiculopathy is located in the nerves of the lower legs, it can cause sciatica.

Other Focal Neuropathies

Patients with diabetes are more commonly affected than nondiabetics by carpal tunnel syndrome (in the fingers) and tarsal tunnel syndrome (in the foot, typically in the heel). These syndromes may occur because of a deposit of carbohydrates and proteinlike material in the canals where the nerves run. The problem may also be caused by medications as well as by blood flow problems.

Damage to the peroneal nerve in the foot can lead to foot drop. This is the inability to extend the foot, causing it to drag when walking.

Diagnosis

Physicians diagnose diabetic neuropathy based on the patient's medical history and physical examination. The most common form of neuropathy, the stocking-glove form, or peripheral sensory neuropathy, is often diagnosed based on history alone. These patients typically complain of numbness, tingling, burning, or a sense that something is in their shoe. In addition, they note that their symptoms increase when they remove their socks and shoes and try to go to sleep. They often complain that the bedclothes bother their feet. This very sensitive feeling is called hyperesthesia.

Early on in this disorder, the nerve conduction studies and electromyograms that are usually done are not helpful and often have normal findings. This is because they measure larger myelinated nerve fibers that are affected much later in the course of the disease. On examination, these patients may have loss of ankle reflexes or changes in sensory testing to stimuli such as vibration and a light touch with nylon microfilaments.

Treatment

Diabetic neuropathy may also cause chronic and sometimes severe pain. People with diabetes may need medications or creams. The first therapy is to tighten glucose control to as near-normal levels as possible. Patients are also counseled to stop smoking and to normalize their blood pressure and lipid levels. Often medications are given at bedtime, when patients' symptoms are typically the worst.

Simple analgesics such as acetaminophen (Tylenol) may be given to patients. The drug tramadol (Ultram), which is a nonnarcotic and not a nonsteroidal anti-inflammatory medication (NSAID), is given if acetaminophen provides insufficient pain relief. Many people do not wish to take narcotics or NSAIDs because of their side effects. The next medication usually tried is in the class of antiseizure or antidepressant medications. Antidepressants such as amitriptyline (Elavil) or nortriptyline (Aventyl or Pamelor) or the antiseizure drug gabapentin (Neurontin) may be used.

When a patient has a lancinating (shooting) form of pain, carbamazepine (Tegretol) is also very helpful. Memantine (Namenda and Axura), a medication currently indicated to treat Alzheimer's disease, has also been found to be effective in reducing neuropathic pain for patients.

If the neuropathy is in a very localized area, topical medications such as capsaicin or lidocaine can be used. As a last resort, narcotics have been used with success.

See also TYPE 1 DIABETES; TYPE 2 DIABETES.

The Diabetes Control and Complications Trial Research Group. "The Effect of Intensive Diabetes Therapy on the Development and Progression of Neuropathy." *Annals of Internal Medicine* 122, no. 8 (April 15, 1995): 561–568.

Petit, William A. Jr., M.D., and Christine Adamec. *The Encyclopedia of Diabetes.* New York: Facts On File, Inc., 2002.

diabetic retinopathy   Disease of the retina of the eye, directly stemming from diabetes mellitus. Diabetic retinopathy is the most common eye disease found among people diagnosed with diabetes. According to the National Institutes of Health (NIH), diabetic retinopathy causes from 12,000–24,000 new cases of blindness each year and is estimated to cause 12 percent of all new cases of blindness each year. It is also the leading cause of adult-onset blindness.

Diabetic retinopathy is at least partially caused by high levels of glucose that result in varying levels of harm to the blood vessels in the retina. Other factors, such as a genetic predisposition to developing the disease, hypertension, smoking, hyperlipidemia, and kidney disease, may worsen the retinopathy.

An early diagnosis, determined by a dilated eye examination and followed by appropriate treatment, could prevent the loss of sight for over 90 percent of patients with diabetes. Because the early stages of the disease produce no symptoms, only an early eye examination will detect possible problems. However, according to the National Institutes of Health, less than half (47 percent) of all patients diagnosed with diabetes have annual eye examinations. In its Healthy People 2010 plan, the federal government has set a goal that 75 percent of all adults with diabetes have a dilated eye examination each year.

The National Diabetes Eye Examination Program offers free eye examinations to patients with diabetes who are over age 65 and on Medicare.

Risk Factors

People with TYPE 1 DIABETES are at greater risk for developing retinopathy than patients with TYPE 2 DIABETES. In fact, almost all patients who have had Type 1 diabetes for 15 or more years have some degree of retinopathy. Patients with Type 2 diabetes who require insulin are also likely to develop retinopathy.

African Americans who have Type 1 diabetes are particularly at risk for developing diabetic retinopathy. In fact, African Americans with diabetes face a 40–50 percent greater risk than Caucasians with diabetes of developing diabetic retinopathy. Hispanics with diabetes, especially Mexican Americans, are also at high risk for developing the condition. It is also possible for children who have diabetes to suffer from diabetic retinopathy, although the risk appears to be low, especially prior to the onset of puberty.

The people with diabetes who are the most likely to suffer from diabetic retinopathy include those who:

- Did not control their diabetes in the first years after diagnosis
- Have had diabetes for 17 or more years
- Experience high blood pressure
- Are African American, Native American, or Hispanic
- Have high cholesterol levels
- Have had gestational diabetes
- Are smokers
- Abuse alcohol
- Have other illnesses, such as kidney disease
- Have a genetic risk for eye disease

Indications of Diabetic Retinopathy

Few symptoms of early diabetic retinopathy are detectable to the patient. This is why screening examinations are so critical. Some early symptoms may be a worsening of peripheral (side) vision or worse color vision. A dilated eye examination performed by an ophthalmologist (a medical doctor who specializes in eye diseases) or an optometrist should reveal the problem. Symptoms may often be mistaken by the patient as minor problems or as signs of aging.

Diagnosis and Treatment

A dilated eye examination will detect diabetic retinopathy, which is why annual eye examinations are crucial for all adults who have been diagnosed with diabetes. Patients with Type 1 diabetes should begin annual eye examinations after having diabetes for five years. In contrast, those with Type 2 diabetes should have a yearly examination beginning the year they are diagnosed. This is due to the fact that many patients with Type 2 diabetes have had metabolic derangements for seven to 12 years prior to diagnosis.

Treatment of Diabetic Retinopathy

If diabetic retinopathy is in the early stages, tight glycemic control may help. This means that the person with diabetes must carefully note glucose levels and respond to significant changes.

When the retinopathy is advanced, laser surgery, which is also known as photocoagulation, may help the patient. The physician uses a special laser to make tiny burns over the surface of the retina and to destroy blood vessels that are growing over the surface of the eye or stop leakage from retinal vessels.

Laser photocoagulation is very successful in most patients who have diabetic retinopathy. This procedure also reduces the risk of blindness in people with diabetic retinopathy by approximately 50 percent. The advantages of laser therapy are that no incision is required and that it can be performed on an outpatient basis. The procedure is best done when the patient's eyesight is still normal or nearly normal. A disadvantage of the surgery is that it does not always resolve the problem.

Sometimes surgery requiring an incision must be performed to preserve vision. The vitrectomy is a surgical procedure that removes old blood and scar tissue from within the eye, all of which have resulted from the disease.

See also EYE PROBLEMS.

For further information, contact:

American Academy of Ophthalmology
P.O. Box 7424
San Francisco, CA 94120-7424
(415) 561-8500
http://www.eyenet.org

National Eye Health Education Program
2020 Vision Place
Bethesda, MD 20892-3655
http://www.nei.nih.gov/nehep

The Diabetes Control and Complications Trial Research Group. "Early Worsening of Diabetic Retinopathy in the Diabetes Control and Complications Trial." *The Archives of Ophthalmology* 116, no. 7 (1998): 874–886.

Fong, Donald S., M.D., and Robin Demi Ross, M.D. *The Diabetes Eye Care Sourcebook.* Los Angeles, Calif.: Lowell House, 1999.

Petit, William A., Jr., M.D., and Christine Adamec. *The Encyclopedia of Diabetes.* New York: Facts On File, Inc., 2002.

dwarfism   A skeletal deformity, usually inherited, that causes below-normal height (usually the individual is less than four feet, 10 inches in height) and often results in other characteristic features, such as a broad forehead, a large head compared with the body, and disproportionately short arms and legs. (Individuals with pituitary dwarfism, however, have arms and legs that are proportional to their bodies.) In rare cases, dwarfism is caused by a growth hormone deficiency. There are an estimated 200 different types of dwarfism. However, the most common form is achondroplasia, which represents about 50 percent of all cases.

It should be noted that some individuals with dwarfism are offended by the term *dwarf,* and they prefer to be known as little people or as a person of short stature. Others, however, do not have a problem with the words *dwarf* or *dwarfism.*

Achondroplasia

The most common form of dwarfism is achondroplasia, which occurs in about one in 15,000 to one in 40,000 births. (Researchers have been unable to narrow the incidence any more precisely than this range.) Most people with achondroplasia are about four feet in height and were born to nondwarf parents of average size. Nearly all (97 percent) of individuals with achondroplasia have a mutation in their fibroblast growth factor receptor (FGFR) *3* gene. Individuals with achondroplasia usually have small stature, large heads, flattened bridges of the nose, short upper arms and legs, and incomplete elbow extensions. Children with achondroplasia are at risk for obstructive apnea (a breathing disorder) and hydrocephalus (enlargement of the brain).

It is important to note, however, that despite these variations from the appearance of the average person, many people with achondroplasia lead normal lives. Additionally, most of them are fertile.

Other Forms of Dwarfism

Although achondroplasia is the most common form of dwarfism, there are other types as well. These include hypochondroplasia, thanatophoric dysplasia (TD), and severe achondroplasia with development delay and ACANTHOSIS NIGRICANS (SADDAN).

People with hypochrondroplasia are of small stature and have bowed limbs. They may have narrowed spines and lumbar lordosis.

Thanatophoric dysplasia is so severe that it is usually fatal. This form of dwarfism occurs in an estimated one of every 60,000 births, and most of these babies die as newborns.

Individuals with SADDAN suffer from chronic seizures and hydrocephalus during infancy. Both their intellectual and motor development is much delayed.

Pituitary dwarfism, which is also known as growth hormone deficiency dwarfism, is caused by a growth hormone deficiency rather than by an inherited defect. (People with pituitary dwarfism were formerly called midgets; however, that term is considered particularly offensive by most people of short stature.)

About 10,000–15,000 people in the United States have pituitary dwarfism. People with pituitary dwarfism have arms and legs that are proportionately sized to their short stature. Sometimes children with pituitary dwarfism are treated with growth hormone. Children born with pituitary dwarfism may grow normally until they are about two or three years old, when their growth lags behind that of other children their own age.

Diseases That May Cause Short Stature

Some medical problems, such as McCUNE-ALBRIGHT SYNDROME, TURNER SYNDROME, and CONGENITAL ADRENAL HYPERPLASIA, may result in dwarfism and short stature. Treatment may help mitigate the growth outcome if the child is treated early enough. Children who experience EARLY PUBERTY are also at risk for short stature. OSTEOGENESIS IMPERFECTA, an inherited condition of brittle bones, may also cause dwarfism, and individuals with this condition usually do not exceed three feet in their final height.

Treatment of Dwarfism

Treatment depends on the nature of the dwarfism. Growth hormone may be used in children whose bones have not yet fused. In a study reported in a 1996 issue of the *Journal of Clinical Endocrinology & Metabolism*, Shohat and colleagues reported on their study of 15 children with achondroplasia and hypochondroplasia who were treated with growth hormone. The children's ages ranged from three to 12 years. The children showed significant growth, particularly the children with hypochondroplasia. The body disproportion did not increase with growth as the researchers had feared it might.

Children and adults with dwarfism may require joint replacement because of early wear and tear on the joints. Some adults have back fusion or neck fusion surgery to strengthen that part of their spine.

Limb lengthening is a controversial form of treatment, in which the bones are cut and pins are inserted to cause new bone growth and lengthening. It is a very painful process that takes at least two years and has not been evaluated as of this writing.

Daily Living

Individuals of short stature need to make many daily adaptations. For example, they may need special tools to help them reach light switches and other common devices. The child or adult may need an expandable wand to enable her to reach the toilet paper holder in bathrooms. Simple stools will enable the child or adult to reach many areas that are too high for their arms. Adaptations will need to be made to cars so that adults can drive. Some experts recommend that air bags be removed from the car, because if activated, they can be very dangerous to adults of small stature.

There are also emotional and psychological pressures upon persons of short stature. Children and adults must face staring from children and adults as well as questions and sometimes negative comments from others. Some people treat persons of short stature as if they were children. During school years, physical education with other children or adolescents may be difficult or even dangerous. Instead, the individual's other talents, in music, art, or other abilities, should be encouraged.

See also GROWTH HORMONE.

For further information on dwarfism, contact:

Little People of America, Inc.
5289 Northeast Elam Young Parkway
Suite F-700
Hillsboro, OR 97124
(888) LPA-2001 (toll-free)
http://www.lpaonline.org

Francomano, Clair A., M.D. "The Genetic Basis of Dwarfism." *New England Journal of Medicine* 332, no. 1 (January 5, 1995): 58–59.

Shohat, M., et al. "Short-Term Recombinant Human Growth Hormone Treatment Increases Growth Rate in Achondroplasia." *Journal of Clinical Endocrinology & Metabolism* 81, no. 11 (1996): 4,033–4,037.

Vajo, Zoltan, Clair A. Francomano, and Douglas J. Wilkin. "The Molecular and Genetic Basis of Fibroblast Growth Receptor 3 Disorders: The Acondroplasia Family of Skeletal Dysplasias, Muenke Craniosynostotis, and Crouzon Syndrome with Acanthosis Nigricans." *Endocrine Reviews* 21, no. 1 (2000): 23–39.

early puberty An earlier-than-normal onset of the body changes that normally occur during adolescence. Early puberty is generally defined as occurring in girls younger than age eight and boys younger than age nine. However, early puberty can occur in children as young as two or three years old. Early puberty is also known as precocious puberty.

Some children are at particular risk for developing early puberty, such as boys with KLINEFELTER SYNDROME and girls with MCCUNE-ALBRIGHT SYNDROME, follicular cysts, or stromal cell ovarian tumors. Early puberty can also be seen in children who have cerebral palsy, NEUROFIBROMATOSIS TYPE 1, CONGENITAL ADRENAL HYPERPLASIA, or fetal alcohol syndrome. In boys, precocious puberty is often due to tumors, radiation therapy, or a hypothalamic disorder with increased secretion of gonadotropin-releasing hormone (GnRH).

If children are under the age of five or six years old, hormones that are administered may help to suppress the puberty. After that age, the physical changes may be difficult or impossible to reverse, although studies have shown that growth in height can be stimulated by medications for at least several years.

In a study of 105 female patients with precocious puberty, reported in a 2003 issue of *Pediatrics,* researchers found that about 12 percent of the patients had other endocrine diseases or disorders, including McCune-Albright syndrome, growth hormone deficiency, hyperinsulinism, HYPOTHYROIDISM, neurofibromatosis, and PITUITARY ADENOMAS. The researchers in this study identified precocious puberty in girls as occurring before age seven or eight years in Caucasian girls and before age six to eight years in African-American girls. (The reason for the discrepancy is that research has

demonstrated that often African-American girls experience normal puberty before Caucasian girls.)

The researchers found that bone ages were advanced by as much as five years in the girls who had at least two signs of pubertal development. Some girls with breast development alone had a bone age that was well advanced for their years. Early puberty is problematic because it means the child's growth will end prematurely and, consequently, these children will attain a height much lower than that of their peers. Though it is not a form of DWARFISM, the short stature of individuals with an early puberty may be in the similar range of individuals who are diagnosed with dwarfism.

Early Puberty and Internationally Adopted Girls

In several cases, some children (especially girls) who were adopted from orphanages in poor countries by parents in North America or Europe have evinced an early puberty. Physicians speculate that the child who was living in an orphanage at a subsistence level and who was then adopted and given all the food she or he needed experienced a surge of growth that may have triggered a change to the brain that caused the onset of the early puberty.

In a 1998 study reported in the *Archives of Disease in Childhood,* Italian researchers studied 19 girls adopted from India by Swedish families and who all experienced an early puberty. The researchers found that hormone treatment to suppress the puberty, which sometimes started at age four, was largely unsuccessful. In general, girls adopted before the age of three are less likely to experience an early puberty than girls adopted at an older age. In addition, girls who have a very dramatic growth spurt within two years of adoption are more likely to experience an early puberty.

Pediatrician and international adoption expert Jerri Ann Jenista, M.D. has stated that children with even subtle indications of an early puberty, such as body odor, any pubic or underarm hair, or acne, should be seen by a pediatric endocrinologist as soon as possible to determine if the child has experienced an early puberty or another illness and what, if anything, can be done to help the child.

Signs and Symptoms

The signs of early puberty are the appearance of body hair in males and females (pubarche), enlarging testicles in males, and breast budding (thelarche) in females. Other signs such as menstruation may develop. In boys, a variety of tests are taken, including a pituitary computerized tomography (CT) scan or a magnetic resonance imaging (MRI) scan as well as tests to ascertain bone age and human chorionic gonadatropin (HCG) level. HCG can be secreted by a Leydig cell tumor. In girls, a pelvic ultrasound is taken. In all children, thyroid function is measured.

Pseudoprecocious puberty can also be caused by the use of exogenous sex steroid hormones.

Psychological Consequences of Precocious Puberty

As might be expected, it can be very difficult for a child to experience an early puberty. A 12-year-old girl has enough difficulty coping with menstrual periods, but at least many of her peers will be going through the same situation at about the same time. In contrast, it is not at all normal for a four- or five-year-old girl to have breasts and menstrual cycles. People can make cruel comments to such children. Children may also need to undergo therapy to help them deal with the behaviors of others. Family therapy may help family members learn how to cope with the actions of others.

Diagnosis and Treatment

In most cases of precocious puberty, the diagnosis is not difficult because a physical examination of the child reveals a sexual maturity beyond the norm for the child's age. In addition, the physician may order a gonadotropin-releasing hormone (GnRH) stimulation test. If the test results are greater than seven to 10 IU/l, the diagnosis of precocious puberty is made. A pelvic ultrasound is usually ordered for girls to rule out an ovarian tumor or cyst or McCune-Albright syndrome.

Boys with suspected early puberty should be tested for androgen levels. If they are elevated, this may indicate the boy has congenital adrenal hyperplasia or a tumor of the adrenal glands. The thyroid level of the child should also be tested. In some cases, hypothyroidism is the cause for early puberty in girls, and treatment with thyroid hormone causes a remission and, for example, the regression of breast development.

Treatment is aimed at maximizing final adult height, avoiding premature menstruation and sexual activity, and treating associated psychosocial issues. Some physicians treat children with early puberty with medications such as luteinizing hormone-releasing hormone (LHRH) agonist drugs.

In a study reported in a 2001 issue of the *Journal of Clinical Endocrinology & Metabolism* by the National Institutes of Health, researchers found that treatment with LHRH agonist medications in girls before the age of eight years and in boys before age nine was effective at improving their final height. The 98 children, including 80 girls and 18 boys with precocious puberty, were treated with deslorelin for two or more years. Although most of the children did grow, they were still shorter than the norm. The researchers also found that even girls with a bone age of 13 years when treatment had started showed improved growth.

See also DELAYED PUBERTY.

Adamec, Christine, and William L. Pierce. *The Encyclopedia of Adoption,* 2d ed. New York: Facts On File, Inc. 2000.

Kaplowitz, Paul B., M.D., Sharon E. Oberfield, M.D., and the Drug and Therapeutics and Executive Committees of the Lawson Wilkins Pediatric Endocrine Society. "Reexamination of the Age Limit for Defining When Puberty is Precocious in Girls in the United States: Implications for Evaluation and Treatment." *Pediatrics* 104, no. 4 (October 1999): 936–941.

Midyett, L. Kurt, M.D., Wayne V. Moore, M.D., and Jill D. Jacobson, M.D. "Are Pubertal Changes in Girls Before Age 8 Benign?" *Pediatrics* 111, no. 1 (January 2003): 47–51.

Oerter Klein, Karen, et al. "Increased Final Height in Precocious Puberty after Long-Term Treatment with

LHRH Agonists: The National Institutes of Health Experience." *Journal of Clinical Endocrinology & Metabolism* 86, no. 10 (2001): 4,711–4,716.

Raffaele, Virdis, et al. "Precocious Puberty in Girls Adopted from Developing Countries," *Archives of Disease in Childhood* 78, no. 2 (1998): 152–154.

eating disorders   Generally refers to either ANOREXIA NERVOSA (self-starvation) or bulimia nervosa, a condition in which the patient binges and then self-induces vomiting. Some patients abuse laxatives. Binge eating disorder is another form of an eating disorder, in which patients eat large quantities of food several times a week, far beyond when they feel full. They may be obese or may be of normal weight. Binge eating disorder is different from bulimia nervosa in that the patients do not induce vomiting. Eating disorders can be difficult to diagnose and treat. Some experts also characterize OBESITY as an eating disorder, while most consider it to be a separate medical problem in its own right.

One unique eating disorder is hyperphagia, an uncontrollable desire to continue eating because of a continuously ravenous and insatiable appetite. This medical problem is rare and is primarily found among individuals with PRADER-WILLI SYNDROME. Some experts report that such patients have extremely elevated levels of GHRELIN, a hormone that controls appetite. The parents or caregivers of patients with Prader-Willi syndrome actually have to lock up the refrigerator and kitchen cabinets or the patient would eat everything in there. These patients are obese.

Eating disorders may cause or worsen existing endocrine problems, such as making diabetic patients more ill. Eating disorders that lead to severe weight loss may also cause AMENORRHEA as well as OSTEOPOROSIS.

There is a fairly high incidence of eating disorders in young patients with TYPE 1 DIABETES, especially females. Early on, these patients realize that by omitting their insulin doses and allowing their glucose levels to run very high, this action puts them in a catabolic state with significant weight loss. Often this manipulation is subtle and vehemently denied by the patient.

Diagnosis and Treatment

Eating disorders are diagnosed via the patient's history and physical examination. The history (often given by others) that reveals symptoms such as excessive eating or refusal to eat, anorexia, nausea, fatigue, and constipation may point to an eating disorder. Physical signs, such as the loss of enamel on the teeth, bruises on the knuckles of the hands, weight loss, the growth of lanugo hair (very fine body hair), and the presence of carotene in the urine (carotenemia) may suggest an eating disorder such as anorexia nervosa.

Treatment is individualized but usually involves the patient's primary care provider, an endocrinologist, a gastroenterologist, and a psychiatrist. In severe cases, patients require hospitalization. Some patients need long-term residential treatment.

See also IMPAIRED GLUCOSE TOLERANCE.

For further information on eating disorders, contact the following organizations:

Academy for Eating Disorders
60 Revere Drive
Suite 500
Northbrook, IL 60062
(847) 498-4274
http://www.aedweb.org

Harvard Eating Disorders Center
55 Fruit Street
YAW 6900
Boston, MA 02114
(617) 726-8470
http://www.hedc.org

National Eating Disorders Association
603 Stewart Street
Suite 803
Seattle, WA 98101
(206) 382-3587
http://nationaleatingdisorders.org

Becker, Anne E., M.D., et al. "Eating Disorders." *New England Journal of Medicine* 340, no. 14 (April 8, 1999): 1,092–1,098.

National Center on Addiction and Substance Abuse at Columbia University. *Food for Thought: Substance Abuse and Eating Disorders.* National Center on Addiction and Substance Abuse at Columbia University, December 2003, New York, N.Y.

Zipfel, Stephan, et al. "Osteoporosis in Eating Disorders: A Follow-Up Study of Patients with Anorexia and Bulimia Nervosa." *Journal of Clinical Endocrinology & Metabolism* 86, no. 11 (2001): 5,227–5,233.

elderly Generally defined as individuals who are age 65 and older. Older people have an increased risk for some endocrine diseases and disorders, such as TYPE 2 DIABETES, OSTEOPOROSIS, and thyroid disease (especially HYPOTHYROIDISM), as well as for some endocrine cancers, such as OVARIAN CANCER and PANCREATIC CANCER.

Undiagnosed endocrine diseases can present serious risks to elderly individuals. For example, the majority of patients experiencing a MYXEDEMA COMA (a thyroid crisis) are older people who were previously not diagnosed with hypothyroidism. This disease may be brought on by the administration of sedating/hypnotic drugs that are given in the hospital to previously undiagnosed elderly, hypothyroid patients.

Diagnosis of Endocrine Diseases in the Elderly May Be Difficult

Sometimes physicians do not realize the significance of signs and symptoms found among older people. For example, patients may complain of joint pain and weakness. Many doctors may attribute these problems to arthritis and aging when they may instead be caused by more unusual diseases and disorders, such as hyperparathyroidism.

Older patients may have serious sleep disorders that have gone unidentified. These disorders may be caused by pineal gland insufficiency, which can be treated with controlled-release melatonin. In a study in Israel of 12 elderly individuals, all of whom complained of chronic insomnia, researchers found below-normal blood levels of the main melatonin metabolite, 6-sulphatoxymelatonin. The subjects were treated for three weeks with controlled-release melatonin and then for three weeks were given a placebo. The patients' sleep efficiency was measured with a wrist actigraphy device.

The researchers found that the sleep efficiency was significantly improved during the period when the patients were taking melatonin compared with when they took the placebo. The researchers concluded, "Melatonin deficiency may have an important role in the high frequency of insomnia among elderly people. Controlled-release melatonin therapy effectively improves sleep quality in this population."

Although it is often true that the first and most obvious diagnosis of a patient is usually the right one, when a patient does not improve with treatment, physicians should explore other possible causes of the medical problem. Many illnesses experienced by older people can be diagnosed and treated.

Ageist Attitudes May Blind Some Physicians to Existing Disease

Ageist attitudes, that older people are supposed to feel ill and that it is normal and acceptable for them to feel sick, may sometimes prevent otherwise competent physicians from exploring a variety of causes of medical complaints from older people. If elderly patients or their caregivers (such as family members) feel that ageist attitudes are preventing the patient from receiving a proper diagnosis and treatment, other physicians should be sought.

Multiple Medical Problems

Sometimes the diagnosis of an endocrine disease means that older patients have an increased risk for experiencing other medical problems. Elderly individuals with diabetes are at risk for thyroid diseases, kidney diseases, eye disorders, cardiac ailments, and other disorders. In one study reported in a 2000 issue of *Clinical Endocrinology*, researchers found that older subjects with subclinical hyperthyroidism were at an increased risk for developing dementia.

Researchers have also found that older women with HYPERTHYROIDISM have a three times greater risk of suffering from FRACTURES than women of the same age with normal THYROID-STIMULATING HORMONE (TSH) levels. These findings were based on a study of 686 white women older than age 65 at four clinical centers in the United States. All the patients had hyperthyroidism, and the patients were a subset of a much larger study of nearly 10,000 patients, the Study of Osteoporotic Fractures Research Group. The study was reported in a 2001 issue of the *Annals of Internal Medicine*. The fracture risk was based on actual fractures experienced by the women over nearly six years and was verified by X-rays.

Medications May Act Differently on Older People

Physicians should realize that medications that may work well in younger people can sometimes cause harm to older people. Additionally, sometimes older people need a different dose of a medication than do younger people.

The kidneys and livers of elderly people often are less efficient than those of younger people, and their overall metabolisms may be much slower, even when no evidence exists of thyroid disease. In addition, some drugs may further exacerbate other existing medical problems. For example, metformin, a medication often used to treat diabetes, can cause lactic acidosis, which is dangerous in patients with renal insufficiency or heart disease.

Signs and Symptoms of Endocrine Disorders May Be Different

Sometimes when older people have endocrine diseases and disorders, they do not have the same symptoms or signs as seen among younger people who have the same disease. For example, older people with hypothyroidism may present with few or no symptoms or with symptoms that are easily overlooked, such as fatigue and general achiness as well as various vague complaints. Older people with thyroid disease often do not have GOITERS, whether they have hyperthyroidism or hypothyroidism.

Older patients with hyperthyroidism may not be hyperactive but, instead, may appear apathetic and depressed (apathetic thyrotoxicosis). Physicians need to realize that the symptoms of older people with thyroid disease may be much more subtle than those found in younger individuals.

Laboratory Tests and Values May Differ in Elderly

When older people have endocrine diseases, some of the laboratory tests used to diagnose them should be different than those used to diagnose younger people. For example, when hypothyroidism is present among older people, often the TSH values may be in the normal range despite the presence of hypothyroidism. Another laboratory test, of free T4 levels, may indicate the presence of hypothyroidism.

Tests for thyroid-releasing hormone (TRH) may also be useful in older women but are not usually valid to diagnose thyroid disease among older men. In general, the older the patient, the less well the pituitary gland responds to a variety of stimuli. This is truer for men than for women.

Other laboratory tests may help to diagnose thyroid disease present in senior citizens, such as a check of the creatine phosphokinase (CPK) levels, which are elevated when thyroid disease is present in older people. Some older people also have anemia with hypothyroidism, which responds to treatment with LEVOTHYROXINE (L-thyroxine), a thyroid supplement.

Treatment May Be Different for Older People

Once illness is determined, the treatment for the medical problem may not be the same as for younger people. For example, doctors may decide that surgery for thyroid disease is too dangerous or not indicated in an older patient. However, it is important to distinguish between whether treatments may be unsafe, and thus should be avoided, and the presence of ageist attitudes among some doctors, who may assume that older people should accept illness as a part of aging.

Older People and Diabetes

An estimated 11 percent of all Americans ages six to 74 years have diabetes. Among Americans age 65 and older, an estimated 20 percent have diabetes, although only about half are aware that they have the disease. Among some racial groups, such as African Americans and Native Americans, diabetes is among the top five causes of death of older people.

According to John R. White Jr. and R. K. Campbell, authors of the chapter on managing Type 2 diabetes in the book *Diabetes Mellitus in the Elderly*, "The [older] patient with diabetes is 25 times more likely to become blind, 17 times more likely to develop kidney disease, 20 times more likely to develop gangrene, and 2 times more likely to suffer a stroke or a heart attack than aged matched cohorts without diabetes. However, recent studies have demonstrated a tight correlation between development and progression of most of the chronic complications of diabetes and strict glycemic control."

Despite the seriousness of diabetes among older individuals, as mentioned earlier, as many as half of all seniors with diabetes do not know they have the disease. Part of the reason is that the signs and symptoms of diabetes in elderly individuals may not be the same as found among younger people. For example, intense thirst is not always present in older people with undiagnosed diabetes.

In addition, rather than frequent urination, which is a common symptom among nonelderly patients with untreated diabetes, older people with diabetes are more likely to experience urinary incontinence. Rather than experiencing intense hunger, older people with undiagnosed diabetes are more likely to have a lack of appetite and to experience weight loss. In addition, older people with undiagnosed diabetes may also present with psychiatric features such as mental confusion, that are misconstrued by physicians and others.

When diabetes is diagnosed in older people, it may also be treated differently by doctors than when the illness is diagnosed in younger people. Physicians may not insist on as tight a glycemic control because very tight glycemic control may be difficult or impossible to achieve in some older individuals. Doctors may also not press patients to lose weight unless they are truly obese. However, as with all other patients, physicians usually urge older patients with diabetes to get regular exercise, particularly recommending walking on a regular basis.

Older patients with Type 2 diabetes may be able to control their illness with oral medications. However, sometimes insulin and other drugs are required to treat the disease as well, depending on its severity. It is also possible for an older person to be diagnosed with Type 1 diabetes (which always requires insulin), although the disease presents in the senior years only very rarely.

People with diabetes (or their caregivers) should test their blood at least several times each day to obtain information that lets them know whether to increase or decrease their glucose levels. This is important for elderly people who may develop hypoglycemia (low blood sugar), which can itself be dangerous, and could lead to falls and injuries. If older individuals are unable to test their own blood, a caregiver (a family member, a staff person at an assisted living facility or nursing home, or another person) should do the tests for the patient and act upon the information that the test provides.

Osteoporosis and Seniors

Middle-aged and younger people may develop OSTEOPOROSIS. However, it is the most dangerous when present among elderly individuals because of the increased risk for bone fractures. In addition, the rate of hospitalization for vertebral fractures caused by osteoporosis increases dramatically with age. For example, among people between the ages of 65–74 in the United States, 6.7 people per 1,000 are hospitalized because of an osteoporotic vertebral fracture. This rate nearly quadruples for people age 75–84, to a rate of 26 people per 1,000. The rate of hospitalization for vertebral fractures rises still higher for people ages 85 and older, with a rate of 39 people per 1,000.

Many people believe that only older women are at risk for osteoporosis. However, older men are at risk as well. In some studies, such as the Rotterdam Study, bone loss in men ages 70–75 was actually worse than the bone loss found among same-aged women.

Some experts believe that bone loss is linked to declining levels of growth hormone among elderly individuals, but studies to date have not borne out this hypothesis. Further studies are needed to determine if administering growth hormone could improve bone density levels in older individuals. However, studies on providing another substance, vitamin D, to elderly individuals who were deficient in vitamin D have demonstrated that bone density can improve with this supplementation. In one study, femoral bone density increased 2–7 percent over 18 months in elderly women given vitamin D, while it declined 4–6 percent in the group that received the placebo.

Osteoporosis is considered primary osteoporosis if no illness or cause can be found for it. It is usually treated with medications such as alendronate (Fosamax) to build up the bones. Other drugs that are prescribed for osteoporosis are risedronate (Actonel), raloxifene (Evista), and calcitonin (Miacalcin).

Osteoporosis is considered to be secondary if other factors have caused this medical problem. Many older people have secondary osteoporosis that was originally caused by hypogonadism, THYROTOXICOSIS, and HYPERPARATHYROIDISM. Some medications, such as GLUCOCORTICOIDS and anticonvulsants, can also cause secondary osteoporosis. Some lifestyle choices, such as alcohol abuse and smoking, can induce secondary osteoporosis as well.

With secondary osteoporosis, a variety of treatment recommendations can be made based on the underlying cause of the osteoporosis. For example, people who smoke should immediately stop smoking. Endocrine diseases and disorders such as hypogonadism, thyrotoxicosis, and hyperparathyroidism can and should be treated. If medications are inducing secondary osteoporosis, physicians may change the drug or lower the dose. For example, if glucocorticoid drugs have caused secondary osteoporosis, physicians may decide to prescribe thiazide diuretics to correct this problem.

Thyroid Disease and the Elderly

Thyroid disease, particularly hypothyroidism, is common among older people. However, as mentioned earlier, the signs and symptoms in older people may be different from those of younger people. In addition, elderly individuals may present with signs and symptoms commonly associated with other diseases of aging, such as mental confusion and paranoia (often associated with Alzheimer's disease or dementia), muscle stiffness (associated with arthritis), and heart irregularities. Older people may also present with depression, which may be masking the underlying problem of hypothyroidism. (Depression may also coexist with thyroid disease.)

Hypothyroidism in the elderly may also coexist with hypertension and hyperlipidemia. In its most severe manifestation, hypothyroidism presents as a myxedema coma, a clinical syndrome with a rapid onset that is potentially fatal to the patient. Almost all individuals who lapse into myxedema are elderly people with hypothyroidism.

Hyperthyroidism (excessive levels of thyroid hormone) is also a problem for some elderly individuals. It too may present differently in older individuals than in younger people. For example, mental decline may be one indicator of hyperthyroidism, which is not seen in middle-aged or younger adults with hyperthyroidism. Weakness is another sign of hyperthyroidism among the aged. The older person with hyperthyroidism may appear listless and depressed, unlike the younger individual with the same disease, who is overactive, nervous, and even manic.

Elderly women with hyperthyroidism have a three times greater risk of having fractures than women of the same age with normal TSH levels. Even a history of having hyperthyroidism is associated with twice the risk of developing fractures.

In general, physicians should treat patients based on their physiological age rather than their chronological age. Some patients who are 70 years old may have no illness, and may be physically fit, at an ideal body weight, and able to tolerate most medications and/or procedures. These patients are what physicians refer to as 70 going on 50.

Obviously, the opposite is also true. A 40-year-old patient may have diabetes mellitus with multiple complications, such as diabetic nephropathy and diabetic neuropathy, and may be unable to tolerate certain medications and/or procedures well. This patient is considered by doctors to be age 40 going on age 70.

See also DIABETES MELLITUS; FRACTURES; TYPE 1 DIABETES.

Bauer, Douglas C., M.D., et al. "Risk for Fracture in Women with Low Serum Levels of Thyroid-Stimulating Hormone." *Annals of Internal Medicine* 134, no. 7 (2001): 561–568.

Boonen, S., J. Aerssens, and J. Dequeker. "Age-Related Endocrine Deficiencies and Fractures of the Proximal Femur. I. Implications of Growth Hormone Deficiency in the Elderly." *Journal of Endocrinology* 149, no. 1 (1996): 7–12.

Boonen, S., J. Aerssens, and J. Dequeker, "Age-Related Endocrine Deficiencies and Fractures of the Proximal Femur. II. Implications of Vitamin D Deficiency in the Elderly." *Journal of Endocrinology* 149, no. 1 (1996): 13–17.

Cooper, James W., ed. *Diabetes Mellitus in the Elderly.* New York: The Haworth Press, 1999.

Garfinkel, D., M. Laudon, and N. Zisapel. "Improvement of Sleep Quality in Elderly People by Controlled-Release Melatonin." *Lancet* 346, no. 8,974 (August 26, 1995): 541–544.

Kalmijn, S., et al. "Subclinical Hyperthyroidism and the Risk of Dementia. The Rotterdam Study." *Clinical Endocrinology* 53 no. 6 (2000): 733–737.

Kandel, Joseph, M.D., and Christine Adamec. *The Encyclopedia of Senior Health and Well-Being.* New York: Facts On File, Inc., 2003.

Kane, Robert L., M.D., Joseph G. Ouslander, and Itamar B. Abrass. *Essentials of Clinical Geriatrics,* 4th ed. New York: McGraw-Hill, 1999.

empty sella syndrome   The syndrome that occurs when the sella turcica, the bony area of the skull that provides the support for the pituitary gland, is not completely filled with pituitary tissue. Empty sella syndrome is divided into primary and secondary types.

With primary empty sella syndrome, it is believed that there is a defect in the diaphragm by the pituitary gland, allowing cerebrospinal fluid to enter and to push the gland aside. No common endocrine abnormalities are seen with primary empty sella syndrome, and it is an X-ray abnormality without significant hormonal sequelae. However, almost all types of pituitary dysfunction have been reported, ranging from single hormone deficiencies to the loss of all anterior pituitary hormonal function.

In the case of secondary empty sella syndrome, the pituitary has been destroyed by surgery, a tumor, an infiltrative process, or radiation therapy. In this syndrome, partial or complete loss of pituitary function often occurs.

See also POSTPARTUM PITUITARY NECROSIS.

Kaufman, B. "The Empty Sella Turcica: A Manifestation of the Intrasellar Subarachnoid Space." *Radiology* 90, no. 5 (1968): 931–941.

endocrine autoimmunity   A condition in which the body mistakenly interprets the actions of an endocrine organ as those of an outside invader and attacks the organ. Sometimes the cause for what triggers an endocrine immunity is known, while other times physicians as well as researchers are unable to identify the cause. GRAVES' DISEASE and HASHIMOTO'S THYROIDITIS are two examples of autoimmune disorders of the thyroid gland. DIABETES MELLITUS is also an autoimmune disorder.

Autoimmune disorders can be difficult to diagnose and treat in their early stages.

Some studies have shown a linkage between an environmental factor and an endocrine autoimmunity. For example, a study reported in a 2000 issue of *Archives of Internal Medicine* compared 132 same-sex twins (264 individuals) and found a significant relationship between smoking and the subsequent development of either Graves' disease or autoimmune thyroiditis (Hashimoto's thyroiditis).

Brix, Thomas, M.D., Kyvik, K. O. and Hegedus, L., "Cigarette Smoking and Risk of Clinically Overt Thyroid Disease." *Archives of Internal Medicine* 160, no. 5 (March 13, 2000): 661–666.

endocrine glands   Ductless glands in the endocrine system that secrete hormones needed for normal functioning as well as for the sustaining of life. These glands work via hormones that are typically secreted into the bloodstream and travel to other organs to have their effects. If the hormones act upon nearby cells, even upon other cells within the same gland, they display the paracrine effect.

The endocrine glands are the following: the adrenal glands, hypothalamus, ovaries, pancreas, parathyroid glands, pineal gland, pituitary gland, testes, thyroid gland, and the thymus. As researchers learn more and more about the human body, all organs in the body can clearly act as endocrine glands, which is to say, they secrete hormones. For instance, the gastrointestinal tract is now known to synthesize and secrete over 40 hormones, many of whose function and operation are still unknown. The heart makes a hormone called atrial natriuretic factor or peptide that is involved in the body's salt and water balance.

endocrinologist   A medical doctor with specialized training who concentrates on treating people with endocrine diseases and disorders such as DIABETES MELLITUS, thyroid diseases, and the full array of other common or rare endocrine problems. A pediatric endocrinologist generally treats patients under the age of 18 years who have endocrine diseases or disorders.

Endocrinologists who treat adults typically complete a three-year post–medical school internship and a residency in internal medicine before training for an additional two to three years in an endocrinology-metabolism-diabetes fellowship program. Pediatric endocrinologists follow a similar course of education and training, but they have a three-year internship and residency in pediatrics. Many endocrinologists who treat adults see some children with endocrine disorders, just as many pediatric endocrinologists will follow their patients into adulthood and past the age of 18 years.

Physicians who complete endocrinology training may sit for board certification for endocrinology/metabolism/diabetes if they have previously passed their internal medicine board examination. This is typically a two-day long examination that tests the physician in all areas of endocrinology and is administered by the American Board of Internal Medicine and its subsidiary boards.

There is great concern that the current number of endocrinologists practicing in the United States is insufficient. In fact, as of this writing, only about 275 physicians are in fellowship training for endocrinology. These new doctors can barely replace the numbers of endocrinologists who are retiring or leaving their practices for other reasons. At the same time, the United States faces a pandemic of diabetes as well as a rapidly aging population that is more susceptible to endocrine disorders such as thyroid disease and osteoporosis. How this situation can be successfully resolved over the short term is unclear.

The two main clinical and research societies that support the endocrinology community are the American Association of Clinical Endocrinologists and the Endocrine Society.

epinephrine   See ADRENALINE.

erectile dysfunction (ED)   The consistent difficulty in achieving or retaining an erection sufficient to achieve a completed act of sexual intercourse. Erectile dysfunction is best viewed as a couple's problem. The patient's partner often prompts the patient to seek medical attention.

According to a 2002 article on erectile dysfunction in *Urology*, 10–20 million men in the United States have ED. In addition, the Massachusetts Male Aging Study found that more than half (52 percent) of men over age 40 had some level of erectile failure. Erectile dysfunction affects a man's quality of life, and many studies have shown that effective treatment of ED significantly improves life quality.

Erectile dysfunction is a distressing problem for most men. Some experts believe that the psychological impact of having erectile dysfunction is more severe than whatever medical problem has actually led to the ED. Even when the erectile problem is solely caused by a medical problem, it still has an emotional effect on the man.

According to Dr. Andre Guay and his colleagues in their article on medical guidelines for treating male sexual dysfunction, published in 2003 in *Endocrine Practice*, "Every man who has some problem with erectile function develops performance anxiety, and determining whether psychological factors are the main problem or merely a minor accompaniment may be difficult."

Causes of ED

There are many causes of erectile dysfunction, including medications, an excessive temporary or chronic consumption of alcohol, or diseases such as DIABETES MELLITUS, hypertension, stroke, prostate surgery, Parkinson's disease, hyperlipidemia, spinal cord disease and/or surgery, coronary artery disease, and seizure disorders. Smoking cigarettes may also impede a man's ability to have an erection.

Some medications can cause or contribute to the development of erectile dysfunction, such as drugs for hypertension, antidepressants, and many others. Even nonprescription medications, such as decongestants or antihistamines, may impede an erection. According to the 2003 update on male sexual dysfunction, published in *Endocrine Practice*, prescription and nonprescription medications cause about 25 percent of erectile problems men experience in the United States.

Men taking hormone therapy for advanced prostate cancer may experience erectile dysfunction until they no longer take the drug, at which time normal sexual functioning will often resume (if they did not have ED before they started taking the hormones). Often the hormones are used after a surgical procedure.

A PROLACTINOMA, or benign tumor of the pituitary gland, may also cause erectile dysfunction, as may rare medical problems such as KALLMANN'S SYNDROME or KLINEFELTER SYNDROME. Hypogonadism (low testosterone levels) can cause ED but usually causes only decreased libido and mild ED. However, some men have very low levels of testosterone and have no problems with erectile dysfunction at all.

When diabetes is the cause of ED (whether it is Type 1 or Type 2 diabetes), the problem is often due to nerve damage caused by diabetic neuropathy as well as premature atherosclerosis, which is more common among men whose levels of glucose are not well-controlled.

Men who have undergone a transurethral resection of the prostate due to benign prostatic hyperplasia (BPH) may also experience erectile dysfunction. This occurs because of nerve damage that occurred during the procedure.

There is often an emotional component to erectile dysfunction, and problems such as depression can lead to ED. Even when the underlying cause for the ED is physical, the man may develop problems with performance anxiety. The combined emotional and physical aspects then make it more difficult for him to attain or maintain an erection.

Diagnosis and Treatment

Primary care doctors typically diagnose and treat erectile dysfunction but may refer the patient to an endocrinologist or urologist. Men with erectile dysfunction are aware that they are having trouble with achieving an erection, and they may seek help from their doctor. However, many men are too embarrassed to discuss this problem with their doctors, not realizing how common this problem is or that it is often reversible with treatment.

The doctor will take a complete medical history to try to ascertain if there may be medical causes of the erectile dysfunction. Some doctors prefer to speak with both the man with erectile dysfunction and his sexual partner to obtain a view of the problem from the perspective of both parties.

During the physical examination, the physician will also examine the man's penis to determine if there are any obvious abnormalities (most commonly, Peyronie's disease). The doctor will also check for obvious signs of testosterone effect (beard, pubic and underarm hair, scalp hair recession, and normal muscle mass) as well as check the testicular size and shape. Most men are embarrassed by such an examination, but they should be reassured that urologists commonly perform many such examinations in a single day.

A rectal examination will also be performed to determine if there is a possible problem with the prostate gland. Problems may include prostatitis, which is an inflammation of the prostate gland that may be caused by an infection, or benign prostatic hyperplasia (BPH), a tissue overgrowth. Both conditions are often treated with prescribed medications. Doctors will also check for indications of prostate cancer with the digital rectal examination and may also order a prostate specific antigen (PSA) blood test.

The PSA test may be ordered routinely because the man is over age 50 and/or he is at risk for prostate cancer or has family members who have had prostate cancer. It may also be ordered if the physician notes the presence of any nodules or excessive tissue growth of the prostate gland. If there is a possibility of cancer, a biopsy will be performed.

The physician may also order laboratory tests, such as a complete blood count, tests of the man's testosterone level, and a urinalysis to check for infection or blood in the urine. If blood testosterone levels are low, the physician may order tests of prolactin, luteinizing hormone, and serum-free testosterone to provide further information. For example, high levels of prolactin indicate a prolactinoma, or pituitary tumor. The doctor may also order tests of glucose level, serum creatinine, cholesterol, and triglycerides. An ultrasound may be ordered as well as other specialized tests, depending on the patient and the doctor.

If any medical problems are identified in the physical examination or by laboratory testing, treating these problems may resolve the erectile dysfunction. For example, low testosterone levels (HYPOGONADISM) may be treated with topical or injected testosterone to normalize the testosterone levels. Better glycemic control may improve erectile function in patients with diabetes. Changing the medications that the patient takes for hypertension may also help to resolve the ED.

Viagra and Other Medications

If a man is diagnosed with erectile dysfunction that is not resolved by treating underlying medical problems, there are many different ways for most men to achieve potency again.

As of this writing, three phosphohodiesterase inhibitors are available on the market to treat erectile dysfunction. They include Viagra (sildenafil), Levitra (vardenafil), and Cialis (tadalafil). All three drugs work via the same mechanism. They inhibit phosphodiesterase (PDE5), and, by doing so, enable an erection. These drugs affect only blood flow and have no direct effect on sexual drive. These medications work within 30–60 minutes and last for four to 12 hours. The drugs cause headaches and flushing in 10–15 percent of the men who use them and also cause nasal congestion in 4–5 percent of men.

None of these drugs should be used if the man is on any medication that contains nitrates (topical, sublingual, or oral). If a man develops chest pains after using one of these drugs and needs medical attention, the treating emergency medical technicians and physicians must be advised that the man used the medication so that they can order medications other than nitrates for the first 24–36 hours of treatment.

When phosphodiesterase inhibitors are ineffective in helping the man to achieve erections, some doctors may prescribe injectable drugs, such as Caverject (alprostadil), Genabid (papaverine), or a combination of three drugs mixed up by the urologist, commonly referred to as trimix. These drugs are injected directly by the man into his penis, which is said to feel like a brief pinch. Urologists teach men how to perform these simple injections. The drug must be injected about 15 minutes before the man anticipates having sex. The erection induced by an injectable drug lasts about an hour.

Another form of alprostadil is available in a pellet called MUSE (Medicated Urethral System for Erection), a drug that is manually inserted into the urethra of the penis and that causes no pain. It is self-dissolving. If the pellet works, the erection will occur within five to 10 minutes of the injection and will last about an hour.

Mechanical Devices

To achieve an erection, some men rely upon mechanical devices such as the vacuum constriction device. It is placed over the penis and pumped up. If the device helps the man achieve an erection, a rubber band–like device is placed around the base of the penis and will help the man to maintain the erection for about 30 minutes. Many men find vacuum devices to be effective, although some complain that it causes their penis to feel cold and strange. Others say that the constriction band hurts them. The man must remove the band after intercourse in order to avoid damage to the penis, up to and including gangrene.

Penile Implants

If other methods for resolving ED are unsatisfactory, some men consider a penile prosthesis that is surgically inserted while the man is under anesthesia. Several different varieties of prostheses are currently available as of this writing, and they vary considerably in their complexity.

With the semirigid or malleable prosthesis, the man will manually change the angle of his penis, depending on whether he wants to have sex or not. When in the down position, the prosthesis is not noticeable unless the man wears very tight-fitting clothes. When he wants to have sex, he simply moves the penis to the up position. According to urologist Paul H. Lange in his chapter on erectile dysfunction in his book *Prostate Cancer for Dummies,* this device is the easiest to use and the most popular type of penile implant among many post–prostate cancer patients.

Another surgically inserted prosthesis uses an inflatable pump that is connected to a cylinder that fits into the penis. The patient presses on his penis to cause the pump to inflate and to achieve an erection. Yet another prosthesis is the three-piece prosthesis, which includes inflatable cylinders and a fluid reservoir. It is activated by the man pressing on an area near his scrotum. This type of implant is the most costly, and it is also considered to be the most effective device.

Penile prostheses can be very expensive (as of this writing, the surgical procedure costs at least $10,000), and they are not always covered by health insurance. In addition, they may last for only five to 10 years, depending on the manufacturer, the type of prosthesis that is implanted, and other factors. If the prosthesis breaks down, a new one can usually be inserted. The area where the prosthesis was inserted can become infected, which usually requires the removal of the entire prosthesis. After healing occurs, a new prosthesis can then be inserted.

The key advantage of the penile prosthesis is that it can often enable the patient to have a normal sex life without the need for taking any drugs such as Viagra. The key disadvantage is that once the penile prosthesis has been inserted, the other, noninvasive methods available to resolve impotence will no longer work.

See also INFERTILITY; MALE REPRODUCTION; TESTOSTERONE.

Althof, Stanley, E. "Quality of Life and Erectile Dysfunction." *Urology* 59, no. 6 (2002): 803–810.

Guay, Andre T., M.D., et al. "American Association of Clinical Endocrinologists Medical Guidelines for Clinical Practice for the Evaluation and Treatment of Male Sexual Dysfunction: A Couple's Problem—2003 Update." *Endocrine* Practice 9, no. 1 (January/February 2003): 77–95.

Lange, Paul H., M.D., and Christine Adamec. *Prostate Cancer for Dummies.* New York: Wiley Publishing, 2003.

Lue, Tom F., M.D. "Erectile Dysfunction." *New England Journal of Medicine* 342, no. 24 (June 15, 2000): 1,802–1,813.

estradiol   The most important form of estrogen released by the body. Estradiol is responsible for female breast development, the growth of the uterus, the placement of body fat, and other functions. Estradiol is secreted from the adrenal cortex, ovarian follicle, and, in a pregnant woman, the placenta. Both males and females synthesize estradiol, which can be measured in the blood.

According to the National Institutes of Health, normal estradiol levels are as follows:

- For premenopausal women: 20–400 picograms per milliliter (pg/ml); the measurement varies according to the time of the menstrual cycle

- For postmenopausal women: 5–25 pg/ml
- For males: 10–60 pg/ml

Some diseases impair the release of estradiol, such as premature ovarian failure and TURNER SYNDROME. Rarely, above-normal levels of estradiol may be detected with an ovarian tumor. Estradiol levels are also important in fertility, and physicians measure these levels when evaluating infertile individuals.

Estradiol is also available as a medication in oral tablets, skin patches, topical creams, and an injectable form. It is used to treat women with estrogen deficiency from a variety of causes. Generally, estradiol is given for the following reasons:

- To reduce menopausal symptoms such as HOT FLASHES
- As replacement therapy in women who are prematurely hypogonadal
- To prevent OSTEOPOROSIS
- To treat vaginal dryness caused by menopause
- To treat some prostate cancers (rare)
- To create female characteristics in biological males prior to and after sexual reassignment surgery.

Risks of Exogenous Estradiol

In addition to its usual physiological effects, estradiol and other forms of estrogen can lead to a prothrombotic state, making the patient more susceptible to blood clots. Such clots may occur in the legs or pelvis and can lead to a pulmonary embolism in the heart, in turn leading to a myocardial infarction (heart attack) or an embolism in the brain, leading to a stroke. Breast cancers that are present in women but that are not yet clinically detectable may have their growth stimulated by the use of exogenous estradiol and other estrogens.

These major adverse effects of estrogens, especially after the report of the Women's Health Initiative, have led to more limited use of estradiol and other estrogens for hormone replacement. These risks are accentuated among smokers.

Estradiol can also increase blood pressure as it stimulates the production of angiotensinogen from the liver, thus leading to increased levels of angiotensin (a very potent constrictor of blood vessels). Estradiol also increases the risk of the development of gallstones and can increase the frequency of headaches, especially in women who are predisposed to migraine headaches. There are some nuisance side effects to estradiol, such as breast tenderness and fluid retention.

Estradiol should not be used in an attempt to decrease macrovascular complications (such as heart attack and stroke) as they may actually increase the risk slightly, especially in the first several years. Estradiol should also not be used in women with a prior history of breast cancer and should be used only with caution in women at high risk of developing breast cancer.

See also ESTROGEN.

estrogen Female hormones, released by the ovaries, that are responsible for female secondary sexual characteristics, hair growth, and other features. Like TESTOSTERONE, estrogens are steroid hormones.

When estrogen levels decline, with advancing age and the onset of MENOPAUSE, some women experience signs and symptoms such as HOT FLASHES (vasomotor symptoms), insomnia, mood swings, and irritability. These women may consult with their physicians about the advisability of taking ESTROGEN REPLACEMENT THERAPY (estrogen alone) or HORMONE REPLACEMENT THERAPY (a combination of estrogen and progesterone). Some women experience an early menopause because their ovaries fail or because they have had the ovaries surgically removed because of a disease such as ovarian cysts or ovarian cancer.

See also ESTRADIOL; FEMALE REPRODUCTION.

Gruber, Christian J., M.D., et al. "Production and Actions of Estrogens." *New England Journal of Medicine* 346, no. 5 (January 31, 2002): 340–352.

estrogen replacement therapy (ERT) Synthetic or natural estrogen hormones given to a woman who is menopausal either due to the natural onset of MENOPAUSE (usually after the age of 45 years or so) or because of the removal of both of her ovaries. Each woman must decide for herself whether to take estrogen, or another type of female hormone replacement medication, after consulting with her physician and considering both the risks and benefits of the medications.

Some studies have indicated that women who take LEVOTHYROXINE (l-thyroxine) for their HYPOTHYROIDISM may need to increase their dosage if they also take estrogen replacement therapy.

See also ESTRADIOL; ESTROGEN; HORMONE REPLACEMENT THERAPY.

Arafah, Baha M., M.D. "Increased Need for Thyroxine in Women with Hypothyroidism During Estrogen Therapy." *New England Journal of Medicine* 344, no. 23 (June 7, 2001): 1,743–1,749.

euthyroid Refers to the physiological state in individuals whose thyroid hormone levels are in balance. In other words, these individuals are neither hyperthyroid (with excessive levels of circulating thyroid hormone) or hypothyroid (with inadequate levels of thyroid hormone). Some individuals have normal levels of thyroid in their blood and yet are ill with thyroid disease, a condition known as EUTHYROID SICK SYNDROME.

euthyroid sick syndrome A condition in which THYROID BLOOD TESTS reveal abnormal results, such as low levels of T3 (triiodothyronine) or T4 (THYROXINE) and typically, but not always, normal levels of thyroid-stimulating hormone (TSH) while the thyroid gland is actually functioning appropriately.

The individual with euthyroid sick syndrome generally has another serious underlying illness such as CANCER, AIDS, ANOREXIA NERVOSA, DIABETIC KETOACIDOSIS, or malnutrition. Some medications, such as corticosteroids, lithium, amiodarone, and propranolol, may affect thyroid blood levels in the absence of thyroid disease. Some patients may be recovering from surgery or from a transplant procedure.

Euthyroid sick syndrome is common among elderly individuals who are hospitalized with a severe illness.

The treatment for euthyroid sick syndrome is oriented to the underlying disease, and thyroid blood tests may be repeated at a later date. Thyroid hormone treatment is generally not begun unless the patient exhibits apparent symptoms of hypothyroidism. In fact, use of thyroid hormone replacement therapy has increased mortality (death) in several clinical trials where it has been administered to gravely ill patients who had abnormal results on their thyroid function tests.

See also GRAVES' DISEASE; HYPERTHYROIDISM.

Camacho, Pauline M., M.D., and Arcot A. Dwarkanathan, M.D. "Sick Euthyroid Syndrome." *Postgraduate Medicine* 105, no. 4 (April 1999): 215–228.

Umpierrez, Guillermo E., M.D. "Euthyroid Sick Syndrome." *Southern Medical Journal* 95, no. 5 (2002): 506–513.

exercise   Regular physical activity to maintain or achieve good health. Nearly all physicians consider regular exercise to be an important part of maintaining good health. Even individuals who are disabled and weak can usually master some simple exercises. Exercise is important to help individuals avoid obesity or to resolve obesity if it is already a problem. Simply walking several times a week may be sufficient to improve the health of many patients with OBESITY and other endocrine diseases and disorders.

In the Diabetes Prevention Program, the study group that walked briskly approximately 150 minutes per week decreased their risk of progressing from IMPAIRED GLUCOSE TOLERANCE (PREDIABETES) to overt DIABETES MELLITUS by 31 percent.

Exercise decreases INSULIN RESISTANCE and improves the glucose levels in patients who have diabetes mellitus. For patients with HYPERLIPIDEMIA, exercise will decrease their triglyceride levels and also increase their high-density lipoprotein (HDL or good CHOLESTEROL) levels.

Losing a significant amount of weight with exercise alone is difficult. However, exercising helps to decrease the overall body fat, including both visceral fat and abdominal obesity.

Tuomilehto, Jaako, M.D., et al. "Prevention of Type 2 Diabetes Mellitus by Changes in Lifestyle Among Subjects with Impaired Glucose Tolerance." *New England Journal of Medicine* 344, no. 18 (May 3, 2001): 1,343–1,350.

eye problems   Disorders of the eye. Some endocrine diseases and disorders cause or contribute to the development of eye diseases. For example, long-term TYPE 1 DIABETES may lead to DIABETIC RETINOPATHY or other eye diseases, up to and including blindness. As many as 24,000 people lose their eyesight in the United States because of diabetic eye disease. Yet experts report that as much as 90 percent of these cases of blindness could have been prevented by regular screening for eye disease. Only about 60 percent of patients with diabetes have an annual dilated eye examination.

Other diseases may cause eye problems. For example, a key feature of GRAVES' DISEASE is bulging of the eyes, or exophthalmos. Not all patients with Graves' disease have this feature of the illness, but many have mild signs or symptoms and do exhibit it.

Patients with DIABETES MELLITUS and/or a history of thyroid disease are more likely to suffer from dry eye syndrome (keratoconjunctivitis sicca), as are women in MENOPAUSE. The illness can cause severe pain and should be treated by an ophthalmologist (medical doctor who specializes in eye disease). The ophthalmologist may treat dry eye syndrome with specialized eyedrops and environmental recommendations (such as advising patients to avoid having heating or air-conditioning vents near their faces and limiting caffeine consumption). Sometimes surgical procedures are also needed. This condition should not be ignored because it can lead to worsened symptoms and even blindness.

For further information on eye diseases, contact the following organization:

American Academy of Ophthalmology
P.O. Box 7424
San Francisco, CA 94120-7424
(415) 561-8500
http://www.aao.org

Bartalena, Luigi, Aldo Pinchera, and Claudio Marcocci. "Management of Graves' Ophthalmopathy: Reality and Perspectives." *Endocrine Reviews* 21, no. 2 (2000): 168–199.

Moss, Scot E., Ronald Klein, M.D., and Klein, Barbara E., M.D. "Prevalence and Risk Factors for Dry Eye Syndrome," *Archives of Ophthalmology* 118, no. 9 (September 2000): 1,264–1,268.

failure to thrive (FTT)   A phrase used to describe the condition of infants or small children up to the age of two years who are not eating adequately and who show markedly poor growth. Such children will rank lower than the fifth percentile for weight at two or more checkups, or show no growth at all while evincing an overall development that is much slower than expected of other children of the same age.

Some children with failure to thrive not only do not grow but may actually lose weight. Untreated FTT may lead to further health problems such as developmental delays.

An estimated 1–5 percent of children younger than age two who are admitted to hospitals are diagnosed with failure to thrive. Children living in orphanages may also experience FTT, especially when they receive the bare minimum of care (such as brief washing, feeding, and changing) and when the caregivers constantly change.

Organic and Nonorganic Failure to Thrive Problems

There are two primary categories of failure to thrive, organic and nonorganic FTT. Organic failure to thrive is caused by a severe chronic medical problem, such as cystic fibrosis, untreated HYPOTHYROIDISM, infection with the human immunodeficiency virus (HIV), or heart disease. Nonorganic failure to thrive is caused by a severe, externally induced factor, such as starvation, maternal drug addiction, or other causes. Extreme cases of abuse and neglect may cause failure to thrive in some children.

Risk Factors

Mothers who are malnourished and/or who are drug abusers are more likely to have children diagnosed with FTT. Poor children are more likely to be diagnosed with FTT than children of other socioeconomic classes.

Symptoms of Failure to Thrive

Infants with FTT generally present with listlessness and apathy and have poor muscular development. Certain behaviors are typical among babies with FTT. For example, according to *The Encyclopedia of Child Abuse*, "Infants suffering from the sensory deprivation associated with FTT often maintain a posture in which the arms are held out, flexed at the elbow with the hands up and legs drawn in. This position of apparent surrender is held for long periods of time."

Diagnosis and Treatment

FTT is diagnosed based on its clinical presentation as well as a comparison of the child's weight and height with the weight and height expected for a child of the same age. Past weights of the child, if known, are also used for a comparison basis.

Physicians also use laboratory tests to screen for infections and metabolic diseases, such as hypothyroidism, that may cause the patient to become lethargic.

If the underlying cause of FTT is organic, the illness is treated. If it is nonorganic, physicians seek to identify and rectify the problem. For example, if abuse or neglect is suspected, the child may need to be removed from the family.

See also CACHEXIA; INFANTS.

Clark, Robin E., Judith Freeman Clark, and Christine Adamec. *The Encyclopedia of Child Abuse*, 2d ed. New York: Facts On File, Inc., 2000.

Zenel, J. A. Jr. "Failure to Thrive: A General Pediatrician's Perspective." *Pediatric Review* 18, no. 11 (1997): 371–378.

familial combined hyperlipidemia An inherited form (autosomal dominant inheritance) of hyperlipidemia with elevated levels of serum CHOLESTEROL and/or triglycerides. Familial combined hyperlipidemia has a variable clinical presentation. One person with the condition may have normal lipid levels, while the next may have elevated cholesterol levels and normal triglycerides, and a third person may have elevated levels of both.

Familial combined hyperlipidemia is linked to an increased risk for cardiovascular disease and for heart attacks if it is not controlled. This condition is also exacerbated by the presence of other illnesses, such as HYPOTHYROIDISM, DIABETES MELLITUS, or alcoholism. In addition, alcoholism may also worsen the condition. Both men and women are at risk for familial combined hyperlipidemia. Patients may develop this condition in adolescence, and treatment should not be delayed.

The gene or genes that cause this condition are unknown as of this writing, but researchers have found familial patterns of occurrence. In the Frederickson classification, this disorder is labeled hyperlipidemia type IIb.

Signs and Symptoms

Patients who are obese and who have had attacks of angina (chest pain) at a young age are suspects and should be screened for familial combined hyperlipidemia. In addition, a family medical history of early heart attacks or HYPERLIPIDEMIA is another indicator of the possible presence of this condition. Typically, there are no cutaneous manifestations.

Diagnosis and Treatment

Patients are diagnosed based on their blood test results as well as a complete medical history. Patients with familial combined hyperlipidemia may have high levels of serum low-density lipoproteins (LDLs) or very low-density lipoproteins (VLDLs), a predominant component of triglycerides. Thus these patients may have elevated levels of total cholesterol and/or elevated triglycerides. They may also have increased apolipoprotein B100 concentrations.

Treatment is aimed at decreasing the levels of cholesterol and triglycerides. Patients are often advised to limit their fat consumption to less than 30 percent of their caloric intake and limit their cholesterol intake to less than 300 mg per day. This generally means that they will eat less beef, chicken, pork, and lamb. Weight loss will also decrease triglyceride levels a bit more than cholesterol levels. Weight loss will typically decrease the total cholesterol levels by 5–20 percent, but typical decreases are 10 percent.

Ingestion of plant stanol esters, now available as spreads, will lower the total cholesterol by 12–17 percent. Alcohol intake should be minimized or prohibited. Exercise is helpful, especially in decreasing VLDL and thus triglyceride levels.

When therapeutic life changes fail to lower the patient's levels to the goal (as often happens, even with the most motivated of patients), pharmacological therapy is generally initiated.

When the triglycerides are less than the desired levels, a statin drug such as simvastatin (Zocor) or pravastatin (Pravachol) is prescribed. If the LDL is not controlled after titration, a second drug, such as nicotininc acid (Niaspan) or ezetimibe (Zetia), is added. This additional drug will provide an 18–26 percent reduction in LDL and a 3–5 percent increase in high-density lipoproteins (HDL).

If the triglycerides are not at goal after beginning the statin drug, nicotinic acid or a fibric acid derivative such as gemfibrozil (Lopid) or fenofibrate (Tricor) is added. Nicotinic acid can decrease the LDL (by 5–20 percent) and the triglycerides (20–50 percent reduction), and it can also increase the HDL by 10–20 percent. The physician and patient must be vigilant for adverse effects, especially myositis and rhabdomyolysis, when these agents (statins and nicotinic acid) are combined. This is especially true among patients with kidney disease or decreased muscle mass and among patients who are elderly.

Bile acid sequestrants such as cholestyramine (Questran) and colestipol (Colestid) are used occasionally. However, they have weak effects on LDL unless used at high doses and may increase triglyceride levels.

Treatment is usually for the remainder of the patient's life.

See also ATHEROSCLEROSIS/ARTERIOSCLEROSIS.

Athyros, V. G., et al. "Atorvastatin Versus Four Statin-Fibrate Combinations in Patients with Familial Combined Hyperlipidemia." *Journal of Cardiovascular Risk* 9, no. 1 (2002): 33–39.

familial dysbetalipoproteinemia A condition also known as type III hyperlipoproteinemia that causes ATHEROSCLEROSIS in the coronary arteries and can lead to coronary artery disease and peripheral vascular disease. It is exacerbated by diabetes, OBESITY, and HYPOTHYROIDISM. These other clinical problems often need to be present to increase the production of the lipoproteins and to lead to the full clinical scenario of familial dysbetalipoproteinemia. This condition occurs in an estimated one in 10,000 individuals and usually does not present until a patient is 20 years old or older. If it is untreated, familial dysbetalipoproteinemia can lead to heart attack, strokes, and blocked arteries to the lower extremities and to the brain (peripheral vascular disease).

Familial dysbetalipoproteinemia, which is inherited as an autosomal dominant defect, is caused by a genetic defect that causes accumulations of remnants of very low-density lipoprotein (VLDL) and chylomicrons with triglyceride and cholesterol concentrations greater than the 90th percentile. Patients have two apo E2 lipoprotein genes that are present. They have lipoproteins that are not appropriately removed from the circulation, as they are abnormal.

Signs and Symptoms

Patients with familial dysbetalipoproteinemia may have fatty skin deposits called XANTHOMAS. Specifically, they may have a tuberoeruptive xanthomata and palmar xanthoma known as xanthomata palmare striatum, which are fatty deposits in the creases of the palms.

Diagnosis and Treatment

A physical examination will reveal the presence of xanthomas. Laboratory tests will show elevated levels of serum total cholesterol and low-density lipoproteins (LDLs) as well as triglycerides. Angiograms will show atherosclerosis.

Patients with concomitant DIABETES MELLITUS and/or hypothyroidism should be aggressively treated to achieve levels as close to normal as possible. Patients are directed to change their diet and reduce the amount of ingested saturated fats and cholesterol. If dietary changes do not cause cholesterol and triglyceride blood levels to drop, physicians may prescribe cholesterol-lowering medications such as HMG CoA reductase inhibitors (statins), nicotinic acid, fibrates, ezetimibe, or some combination of several drugs.

familial hypercholesterolemia (FH) An inherited predisposition to high levels of blood cholesterol, first described by C. Muller in 1939. The heterozygous form of familial hypercholesterolemia is common, and it affects an estimated one in 500 individuals. According to an article on cardiovascular disease in a 2003 issue of the *New England Journal of Medicine*, over 600 mutations in the low-density lipoprotein (LDL) receptor gene have been linked to this disorder. In contrast, the severe homozygous form of familial hypercholesterolemia affects only one per 1 million individuals. Most of these individuals die in childhood from a heart attack (myocardial infarction).

Individuals with heterozygous FH have an increased risk for heart attacks at an early age (by age 20) because of their severe ATHEROSCLEROSIS (clogged arteries). Men with this condition are more likely to have early heart attacks than women with familial hypercholesterolemia. According to Dr. Evan Stein and his colleagues in an article on hypercholesterolemia in a 1999 issue of the *Journal of the American Medical Association*, among males with untreated FH, 5 percent have clinically overt coronary artery disease by age 30. The risk increases to 20 percent by age 40 and more than doubles to 50 percent by age 50.

In most cases, changing the diet has only a minimal effect on people with FH. These individuals must also take cholesterol-lowering medications to control the condition.

Men and women are both at risk for FH. Children and adolescents can also present with this medical problem. Stein and his colleagues studied adolescent boys ages 10–17 years with FH at 14 pediatric outpatient clinics in the United States and Finland. In one group, there were 63 intervention subjects (patients who took lovastatin to lower their cholesterol levels) and 59 who took the placebo. In another group, there were 61 intervention subjects and 49 who took the placebo drug. The researchers found that lovastatin was effective at lowering cholesterol and did not impair growth and development among the boys who took the medication.

The researchers also looked at the family history of their study subjects. They found that the mother passed on the FH in 56 percent of the cases and the father in 44 percent. They also found that, among the parents, the average age of onset of coronary artery disease was 37. Eight of the subjects had fathers who had died of CAD, and their average age of death was 39 years.

Signs and Symptoms

The presence of XANTHOMAS (lipoprotein deposits under the skin) is one sign of hypercholesterolemia, as are cholesterol deposits that are found in the eyelid area (xanthelasmas). However, many patients with xanthelasmas also have normal cholesterol levels.

Diagnosis and Treatment

Diagnosis is made by taking a careful medical history, including any early-age heart attacks in close family members, such as among parents or siblings. Laboratory testing will show that patients with familial hypercholesterolemia have elevated levels of total cholesterol that are greater than 300 mg/dl in adults and greater than 250 mg/dl in children. They also have elevated levels of low-density lipoproteins (LDLs), typically greater than 200 mg/dl. In addition, the patients have normal or mildly increased triglyceride levels. In addition, protein electrophoresis may be abnormal, as may the results of heart function studies, such as stress tests.

Although changing the diet alone will probably not resolve FH, it can help improve the situation. As a result, patients with FH are urged to decrease their consumption of fat to less than 30 percent (less than 10 percent as saturated fat) of all the calories consumed. Patients are also encouraged to exercise, which will help them lose weight and by doing so, lower their cholesterol levels.

Diet and exercise will not bring the hypercholesterolemia under control, and these patients will require several medications. Typically, patients are treated with high doses of statin medications as well as with bile acid sequestrants or cholesterol absorption inhibitors.

See also CHOLESTEROL; FAMILIAL COMBINED HYPERLIPIDEMIA; FAMILIAL DYSBETALIPOPROTEINEMIA; FAMILIAL HYPERTRIGLYCERIDEMIA.

Nabel, Elizabeth G., M.D. "Cardiovascular Disease." *New England Journal of Medicine* 349, no. 1 (July 3, 2003): 60–72.

Ronzio, Robert A. *The Encyclopedia of Nutrition and Good Health.* New York: Facts On File, Inc., 1997.

Stein, Evan A., M.D. "Efficacy and Safety of Lovastatin in Adolescent Males with Heterozygous Familial Hypercholesterolemia: A Randomized Controlled Trial." *Journal of the American Medical Association* 281, no. 2 (January 13, 1999): 137–144.

familial hypertriglyceridemia   An inherited autosomal dominant disorder that causes moderately high levels of very low-density lipoprotein (VLDL) in the blood and occurs in an estimated one in 300 individuals in the United States. Familial hypertriglyceridemia is also known as type IV hyperlipoproteinemia in the Frederickson classification.

This elevation of VLDLs causes an increased risk for patients to develop PANCREATITIS, heart disease, and OBESITY. It is also associated with hypertension, hyperuricemia, HYPERGLYCEMIA, and INSULIN RESISTANCE. The condition may be worsened by HYPOTHYROIDISM, DIABETES MELLITUS, and the use of estrogen therapy in an affected postmenopausal female.

Familial hypertriglyceridemia does not usually become apparent until after puberty or young adulthood. Patients are at risk for this dyslipidemic syndrome if either parent was diagnosed with hypertriglyceridemia or if there is a history of premature heart disease (clinical heart disease occurring before age 50). The condition is caused by a mutation in the lipoprotein lipase enzyme.

Diagnosis and Treatment

Hypertriglyceridemia is easily diagnosed by obtaining a fasting lipid profile from the patient. This should include total cholesterol, high-density lipoprotein, and triglycerides levels.

Patients typically have elevated triglyceride levels in the 200–500 mg/dl range with lower-than-normal high-density lipoproteins (a condition called hypoalphalipoproteinemia). They also have normal or modestly elevated total cholesterol or LDL cholesterol. Typically, LDL levels cannot be measured accurately as is done with most standard lipid profiles but, instead, must be measured directly with radioimmunoassay.

The first therapy is good medical nutrition therapy, with attention to lowering the carbohydrate content in meals. Alcohol is removed from the diet. Exercise will help tremendously as well. The intent of the nutrition and exercise is to have patients get their weight as close to ideal as possible. However, often diet and exercise are inadequate and pharmacological therapy is employed as well.

The first-line medication therapy is usually a fibric acid derivative, such as gemfibrozil (Lopid) or fenofibrate (Tricor) or a form of nicotinic acid, such as an intermediate-release product like Niaspan. If the patient's triglyceride level is in the lower range of 200–350, then HMG CoA reductase inhibitors are often employed, such as simvastatin (Zocor), pravastatin (Pravachol), atorvastatin (Lipitor), lovastatin (Mesvacor), or fluvastatin (Lescol-XL). Bile acid sequestrants are to be avoided in these patients, because they may actually increase the triglyceride levels.

In postmenopausal women, estrogen therapy may need to be discontinued. Younger woman taking ORAL CONTRACEPTIVES may need to discontinue them.

The aim of the doctor is for the patient to have the condition corrected as much as possible. Patients with diabetes need to attain a normal hemoglobin A1c, and patients with hypothyroidism need to achieve normal thyroid-stimulating hormone (TSH) levels.

familial hypocalciuric hypercalcemia (FHH) A hereditary (autosomal dominant) form of hypercalcemia in which the individual has high blood levels of calcium, while at the same time, he or she has low urinary calcium levels and normal levels of parathyroid hormone in the blood. Parathyroid hormone is produced by the parathyroid glands and it regulates calcium levels in the bloodstream.

The basic cause of familial hypocalciuric hypercalcemia is an inactivating mutation in the calcium-sensing receptor gene, which typically causes fewer calcium receptors that are expressed on parathyroid tissue and in the kidney. Thus, in the parathyroid glands, which are the glands located behind the thyroid, this defect causes the gland to be exposed to higher-than-normal levels of calcium to the appropriately suppressed parathyroid hormone secretion. At the same time, in the kidney, excessive calcium is absorbed.

Most people with familial hypocalciuric hypercalcemia have no signs or symptoms at all and do not require any treatment. Doctors must carefully differentiate these patients from those with true primary hyperparathyroidism, as patients with familial hypocalciuric hypercalcemia do not require surgery. If the physician does not measure the urinary calcium levels, he or she could misdiagnose patients with FHH, as patients may have high-normal or even slightly elevated intact parathyroid hormone levels.

See also HYPERCALCEMIA; HYPERPARATHYROIDISM; PARATHYROID CANCER.

feedback loops A complex process, key to the functioning of endocrine glands, in which sensors recognize changes to the individual or to the environment and, as a result, cause higher or lower levels of hormones to be secreted.

Feedback loops are analogous to a thermostat or other device that seeks to maintain a certain homeostatic level. For example, say a thermostat in a house is set at 70 degrees. When the inside temperature falls below that temperature, the change causes a sensor to order the heat to turn on. If a home has both heat and air-conditioning, the thermostat was set at 70 degrees, and the temperature rose to 71 degrees, the air-conditioning would come on.

Similarly, if the blood levels of hormones rise to a given level, feedback loops will send a message to the body to cut back on their production. If they fall below a certain level, feedback loops enable an increase in their production. For instance, cells within the pancreas measure or sense the ambient glucose concentration in the blood. Then the beta cells of the pancreas secrete an appropriate amount of insulin while the alpha cells secrete an appropriate amount of glucagons to maintain the glucose level at the appropriate level for that person. With damage to the beta cells, resulting in diabetes mellitus, this loop is disrupted and the blood glucose level rises.

Feedback loops control the increase and decrease of such HORMONES as T4 and T3 (thyroid hormones), cortisol, estradiol, and others. The usual hierarchy is as follows. If the cortisol levels dip to a less-than-adequate level, the hypothalamus perceives this drop. The production of corticotropin releasing hormone (CRH) is then increased, which in turn increases the synthesis of adrenocorticotropic hormone (ACTH) from the pituitary gland. This action stimulates the adrenal gland to produce and release more cortisol. The reverse process also occurs. If the cortisol levels rise too high, this feedback travels back to the hypothalamus, which decreases the production of CRH and so on.

When patients have hypothyroidism, there are inadequate levels of T3 and T4 in the bloodstream. These low levels of thyroid hormones are perceived by the hypothalamus, which decreases the levels of thyrotropin-releasing hormone (TRH). This, in turn, causes a decrease in the level of thyroid-stimulating hormone (TSH) that the pituitary gland produces. Thus, damage to the hypothalamus or the pituitary gland can dramatically upset these normal feedback loops and lead to endocrine diseases. This is also why physicians usually order the laboratory levels of several hormones to be tested at the same time. In a healthy person, hormonal levels all exist in balance with each other.

female reproduction   The process of creating a pregnancy and, about nine months later, bearing a live child. Reproduction can be impaired by a wide variety of conditions affecting the endocrine glands as well as other organs in the body. For example, the ovaries must produce an egg for a pregnancy to occur, and some woman do not ovulate regularly or at all (ANOVULATION). Some women do not have a uterus that can carry a child. Sometimes, even when the woman's and the man's reproductive systems appear healthy to their respective physicians, no pregnancy occurs.

Couples seeking to attain pregnancy report that unexplained infertility is an extremely upsetting situation. However, amazing progress has been made in reproductive technologies, allowing many women to achieve pregnancies once thought to be impossible. Women may be advised to take medications to stimulate ovulation or other drugs needed to achieve pregnancy, or they may become pregnant by way of in vitro fertilization.

Endocrine diseases can impede the course of a normal pregnancy. For example, some women develop GESTATIONAL DIABETES, which is diabetes that occurs only during pregnancy. Such women must be carefully followed by their physicians during their pregnancies to help ensure a normal pregnancy and the delivery of a healthy child. Some endocrine diseases, such as untreated HYPOTHYROIDISM, can cause an otherwise healthy woman to have great difficulty achieving a pregnancy. Once her thyroid levels are normalized, the woman may be able to become pregnant.

See also AMENORRHEA; BREAST-FEEDING; FERTILITY; INFERTILITY; MALE REPRODUCTION; PREGNANCY; REPRODUCTIVE ENDOCRINOLOGY.

fertility   The ability to create a pregnancy that results in the delivery of a live child. If they have normal fertility, an estimated 93 percent of couples should be able to achieve a pregnancy after 12 months of unprotected intercourse. The inability to achieve a pregnancy is the definition of INFERTILITY.

For most women, fertility declines markedly after age 35–40 years. They may require assisted reproductive techniques from specialized clinics, such as in vitro fertilization or donated embryos, to achieve a pregnancy and a birth. Unfortunately, these techniques do not always succeed. Fertility also declines in men as they age, although many men can continue to father children well beyond the age of 40. Sometimes infertile couples or single individuals who desire to parent a child but cannot create a pregnancy will hire a surrogate mother. Others will adopt a child from their own country or another country.

Sexually transmitted diseases, heavy drug or alcohol use, and other factors may impair fertility for both men and women. Endocrine diseases such as HYPOTHYROIDISM, CUSHING'S DISEASE, HYPOGONADISM, and POLYCYSTIC OVARY SYNDROME can also impair fertility.

See also FEMALE REPRODUCTION; MALE REPRODUCTION; PREGNANCY; REPRODUCTIVE ENDOCRINOLOGY.

follicle-stimulating hormone (FSH) A hormone released by the anterior pituitary gland as directed by the HYPOTHALAMUS GLAND. In women, this hormone stimulates ovulation to occur and also causes the release of ESTRADIOL. In men, FSH stimulates the production of sperm. Estradiol in women and testosterone in men are the hormones that feed back to the pituitary and hypothalamus and help to maintain an appropriate balance.

Like other pituitary hormones, FSH is secreted in a pulsatile fashion. Levels of FSH need to be assessed by physicians who have knowledge of the clinical situation of the patient as well as the concurrent estradiol or testosterone levels or semen analysis.

When adult women present with menstrual difficulties, such as the failure to menstruate (AMENORRHEA) or with infrequent menstruation (oligomenorrhea), physicians will measure levels of FSH, LUTEINIZING HORMONE (LH), and possibly other hormone levels. The normal FSH blood levels of a premenopausal woman, according to the NATIONAL INSTITUTES OF HEALTH, is five to 30 international units per liter (IU/l), although the midcycle peak may range from 10–60 IU/l.

Physicians may also decide to test the FSH levels if a woman has (or is suspected of having) OVARIAN CYSTS or MULTIPLE ENDOCRINE NEOPLASIA, type 1 (MEN 1). With primary ovarian or testicular failure, the FSH level will be increased and the estradiol or testosterone levels will be elevated. When a hypothalamic or a pituitary problem is present, the FSH level will be inappropriately low.

Some endocrine disorders associated with abnormal FSH blood test results include the following: HASHIMOTO'S THYROIDITIS, HYPOPITUITARISM, POLYCYSTIC OVARY SYNDROME, POSTPARTUM PITUITARY NECROSIS (pituitary failure after childbirth), and TURNER SYNDROME.

fractures Breaks in the bones. People who have OSTEOPOROSIS have a low bone density and also experience a greater risk of developing fractures than do others. In addition, individuals with OSTEOMALACIA, another low-density BONE DISEASE, also have an increased risk for suffering from bone fractures.

Endocrinologists differentiate between fragility fractures and other fractures. Fragility fractures are those that occur with minimal or no trauma and are clearly a sign of decreased bone strength. This decreased bone strength is typically due to decreased bone density usually associated with microarchitectural abnormalities of the bone. Radiographic fractures are those seen on X-rays but that are not clinically significant to the patient. In contrast, a broken arm or leg that occurs in an accident is usually severely painful to the patient, who actively seeks treatment for the problem.

Some endocrine diseases are linked to a greater risk for fractures. For example, a large study, the Study of Osteoporotic Fractures, demonstrated that elderly women with HYPERTHYROIDISM have a three times greater risk of having fractures than women of the same age with normal thyroid-stimulating hormone (TSH) levels. A past history of having hyperthyroidism, among women who currently had normal thyroid levels, was associated with twice the risk of developing fractures.

Research has shown that women taking 3-hydroxy-3-methylglutaryl coenzyme A (HMG CoA) reductase inhibitor medications, also known as statins, for hyperlipidemia have a lower risk of suffering from hip and nonspine fractures. Statins apparently stimulate bone formation and enhance bone strength.

See also ELDERLY; OSTEOPENIA.

Bauer, Douglas C., M.D., et al. "Risk for Fracture in Women with Low Serum Levels of Thyroid-Stimulating Hormone." *Annals of Internal Medicine* 134, no. 7 (2001): 561–568.

Bauer, Douglas, M.D., et al. "Use of Statins and Fracture: Results of 4 Prospective Studies and Cumulative Meta-Analysis of Observational Studies and Controlled Trials." *Archives of Internal Medicine* 164, no. 2 (January 2004): 146–152.

galactorrhea   Breast milk production in nonnursing women. Hyperprolactinemia, the excess production of prolactin from the lactotrophs in the anterior pituitary gland, is the most common cause of galactorrhea.

PROLACTINOMA is a benign cause of hyperprolactinemia that can lead to galactorrhea. Other causes of excess prolactin can also lead to breast milk production, for example, HYPOTHYROIDISM, the chronic excessive stimulation of the breast or nipple, or drugs that reduce the production of dopamine in the brain, such as certain antipsychotic drugs (haloperidol and risperidone) and the antiemetic drug metoclopramide. The galactorrhea usually resolves with successful treatment of the underlying illness.

See also PROLACTIN.

gastric surgery for weight loss   An elective surgery and the most effective form of weight reduction surgery (also known as bariatric surgery). It is performed on some morbidly obese patients who have failed to lose weight with diet and exercise regimens and whose health is seriously compromised. Many patients who have gastric bypass surgery also have TYPE 2 DIABETES and hypertension prior to the procedure. They are also at risk for developing heart disease and stroke. The surgery usually improves these conditions, in many cases bringing glucose and blood pressure levels to normal.

In a study reported in a 2003 issue of the *Annals of Surgery*, the researchers evaluated 191 patients with Type 2 diabetes and who underwent laparoscopic Roux-en-Y gastric bypass surgery. Most patients lost about 100 pounds. A dramatic percentage (83 percent) experienced a normalization of their blood glucose levels and thus a reversal of

their diabetes after the weight loss caused by the surgery. The remaining 17 percent showed marked improvements of their glucose levels.

Most patients who choose gastric bypass surgery are females. Many physicians who perform gastric bypass surgery require prospective patients to undergo psychological evaluations. This is done to ensure that patients are emotionally stable and that they understand that the procedure is not reversible, should they be unhappy with their new inability to eat large quantities of food. In addition, these patients require a comprehensive evaluation, including, but not limited to, cardiac stress testing, pulmonary function testing, sleep studies, and complete laboratory evaluations.

In general, physicians restrict weight reduction surgery to adult patients with a BODY MASS INDEX (BMI) of 40 or greater. However, in some cases, the procedure will be performed in patients whose BMI is 35 or greater when they have other significant health problems (such as diabetes) that would be improved with extensive weight loss.

Gastric bypass surgery allows digestion to occur. However, patients can eat only small quantities because of the shrunken size of the stomach. If they revert to past habits of consuming large amounts of food, they become severely nauseated and experience stomach upset and vomiting.

Benefits of Surgery

In addition to the general benefits of a considerable weight loss in obese individuals, these patients usually show an improvement in their menstrual regularity, FERTILITY, and overall hormonal balance. Women can become pregnant after having gastric bypass surgery, although physicians recommend that women wait at least a year after surgery before they seek to conceive a child.

Of interest is that some patients who have had gastric surgery experienced a change in their GHRE-LIN levels. Ghrelin is a hormone released by the stomach that affects hunger and a feeling of fullness after eating (satiety). In a study reported in a 2002 issue of the *New England Journal of Medicine,* researchers compared the ghrelin levels of individuals who lose weight through dieting after six months on a low-calorie, low-fat diet, with patients who lost weight from gastric surgery. They found that the gastric surgery patients had significantly lower levels of ghrelin. In a seemingly self-defeating manner, the dieters' ghrelin levels actually went up when they dieted.

Said the researchers, "In summary, 24-hour plasma ghrelin levels increase in response to diet-induced weight loss, suggesting that ghrelin may play a part in the adaptive response that limits the amount of weight that may be lost by dieting. We also found that ghrelin levels are abnormally low after gastric bypass, raising the possibility that this operation reduces weight in part by suppressing ghrelin production."

Disadvantages to Gastric Bypass Surgery

Gastric bypass surgery comes with disadvantages. For example, patients may develop serious vitamin and mineral deficiencies, particularly of vitamin B12, as well as of iron, folate, and calcium. Some patients develop gallstones after surgery as well as other digestive ailments.

The surgery is a serious one, and some fatalities have occurred. However, with proper preoperative selection and evaluation of patients, operative and perioperative mortality should be less than 1 percent. This percentage needs to be contrasted with the nearly 33 percent death rate over 10 years in those obese patients who do not have the surgery.

Adolescents and Gastric Bypass Surgery

Some adolescents are severely obese, and they may seek gastric bypass surgery. However, this procedure is controversial in adolescents, and most health insurance companies will refuse to pay for it. According to an article in a 2003 issue of the *Wall Street Journal,* an estimated 150 adolescents in the United States have had gastric bypass surgery,

compared with an estimated 100,000 adults who have weight reduction surgery in a year.

Physicians who perform gastric bypass surgery generally require adolescents to be more obese than their adult counterparts in order to be considered for this surgery or to have a BMI of greater than 40 accompanied by a serious medical problem, such as diabetes mellitus or hypertension.

See also OBESITY.

For further information on gastric bypass surgery, contact the following organizations:

American Society for Bariatric Surgery
7328 West University Avenue
Suite G
Gainesville, FL 32607
(352) 331-4900
http://www.asbs.org

American Society of Bariatric Physicians
5453 East Evans Place
Denver, CO 80222
(303) 770-2526
http://www.asbp.org

Cummings, David E., M.D., et al. "Plasma Ghrelin Levels After Diet-Induced Weight Loss or Gastric Bypass Surgery." *New England Journal of Medicine* 346, no. 21 (May 23, 2002): 1,623–1,630.

Minocha, Anil, M.D., and Christine Adamec. *The Encyclopedia of Digestive Diseases and Disorders.* New York: Facts On File, Inc., 2004.

Schauer, P. R., et al. "Effect of Laparoscopic Roux-en Y Gastric Bypass on Type 2 Diabetes Mellitus." *Annals of Surgery* 238, no. 4 (2003): 467–485.

Winslow, Ron, and Rhonda L. Rundle. "For Obese Teens, A Radical Solution: Stomach Surgery." *Wall Street Journal* CCXLII, no. 69 (October 7, 2003): A1, A15.

gastrinomas   Tumors that typically occur in the pancreas or duodenum and that secrete excess gastrin, a hormone necessary for the production of acid in the stomach. The excessive gastrin triggers an overproduction of digestive acids. Gastrinomas are a characteristic feature of Zollinger-Ellison syndrome, a condition first discovered by Drs. Zollinger and Ellison in 1955. One or multiple tumors may be present.

Patients with gastrinomas usually present with excessive peptic ulcer disease (in about 90 percent of cases). However, very few patients with peptic ulcers have gastrinomas. Patients also present with malabsorption plus weight loss and dumping syndrome, a condition that occurs when food enters the small intestine too rapidly. Common symptoms are abdominal pain and diarrhea as well as large amounts of fat in the stool.

Gastrinomas also sometimes contain and secrete other hormones, including adrenocorticotropic hormone (ACTH), INSULIN, GLUCAGON, vasoactive intestinal peptide (VIP), 5-hydroxyindole-acetic acid (HIAA), and melanocyte-stimulating hormone (MSH). About 40–50 percent of gastrinomas are malignant (cancerous), and about 25 percent are associated with MULTIPLE ENDOCRINE NEOPLASIA (MEN) syndrome. Many gastrinomas are multifocal. Of those that are malignant, greater than 50 percent have already metastasized (spread) by the time the condition is diagnosed.

Gastrinomas are most common in individuals 35–65 years of age. They occur slightly more commonly in males than in females.

When gastrinomas are suspected, serum levels of gastrin and gastric acid output are both measured. The patient's medical history is extremely important as other conditions (such as kidney failure, antral G cell hyperplasia, retained antrum syndrome, and some medications) can also lead to elevated gastrin levels.

Once the biochemical diagnosis is performed, attempts are made to localize the tumor. Often nuclear medicine studies with octreotide are used. An endoscopic ultrasound may be useful in locating tumors. Computerized tomography (CT) scans and magnetic resonance imaging (MRI) scans can be used to look for metastases, but they are not usually sensitive enough to locate the small, primary tumors.

Patients with gastrinomas can be treated with a combination of medications (histamine-2 blockers and proton pump inhibitors) and octreotide. The indications for surgery have become more controversial. Surgery is used for early and easily localized disease, when medical therapy has failed, or in metastatic disease for palliative (pain relief) purposes. Chemotherapy may also be employed if the cancer has spread.

genetic risks The probability of inheriting a disease because it is present in other family members such as parents and/or siblings. If a disease is particularly linked to a genetic risk, it will often have the word "familial" as part of the name of the medical problem, such as with FAMILIAL HYPERCHOLESTEROLEMIA or FAMILIAL COMBINED HYPERLIPIDEMIA. The likelihood of becoming ill with many diseases and disorders, such as DIABETES MELLITUS, hypertension, and thyroid disease, includes genetic components. However, in most cases, people who have genetic risks for a disease can mitigate the chances of developing the disease. For example, people at risk for developing hypertension can exercise, maintain a healthy weight, and eat a nutritious diet.

People at risk for TYPE 2 DIABETES can maintain a normal weight and eat a balanced diet, which will often stave off diabetes permanently or until the individual is elderly.

genetic short stature The attainment of below-normal height but with proportional features, such as arms and legs that are proportional to the person's height. Genetic short stature occurs because the individual was born to individuals who were of short stature themselves or who carry a gene for short stature. Thus the person has inherited a genetic predisposition to a small size. Genetic short stature is not the same as dwarfism, which brings other characteristic facial features, such as a large head and high forehead.

Sometimes physicians will administer GROWTH HORMONE to individuals who would not otherwise reach the norm for height among their peers. However, this is considered controversial therapy by many physicians.

See also DWARFISM.

gestational diabetes (GDM) Diabetes that is diagnosed during pregnancy, typically in the second or third trimester.

The cause of gestational diabetes is unknown, although experts speculate that the many hormonal changes that are experienced during pregnancy are a factor. Women who develop GDM may also have a genetic predisposition to the development of diabetes mellitus and the stress of the pregnancy may be allowing the problem to manifest itself. Another argument in favor of a genetic component to GDM is that women who were born to mothers who had GDM will present with GDM more frequently than women born to mothers not afflicted with the condition.

Women with gestational diabetes have a dramatically higher risk of developing Type 2 diabetes 15–20 years after the onset of GDM. This risk is the highest among Hispanic, Native-American, and African-American women who have had gestational diabetes.

Other risk factors for developing GDM are age (women over age 30 have a greater risk than younger woman) and the number of children that a woman has borne (the risk increases with each subsequent pregnancy).

Other risk factors for experiencing GDM include:

- A family history of diabetes
- Gestational diabetes with previous pregnancies
- Previous births of very large infants (heavier than 9 pounds)
- Prior problem pregnancies (either stillbirths or miscarriages)

Screening Pregnant Women for GDM

All pregnant women should be screened for risk factors for GDM in their first prenatal visit, according to the AMERICAN DIABETES ASSOCIATION. Physicians should consider if risk factors such as obesity, a previous history of GDM, or a family history of the disease are present. If a woman is believed to be at high risk, she should be screened prior to any planned pregnancy or very early in the pregnancy as well as at intervals throughout the pregnancy, at the discretion of the obstetrician. Typically, this screening is performed by measuring the woman's blood glucose levels or with a glucose tolerance test.

All women should be rescreened for GDM between the 24th and 28th weeks of pregnancy, unless they lack all risk factors for GDM.

Diagnosis and Treatment

The diagnosis is made either by an in-office glucose test if the glucose levels are very high or by a formal glucose tolerance test performed by a laboratory. The screening test done at 24–28 weeks of pregnancy is followed by a formal glucose tolerance test to make the diagnosis of gestational diabetes.

If testing confirms GDM, women should be referred to a diabetes care team within 48 hours of the initial diagnosis so they can receive complete information and recommendations on their particular cases. This team should include, at a minimum, the obstetrician, an endocrinologist, and a registered dietitian. Most women with GDM should also learn how to test their own blood and use the information from blood glucose testing to make appropriate meal-planning and health decisions. In very mild cases of GDM, changes in caloric and carbohydrate intake can control the diabetes. In other cases, INSULIN is required. Most experts believe that women with GDM who require insulin should test their blood at least two to four times per day.

In other cases (about 30–60 percent) insulin is required. As the pregnancy progresses, women may need higher doses of insulin. Several studies have shown the efficacy of oral hypoglycemia medications in the treatment of GDM. However, as of this writing, none of the oral medications have been approved by the Food and Drug Administration (FDA) for use in pregnancy; thus, the only approved therapy other than nutrition and exercise is injected insulin.

Lifestyle changes will also be recommended to women with GDM. Nearly all women with GDM need to eat three meals and three snacks per day at regular intervals, with a small breakfast to avoid developing a midmorning HYPERGLYCEMIA. The physician may also prescribe an exercise plan that includes non-weight-bearing types of exercises, such as walking or bicycling.

After Delivery

In most cases, women with GDM are no longer diabetic after the delivery of their babies. Only about 10–15 percent of women with GDM have persistent diabetes immediately after delivery. Despite this, women who have had GDM must continue to monitor their blood glucose levels for at least several weeks after being discharged from the hospital. All women with GDM should have a follow-up glucose tolerance test six to eight weeks postpartum to ensure that they no longer have diabetes and to gauge their current and future risk of the development of diabetes.

Women with GDM are also usually encouraged to breast-feed their babies. In addition to the many known benefits of BREAST-FEEDING accruing to both the mother and the infant, breast-feeding may also help to improve the mother's own insulin status. In addition, it may also help her to lose weight, which should further decrease her future susceptibility to developing Type 2 diabetes.

See also DIABETES MELLITUS; PREGNANCY; TYPE 2 DIABETES.

Kjos, Siri L., and Tomas A. Buchanan, M.D. "Gestational Diabetes Mellitus." *New England Journal of Medicine* 341, no. 23 (December 2, 1999): 1,749–1,756.

Langer, Oded, M.D., et al. "A Comparison of Glyburide and Insulin in Women with Gestational Diabetes Mellitus." *New England Journal of Medicine* 343, no. 16 (October 19, 2000): 1,134–1,138.

Petit, William A. Jr., and Christine Adamec. *The Encyclopedia of Diabetes.* New York: Facts On File, Inc., 2002.

ghrelin A protein hormone discovered in 1999 in Japan. It is synthesized in the stomach and duodenum and consists of 28 amino acids. Ghrelin is the first hormone that clearly links the gastrointestinal tract, the pituitary gland, and the hypothalamus.

Ghrelin, which increases food intake in rats and humans, is the first hormone that has been found to stimulate appetite and appears to be involved with the regulation of appetite and weight. Ghrelin levels can be measured in the bloodstream. In addition, ghrelin seems to bind to the growth hormone-releasing receptor and to have a role in the secretion of growth hormone.

After standard dieting, ghrelin levels increase and again decline with refeeding. In patients who have undergone GASTRIC BYPASS SURGERY, ghrelin levels are decreased. This may be part of the reason why this procedure has the best track record in terms of patients maintaining their weight loss over years. Some studies indicate that people with PRADER-WILLI SYNDROME have abnormally high levels of ghrelin, which may account for their ravenous and uncontrollable appetites.

Experts and clinical researchers are studying the impact of ghrelin and hope to develop an antighrelin type of medication that will help combat the epidemic of OBESITY currently seen in the United States, Canada, and other developed countries.

See also GROWTH HORMONE.

Ariyasu, Hiroyuki, et al. "Stomach Is a Major Source of Circulating Ghrelin, and Feeding State Determines Plasma Ghrelin-Like Immunoreactivity Levels in Humans." *Journal of Clinical Endocrinology & Metabolism* 86, no. 10 (2001): 4,753–4,758.

Cummings, D. E., et al. "Plasma Ghrelin Levels after Diet-Induced Weight Loss or Gastric Bypass Surgery." *New England Journal of Medicine* 346, no. 21 (2002): 1,623–1,630.

Wren, A. M., et al. "Ghrelin Enhances Appetite and Increases Food Intake in Humans." *Journal of Clinical Endocrinology & Metabolism* 86, no. 12 (2001): 5,992–5,995.

gigantism A condition caused by excessive secretion of growth hormone, usually due to a tumor of the pituitary gland. The tallest man ever recorded was the late Robert Wadlow, at 8 feet, 11 inches in height. The tallest woman (who is still alive, as of this writing) is 7 feet, 5.5 inches. A photograph of the tallest living woman is provided in a 1999 issue of the *Journal of Clinical Endocrinology & Metabolism.*

For gigantism to occur, the excess growth hormone must be secreted prior to the closing of the growth plates (epiphyses) in the bones. The excess growth hormone can result from a pituitary tumor, hypersecretion of growth hormone-releasing hormone (GHRH) from the hypothalamus, or a deficiency of SOMATOSTATIN in the neural pathways in the hypothalamus leading to the pituitary gland. Gigantism can accompany the following endocrine disorders: McCUNE-ALBRIGHT SYNDROME, CARNEY

COMPLEX, NEUROFIBROMATOSIS, and MULTIPLE ENDOCRINE NEOPLASIA (MEN) syndrome type 1. It can also occur with optic nerve tumors.

The symptoms of gigantism are similar to those seen with acromegaly, in which the excess growth hormone is secreted after the growth plates in the bones have closed, causing patients to have enlarged hands and feet, excess sweating (hyperhydrosis), coarse facial features, and prognathism (jaw protrusion). Most children with increased growth do not have gigantism and are more likely to have genetic tall stature, HYPERTHYROIDISM, or genetic abnormalities such as Soto, Weaver, Marshall-Smith, and XYY syndromes.

To diagnose gigantism, initially insulin-like growth factor 1 (IGF-1) is measured as well as IGF binding protein 3. The gold standard is the glucose suppression test. In this test, the patient is given oral glucose, and then serial growth hormone levels are measured. In patients with normal growth hormone physiology, the growth hormone will decrease to a level of less than 2 ng/dl. If ectopic GHRH secretion is suspected, this can be measured in the blood. As with all endocrine disorders, once there is biochemical evidence of a disorder, imaging of the pituitary and hypothalamus with MAGNETIC RESONANCE IMAGING (MRI) or COMPUTERIZED TOMOGRAPHY (CT) is indicated. If imaging reveals the presence of a pituitary or hypothalamic tumor or structural lesion, surgical intervention is the best approach. This can be followed by medication and radiotherapy.

BROMOCRIPTINE (Parlodel), octreotide (Sandostatin and Sandostatin LAR), lanreotide, and pegvisomant may be utilized to treat patients with gigantism, and combinations of medications are often used. Radiotherapy in children often leads to pituitary failure and the need for multiple hormone replacement therapies.

See also ACROMEGALY; PITUITARY GLAND.

Eugster, Erica A., and Ora H. Pescovitz. "Gigantism." *Journal of Clinical Endocrinology & Metabolism* 84, no. 12 (1999): 4,379–4,383.

glucagon A hormone secreted by the alpha cells of the pancreas. Glucagon acts in the liver to increase the glucose level in the blood by stimulating stored glycogen to break down as well as by stimulating the synthesis of new glucose from other precursors. However, some individuals, such as those who are severely alcoholic and/or malnourished, do not have stored glycogen readily available to them, and thus the glucagon cannot act properly in their cases.

Patients who have had Type 1 diabetes for five or more years will still have glucagon in their pancreas. However, they will lose the ability to secrete glucagon when they become hypoglycemic, thus rendering them more likely to develop hypoglycemia again.

In an emergency, glucagon may be administered by intramuscular injection to patients with diabetes and severe hypoglycemia who cannot eat or drink. The injected glucagon will work within 15–20 minutes to increase the blood glucose level. Thus, the glucagon injection is a critical tool for use at home, in the field, and even in the hospital if an intravenous line cannot be placed to give glucose. The one side effect of a glucagon injection is mild-to-moderate nausea.

On very rare occasions, the pancreas can produce tumors—glucagonomas—that secrete excessive glucagon that can cause HYPERGLYCEMIA, nausea, and rash. Cancerous tumors can also, rarely, produce glucagons. An antidiabetic medication, pramlintide (Symlin) exerts part of its effect by suppressing the surge in endogenous glucagon that occurs after meals in patients with diabetes.

See also DIABETES MELLITUS; HORMONES.

glucagonoma An extremely rare, slow-growing neuroendocrine tumor, usually malignant (in 80 percent of the cases), of the alpha 2 islet cells of the pancreas, the organ that secrets both INSULIN and GLUCAGON. It is most likely to occur after the age of 55. Since Dr. S. W. Becker's first description of a glucagonoma in 1942, fewer than 300 glucagonomas have been described worldwide.

Individuals with MULTIPLE ENDOCRINE NEOPLASIA, type 1 have an increased risk for developing glucagonomas, although they are rare in these individuals as well. This type of tumor may also spread to the liver. The tumor may also cause impaired glucose tolerance or overt HYPERGLYCEMIA. It also causes a special type of skin lesion called a necrolytic migratory erythema, in which the skin is hypersensitive to pressure and friction.

Symptoms of a glucagonoma include the following:

- A skin rash present on the face, abdomen, buttocks, or legs, which may be scaly and crusty
- Inflammation of the tongue and mouth
- Unexplained weight loss
- Frequent urination (polyuria)
- Extreme thirst
- Nighttime urination (nocturia)
- Increased appetite
- Thromboembolic disorders (blood clots, pulmonary embolism)

Doctors who suspect that a patient may have a glucagonoma will measure blood levels of glucagon with a concurrent glucose level. The patient will also have an abnormal result on the glucose tolerance test and will have an elevated fasting glucose level. Once the biochemical diagnosis of a glucogonoma is made, imaging studies may be done to try and localize the tumor for the surgeon. Computerized tomography (CT) will often show the presence of the tumor within the pancreas.

The only treatment as of this writing is surgery because glucagonomas do not respond to chemotherapy or radiation treatment. Octreotide (Sandostatin) may be used to decrease symptoms.

glucocorticoids The name given to the steroids that help to maintain blood glucose levels. It is often used interchangeably with the term *steroid*. Glucocorticoid medications such as prednisone (Deltasone, Metiorten, Sterapred, Pediapred), dexamethasone (Decadron), and cortisone acetate (Cortef) are used to treat many inflammatory conditions such as asthma, ulcerative colitis, and rheumatoid arthritis. They are also used to treat ADDISON'S DISEASE.

When glucocorticoids are given in excess quantity for any reason, it can lead to CUSHING'S SYN-DROME, with increased blood pressure and glucose, centripetal redistribution of body fat (especially around the abdominal area), and a "moon face."

The term glucocorticoid was devised when these compounds were first being analyzed and segregated by their abilities to maintain blood glucose levels (glucocorticoids) or to maintain blood pressure and salt and water balance (mineralocorticoids). Most of these compounds have both glucocorticoid and mineralocorticoid capabilities, with the exception of dexamethasone, which has no mineralocorticoid effect.

Other examples of oral glucocorticoid medications include:

- Betamethasone (Celestone)
- Methylprednisone (Meprol)
- Triamcinolone (Aristocort)

glucose intolerance Refers to a condition in which glucose levels are higher than normal but lower than the level used to determine DIABETES MELLITUS. Glucose intolerance is determined by the two-hour ORAL GLUCOSE TOLERANCE TEST. In this test, the patient's blood is assessed after one hour and then again an hour later. Glucose intolerance is defined as a glucose level greater than 140 mg/dl but less than 199 mg/dl.

Often patients with glucose intolerance have HYPERLIPIDEMIA or OBESITY. Women with this condition may also have POLYCYSTIC OVARY SYNDROME.

Patients may progress to diabetes. They also have an increased risk for cardiovascular disease such as heart attack and stroke.

goiter A general term that implies an enlargement of the thyroid gland without any determination as to the cause for the enlargement or whether the thyroid function is low, normal, or high. Goiters may be seen in patients with HYPOTHYROIDISM (below-normal levels of thyroid hormone), HYPERTHYROIDISM (excessively high levels of thyroid hormone), and even sometimes among patients who have a completely normal thyroid function.

A symmetrical goiter (an enlargement on both sides of the neck) is common among patients with hypothyroidism, THYROIDITIS, or GRAVES' DISEASE. An asymmetrical goiter is typically due to multiple nodules and/or thyroiditis. Elderly patients with thyroid disease are less likely to have goiters than younger patients with thyroid problems.

Before the twentieth century, goiters were often caused by a severe deficiency in iodine, which then led to hypothyroidism. Today, iodine deficiency is very rarely a cause of thyroid disease in the United States, Canada, and other developed countries. However, iodine deficiency continues to cause goiters and thyroid disease in developing countries around the globe.

Signs and Symptoms

Often there are no symptoms of goiter other than an enlarged neck, a sign that is often overlooked by patients and even by some medical doctors if the enlargement is not prominent. Other symptoms that may occur are dysphagia (difficulty swallowing) and a change in the patient's voice, which becomes weaker and more hoarse. Some patients may also have difficulty breathing because of the size of the goiter.

Diagnosis and Treatment

Goiters are evaluated for two reasons. The first is structural. If a dominant nodule is present within a goiter, the next best step is a fine-needle aspiration to check for malignancy. If a patient has a diffuse goiter causing structural symptoms, such as problems with swallowing (dysphagia) or pain, often surgery is the best option, unless an underlying cause can be treated. The second reason for evaluating a goiter is functional. If a gland is enlarged due to primary hypothyroidism, with decreased thyroid hormone and increased thyroid-stimulating hormone (TSH) levels, it is best treated with thyroid hormone replacement therapy. This therapy will normalize the TSH levels and lead to shrinkage of the goiter. Thus, a variety of tests are used in this diagnostic process, including blood tests for thyroid hormone levels, ultrasound, and radionuclide scan. All tests do not have to be performed in all patients.

Each patient's evaluation should take place after a medical history is taken and a physical examination is performed. This way the appropriate tests may be done in the appropriate order to avoid wasting the patient's time and money and to lead to an expedient diagnosis.

See also HASHIMOTO'S THYROIDITIS.

gonadal disorders   See HYPOGONADISM.

gonadotropin deficiency   See HYPOGONADOTROPISM.

Graves' disease   The most common cause of HYPERTHYROIDISM, an excessive level of thyroid hormone circulating in the body. This thyroid disease was named after Irish physician Robert Graves in 1835. Graves' disease is an autoimmune disease, which means that the immune system mistakenly attacks the body rather than foreign invaders such as bacteria or viruses. In addition to hyperthyroidism/THYROTOXICOSIS, Graves' disease may cause exopthalamos (severely bulging eyes) or other eye findings. Rarely, it may cause a rash.

Researchers have demonstrated that the cause of Graves' disease is the stimulation of the thyroid gland by a thyroid-stimulating immunoglobulin. Some researchers have also noted that extremely stressful events (such as a death in the family, losing a job, or another extreme stressor) may sometimes precede the development of Graves' disease. This has led experts to speculate that stress may trigger the disease to develop among susceptible individuals. However, most studies that have carefully looked at this issue have failed to show a convincing link between stress and the subsequent development of Graves' disease.

Graves' disease also has a strong genetic component. The illness may be discovered because of the characteristic GOITER (thyroid enlargement), which causes the patient's neck to become noticeably swollen and disproportionate to the head and the rest of the body. In addition, the patient's wide-open staring gaze and bulging eyes are other common indications of the disease.

Risk Factors

Graves' disease is much more common in females; women have about five times the risk of developing the disease as do men. Children and adolescents can also develop Graves' disease, although it is more frequently seen among adults. Often coexisting diseases and medical conditions are also seen in patients who have Graves' disease, including TYPE 1 DIABETES, ADDISON'S DISEASE, and pernicious anemia.

Signs and Symptoms of Graves' Disease

The following signs and symptoms are usually seen in patients with Graves' disease (some of these are also seen in patients with hyperthyroidism but who do not have Graves' disease):

- A goiter that is visible and palpable (can be felt by a physician)
- Eye problems (feeling of grittiness or irritation in the eye or other eye symptoms)
- Bulging, eye-popping appearance
- Heat intolerance
- Weight loss (when the patient is not seeking to lose weight); however, about 10 percent of patients gain weight
- Itching skin
- Excessive thirst
- Rapid heartbeat
- AMENORRHEA (no menstrual periods) in women
- Loss of sex drive

Diagnosis and Treatment

If the physician suspects that Graves' disease is present, based on the patient's appearance and the presence of hyperactive symptoms (such as an elevated blood pressure and pulse and overall extreme nervousness), the doctor will almost invariably order a thyroid-stimulating hormone (TSH) test to check for the levels of thyroid in the patient's bloodstream. Unusually low levels of TSH are indicative of hyperthyroid disease.

Unless the patient is pregnant, doctors will also usually order thyroid radionuclide studies to determine whether Graves' disease or THYROIDITIS may be causing the patient's hyperthyroidism.

Treatment is often first given in the form of antithyroid medications, such as propylthiouracil or Tapazole (methimazole). If these drugs fail to bring the patient's thyroid levels down to within normal levels, radioactive treatments may be given to the patient. Surgery, which usually involves a nearly total removal of the thyroid gland, may become necessary, although surgery is not generally used as a common treatment for Graves' disease in the United States.

Ophthalmologists treat the eye complications that are caused by Graves' disease, often with glucocorticoid medications or with external X-ray therapy. Barbara Bush, former first lady, suffered from eye complications caused by Graves' disease and she was treated with orbital radiation therapy and glucocorticoid medications. The late actor Marty Feldman, also noted for his extremely bulging eyes, suffered from Graves' ophthalmopathy.

Patients with severe eye problems caused by Graves' disease may need surgery. Fortunately, severe eye disease is rare. Older men have a higher risk than other patients for developing serious eye complications of the disease, and Caucasians have a higher risk of developing eye complications than individuals of other races. In addition, patients with Graves' disease who smoke have a greater risk for developing eye complications of the disease.

Pregnancy and Graves' Disease

Graves' disease is the most common form of hyperthyroidism identified during pregnancy, representing about 85 percent of all cases found during that period. When present, the signs and symptoms of Graves' disease usually appear in the first trimester or after the delivery of the baby. Graves' disease must be treated in the pregnant woman because she is at risk for excessive weight loss and for the development of congestive heart disease. The fetus is also at risk, for premature birth, fetal tachycardia, and severely slowed growth.

Treatment of Graves' disease during pregnancy is generally in the form of beta-blocker drugs rather than radioiodine, which can be dangerous to the developing fetus. Doctors may also treat the pregnant woman or new mother with propylthiouricil (PTU). It is less likely to cross into the placenta than other drugs, and it is also less likely to appear in breast milk than are other antithyroid medications.

See also HASHIMOTO'S THYROIDITIS; THYROID BLOOD TESTS; THYROID-STIMULATING HORMONE; THYROID STORM.

For further information on Graves' disease, contact the following organization:

National Graves' Disease Foundation
P.O. Box 1969
Brevard, NC 28712
(828) 877-5251
http://www.ngdf.org

Imrie, Helen, et al. "Evidence for a Graves' Disease Susceptibility Locus at Chromosome Xp11 in a United Kingdom Population." *Journal of Clinical Endocrinology & Metabolism* 86, no. 2 (2001): 626–630.

Rivkees, Scott A., Charles Sklar, and Michael Freemark. "The Management of Graves' Disease in Children, With Special Emphasis on Radioiodine Treatment." *Journal of Clinical Endocrinology and Metabolism* 83, no. 11 (1998): 3,767–3,777.

Weetman, Anthony P., M.D. "Graves' Disease." *New England Journal of Medicine* 343, no. 17 (October 26, 2000): 1,236–1,248.

growth disorders   Medical problems that are often caused by either inadequate or excessive levels of growth hormone. The underlying cause is often a problem with the pituitary gland.

Growth hormone deficiency refers to lower-than-normal levels of circulating growth hormone and results in short stature, such as DWARFISM. When ACROMEGALY occurs before puberty, it leads to excessive growth and GIGANTISM.

See also GENETIC SHORT STATURE; GROWTH HORMONE.

growth hormone (GH)   A protein hormone synthesized by the PITUITARY GLAND that enables individuals to grow to an adult height. Of the seven anterior pituitary hormones, GH is produced in the greatest amounts. Growth hormone is secreted throughout life, although the amount that is secreted decreases as individuals age. Most of the effects of GH are mediated by insulin-like growth factor 1.

In addition to leading to the linear growth of a child, growth hormone also helps with the breakdown of fat (lipolysis), stimulates protein synthesis, and helps the body to retain needed sodium and water. Growth hormone is produced by individuals at all ages because it is also needed for the body to repair microscopic tissue damage properly. Peak levels of growth hormone production usually occur in the evening, when individuals are asleep.

A tumor of the pituitary gland may cause an excessive production of growth hormone, resulting in GIGANTISM if it occurs before puberty and is not treated and ACROMEGALY if it occurs after puberty. An insufficiency of growth hormone, on the other hand, may cause short stature or may cause some rare cases of DWARFISM. (Dwarfism is usually caused by a genetic mutation rather than by a lack of growth hormone.)

It is controversial, but some children—especially males—who are below normal in height have been treated with growth hormone. Although growth hormone does not make them become tall, it generally allows them to achieve a greater height than they otherwise would have attained. If administered, growth hormone must be given to children prior to the onset of puberty and before the endplates in their bones (the epiphyses) close for the best effect.

Some examples of growth hormones that are used include:

- Genotropen
- Norditropen
- Humatrope
- Serostim

Growth hormone is also sometimes used in adults who have growth hormone deficiency. It will help to increase their strength and muscle mass, decrease their percentage of body fat, increase their bone density, and in general, increase their overall sense of well-being.

See also AIDS; DELAYED PUBERTY; EARLY PUBERTY; GROWTH DISORDERS; GROWTH HORMONE DEFICIENCY.

For further information, contact the following organization:

Human Growth Foundation
997 Glen Cove Avenue
Suite 5
Glen Head, NY 11545
(800) 451-6434 (toll-free)
http://www.hgfound.org

Cohen, Pinchas, et al. "Effects of Dose and Gender on the Growth and Growth Factor Response to GH in GH-Deficient Children: Implications for Efficacy and Safety." *Journal of Clinical Endocrinology & Metabolism* 87, no. 1 (2002): 90–98.

Drake, W. M., S. J. Howell, and S. M. Shalet. "Optimizing GH Therapy in Adults and Children." *Endocrine Reviews* 22, no. 4 (2001): 425–450.

growth hormone deficiency (GHD)   A condition that exists when the pituitary gland fails to produce sufficient growth hormone, either due to a primary pituitary lesion or a problem with the hypothalamus. When GHD occurs in children, growth failure and short stature occur.

All humans, including even elderly adults, require some level of growth hormone to function at optimal levels. Growth hormone (GH) helps to maintain normal protein synthesis and thus helps maintain normal muscle and bone mass. Adults with GHD have decreased muscle mass and increased fat mass. They have poor lipid profiles, low high-density lipoprotein (HDL) levels, and high low-density lipoprotein (LDL) levels. These persons also appear to have increased mortality from cardiovascular causes.

Measurements of heart function are improved with GH replacement therapy. In addition, markers of endothelial inflammation, such as C-reactive protein, are higher in patients with GHD than in controls. Adults with GHD have more psychological distress and depression that seems to decrease when their GH is replaced. Thus, even in adults, GHD can be treated with recombinant subcutaneous growth hormone.

The cells that make GH in the anterior pituitary, the somatotrophs, are perhaps the most sensitive to damage. The causes of deficiencies in all of the other pituitary hormones can also cause growth hormone deficiency. However, isolated GH deficiency can also occur. Thus, in adults, the causes of GHD include trauma, vascular accidents, surgery (for trauma, pituitary tumors, or other tumors), and radiation therapy.

Diagnosis
Growth hormone deficiency should be suspected in all patients with pituitary failure or pituitary tumor. The usual screening test is a measurement of fasting levels of insulin-like growth factor 1 (IGF-1). If this level is abnormally low, further testing can be performed to attempt to stimulate the anterior pituitary gland to produce GH. Typically, drugs such as clonidine, L-dopa, growth hormone-releasing factor (GHRH or GHRF), and the amino acid L-arginine can be used.

The gold standard test for growth hormone deficiency is the insulin tolerance test. In this test, a graded amount of intravenous insulin is given to induce hypoglycemia purposely. Growth hormone is one of the counterregulatory hormones, and the anterior pituitary should produce increased levels of growth hormone in response to the induced hypoglycemia. A lack of this response would indicate GHD. This test is typically done in an outpatient area of the hospital or may be done in an endocrinologist's office. It must be performed with caution, however, especially among patients who may be at risk for heart problems. Hypoglycemia could provoke angina or even a heart attack in a person with pituitary insufficiency or even an isolated growth hormone deficiency.

Treatment
Growth hormone deficiency in adults can be treated with the use of daily recombinant growth hormone via subcutaneous injection. The doses used are often less than those used to treat children with growth hormone deficiency and short stature. Progress is monitored by evaluating the patient's sense of well-being, muscle and fat mass, IGF-1 levels, bone density, and other parameters.

GHD treatment among adults is controversial. As of this writing, experts feel that not all adults with GHD should be treated. However, treatment is certainly a consideration in patients with GH deficiency.

Each case should be evaluated by the patient's primary care physician, in conjunction with an endocrinologist, to determine what is best for the individual.

Overtreatment with growth hormone can lead to signs and symptoms of acromegaly and a worsening of diabetes. In patients with previous malignancies, the use of growth hormone is controversial and typically is not used.

See also DELAYED PUBERTY; DWARFISM; GROWTH HORMONE.

Cook, David M., M.D. "Shouldn't Adults with Growth Hormone Deficiency Be Offered Growth Hormone Replacement Therapy?" *Annals of Internal Medicine* 137, no. 3 (2002): 197–201.

DeBoer, H., et al. "Clinical Aspects of Growth Hormone Deficiency in Adults." *Endocrine Review* 16, no. 1 (February 1995): 63–86.

Frohman, L. A. "Controversy About Treatment of Growth Hormone-Deficient Adults: A Commentary." *Annals of Internal Medicine* 137, no. 3 (2002): 202–204.

Isley, William L., M.D. "Growth Hormone Therapy for Adults: Not Ready for Prime Time." *Annals of Internal Medicine* 137, no. 3 (2002): 190–196.

gynecomastia The benign enlargement of the male breasts, which may be painful, and may be caused by a hormonal imbalance or by hormone therapy, such as that taken to combat advanced prostate cancer. Gynecomastia is the development of true breast tissue that extends out from the nipple. It must often be differentiated from pseudogynecomastia, which is often secondary to obesity, and is a condition of increased fatty deposits in and around the nipple area, suggesting the appearance of gynecomastia.

If gynecomastia is suspected, the physician must first be sure that it is not male breast cancer, which does occur. If the tissue is hard and nonmovable, the patient generally needs a mammogram and a surgical consultation for a biopsy and/or excision.

Gynecomastia is sometimes seen in newborns for two to four weeks, as they have been exposed to high levels of circulating estrogens from the mother. It can also be seen in pubertal teenage boys and is transient.

As a true pathological condition, gynecomastia is most common in men ages 50 and older. It can affect one or both breasts. The hormonal causes typically involve a disruption of normal hormone balance. There are generally below-normal levels of male hormone (androgen) production or increased female hormones (estrogen). These hormones are synthesized in both the male testes and the adrenal glands. Thus, in men, primary or secondary gonadal (testicular) failure, hyperthyroidism, and hormonal enzyme abnormalities (increased aromatase activity) may each lead to the development of gynecomastia.

Tumors of the testes (germ cell/Leydig's cell/Sertoli's cell tumors), adrenal tumors (benign adenomas and carcinomas), and tumors elsewhere can also cause gynecomastia. Severe liver disease, kidney failure, and starvation can lead to gynecomastia. Multiple drugs can also cause gynecomastia, including but not limited to estrogens, antiandrogens (used to treat cancers), antiulcer drugs (cimetidine, ranitidine, and omeprazole), alcohol, narcotics, marijuana, digtoxin, some angiotensin-converting enzyme (ACE) drugs, and spironolactone. Some syndromes, such as Kallmann's syndrome, as well as rare tumors and enzyme deficiency disorders can also lead to gynecomastia. Gynecomastia is very common among males with KLINEFELTER SYNDROME.

Treatment is aimed at removing the stimulus that led to the breast development. Treatment of the underlying cause will often resolve the gynecomastia. For example, when males with Klinefelter syndrome are treated with testosterone replacement therapy, the gynecomastia often abates. If treatment is impossible and the breast tissue is uncomfortable or cosmetically disturbing, mastectomy surgery may be performed.

See also HORMONES; HYPOGONADISM.

Braunstein, G. D. "Diagnosis and Treatment of Gynecomastia." *Hospital Practice (Office Edition)* 28, no. 10A (1993): 37–46.

Hashimoto's thyroiditis   An autoimmune form of hypothyroidism in which the immune system attacks the thyroid gland. This disorder is also known as chronic thyroiditis, chronic lymphocytic thyroiditis, struma lymphomatosa, lymphadenoid goiter, and autoimmune thyroiditis.

Hashimoto's thyroiditis is the most common cause of below-normal thyroid levels in areas of the world with adequate iodine in the diet. In countries where there is inadequate iodine in the diet, it is the iodine deficiency that causes the hypothyroidism (without iodine, thyroid hormone cannot be produced naturally). Hashimoto's thyroiditis is a slowly progressive form of thyroid failure that may or may not be associated with a GOITER. Other variants of Hashimoto's thyroiditis are painless lymphocytic thyroiditis or postpartum thyroiditis, both of which can progress to HYPOTHYROIDISM that is indistinguishable from Hashimoto's thyroiditis.

Japanese physician H. Hashimoto first described Hashimoto's thyroiditis in 1912. Other researchers subsequently identified the specific autoimmune antibodies causing the condition in 1956.

Risk Factors

There is a genetic predisposition to Hashimoto's thyroiditis. In addition, individuals with other autoimmune conditions, such as GRAVES' DISEASE and TYPE 1 DIABETES, have an increased risk for developing Hashimoto's thyroiditis, as do individuals with TURNER SYNDROME and Down syndrome.

Women have a five to 10 times greater risk than men of developing the disease, and women between the ages of 50 and 60 years are the most at risk. Hashimoto's thyroiditis occurs in up to 5 percent of adults in the United States and other developed countries. Sometimes the disease is linked to a familial predisposition. An estimated 50 percent of first-degree relatives (parents and siblings) of individuals with Hashimoto's thyroiditis also have thyroid autoantibodies and may develop the disease.

Often the patient is not diagnosed for years after the onset of Hashimoto's thyroiditis. This occurs because the initial symptoms are subtle and can be easily confused with those of many other conditions.

Graves' disease is another autoimmune thyroid disease, but it causes HYPERTHYROIDISM (excessive levels of thyroid) rather than hypothyroidism. Individuals who have Hashimoto's thyroiditis usually have the symptoms and signs of hypothyroidism, although some individuals have no symptoms until the disease is more advanced. When symptoms are present, they may include some or all of the following:

- Cold intolerance
- Slowed movements
- Lethargy/fatigue
- Unexplained weight gain
- Constipation
- Presence of a goiter
- Dry skin
- Heavy menstrual periods or irregular periods
- Greater difficulty with thinking
- Joint stiffness/muscle aches and cramps
- Brittle nails and dry, coarse hair

In almost all cases of Hashimoto's thyroiditis, with or without the presence of a goiter, the changes in the thyroid are painless. If pain occurs, the physician must consider other diagnoses, such as subacute thyroiditis or de Quervain's thyroiditis.

Diagnosis and Treatment

Physicians who suspect the presence of Hashimoto's thyroiditis will order laboratory tests of thyroid functioning, including a free T4 test and a serum thyroid-stimulating hormone (TSH) test. These tests will reveal if the patient is hypothyroid. Generally, an elevated TSH serum level and a low-normal or below-normal free T4 level indicate hypothyroidism.

If early enough in the course of the disease, a blood test can measure the levels of antibodies to peroxidase, antiperoxidase, or anti-thyroid peroxidase (TPO) antibodies. Peroxidase is an important enzyme in the thyroid gland. It is the protein to which the immune system reacts in some cases. Thus, the anti-TPO antibodies damage the thyroid by attacking the enzyme and causing hypothyroidism. Why the enzyme is attacked is unknown. This is a much more specific test than previously used to measure antimicrosomal antibodies and antithyroglobulin antibodies. If the process has gone on for a long time, the level of these antibodies may be quite low.

The anti-TPO antibody test is not 100 percent specific for Hashimoto's thyroiditis, as these antibodies can also be detected in other forms of thyroiditis as well as Graves' disease. However, if the cause of the hypothyroidism is not primary (due to destruction of the thyroid gland) but is secondary or tertiary, as in PITUITARY FAILURE or hypothalamic dysfunction, patients will have low levels of free T4 and inappropriately normal or low levels of TSH.

Patients with the presence of anti-TPO antibodies will progress to overt Hashimoto's thyroiditis at the rate of about 5 percent per year. If a technetium thyroid scan is done, patchy or heterogeneous uptake is typically seen. Usually iodine uptake studies are not ordered, however, as the blood tests are usually sufficient to confirm the diagnosis.

Because the thyroiditis or inflammation in the thyroid gland occurs at different rates in different areas, the gland may feel as if there are nodules present. On ultrasound examination, nodules may be seen. Hashimoto's thyroiditis can coexist with many other forms of thyroid dysfunction. A significant number of patients who first develop Graves' disease can go on to develop Hashimoto's thyroiditis later. This can also happen in the reverse sequence (Graves' disease first, then Hashimoto's thyroiditis later) but is much more rare.

Patients with Hashimoto's thyroiditis are usually treated with levothyroxine in a dose that is sufficient to maintain normal functioning. However, if there is no indication of hypothyroidism (in a patient who has antiperoxidase antibodies and normal thyroid function tests), doctors may instead follow the patient on a regular basis. Ultimately, the patient will need to take levothyroxine as the disease progresses further.

Endocrinologists will usually treat all of the following patients: those who have an abnormal TSH level, those with a borderline TSH level and no symptoms, those with an enlarged thyroid with the presence of antibodies, and also sometimes those patients with coexisting nodules even with normal thyroid function.

In rare cases, patients will need surgery because of the compression of the trachea caused by a goiter.

See also THRYOID BLOOD TESTS; THYROIDITIS.

Dayan, Colin M., M.D., and Gilbert H. Daniels, M.D. "Chronic Autoimmune Thyroiditis." *New England Journal of Medicine* 35, no. 2 (July 11, 1996): 99–107.

Rose, Noel R., M.D., and Patrizio Caturegli, M.D. "Chronic Lymphocytic Thyroiditis," in *NORD Guide to Rare Disorders: The National Organization for Rare Disorders.* Philadelphia, Pa.: Lippincott Williams & Wilkins, 2003, 329.

hermaphroditism   Very unusual condition in which both male and female sex organs are present at birth. In one example of such a condition, Dr. Eric M. Pachter and his colleagues described a "true hermaphrodite" in a 1998 issue of *Urology.* The newborn child had an XX karyotype (normal males have both an X and a Y chromosome). The child had a vagina, partial uterus, and tissue that resembled an ovary as well as such male body parts as a vas deferens, spermatic cord, and an intrascrotal testicle. Because of the XX karyotype, the female gender was assigned to the child, and the doctors performed a right orchiectomy (removal of the testicle). Feminizing genital surgery was planned for the future. The doctors also noted that patients such as this child have potential for future fertility.

In past years, parents were advised to raise the child with hermaphroditism as a female. Some children who were raised as females but never told about their hermaphroditism eventually chose to assert their masculine identities. The malleability of male/female identity may have more to do with DNA than with environmental influences, even when the child has inherited both sexual characteristics.

Currently, some experts suggest delaying the gender choice in children with hermaphroditism until the child is at least two years old, while others believe the decision should be delayed until the child is old enough to participate in the decision. (It is difficult to understand how the gender choice could be delayed much beyond early childhood since gender identities are important, even to small children.)

According to Steven E. Lerman and his colleagues in an article on ambiguous genitalia in children, "Sexual identity is thought to be largely a conditioning process that is firmly established by 2 years, 6 months of age. For this reason, any attempt to change the sex of rearing beyond this age should be undertaken only when the initial sex assignment has clearly been wrong, and psychiatric assessment unequivocally indicates that sex reassignment is in the best interest of the child; ongoing psychiatric support may be necessary." The doctors also noted that when gender reassignment occurs at an age older than two-and-a-half years, there is a greater risk of maladjustment.

See also HYPOGONADISM; KLINEFELTER SYNDROME.

Lerman, Steven E., Irene M. McAleer, and George W. Kaplan. "Sex Assignment in Cases of Ambiguous Genitalia and Its Outcome." *Urology* 55, no. 1 (2000): 8–12.

Pachter, Eric M., Mark Horowitz, and Kenneth I. Glassberg. "True Hermaphrodite." *Urology* 52, no. 2 (1998): 318–319.

hirsutism in women   The excess growth in women of the stiff, pigmented hairs that are normally found in males in areas that are androgen dependent, such as on their face, chest, and on the abdomen. These hairs are known as terminal hairs.

Some experts estimate that as many as 10 percent of all women in the United States have experienced hirsutism at some point in their lives.

Hirsutism in women is usually caused by an endocrine disorder. Women normally have some male hormones, and hirsutism is caused by excessive amounts or overactivity of male hormones (androgens). This overproduction may stem from the ovaries or the adrenal glands. Rarely, it may be caused by tumors of these glands. Hirsutism is commonly seen in patients with polycystic ovary syndrome (PCOS). It is also sometimes seen in patients with congenital adrenal hyperplasia.

Hirsutism can also be caused by an excessive intake of exogenous androgens, as is sometimes seen among female bodybuilders.

The excessive activity of the 5-alpha reductase enzyme at the hair follicle, which causes the conversion of testosterone to dihydrotestosterone, may be responsible for the hirsutism.

Women who are Asian or Native American rarely develop hirsutism, while women whose families stem from the southern Mediterranean are more likely to develop the problem. Patients with hirsutism may be treated with medications, such as ORAL CONTRACEPTIVES, that decrease the level of androgens. The symptoms may also be treated with electrolysis hair removal as well as with cosmetic creams.

See also ACROMEGALY; ANDROGEN EXCESS; CONGENITAL ADRENAL HYPERPLASIA; INFERTILITY; POLYCYSTIC OVARY SYNDROME.

homocysteine   An intermediary amino acid formed when methionine is converted to cysteine. HOMOCYSTINURIA or severe hyperhomocystinuria is a rare autosomal recessive organic aciduria (acid in the urine) that is typically diagnosed in infancy, causing failure to thrive and developmental delays, premature severe ATHEROSCLEROSIS, eye problems, and OSTEOPOROSIS. Homocysteine has direct effects that accelerate atherosclerosis and clotting. Depending upon the population that is tested, the range of homocysteine can vary from about 5–15 micromoles per liter.

Mild-to-moderate elevations of homocysteine occur in about 6 percent of the population in the

United States and are an independent risk factor for atherosclerosis and venous thromboembolic phenomenon. Deficiencies of folic acid, vitamin B12, or vitamin B6 can lead to increased levels of homocysteine. Homocysteine levels will decrease in most patients as oral folate intake is increased to the level of 400 mcg per day.

In one trial, 158 healthy siblings of 167 patients with premature atherosclerosis were given 5 mg of folic acid and 250 mg of vitamin B6 daily. In these patients, the homocysteine levels decreased from 14.7 to 7.4 micromoles per liter.

A number of retrospective studies have shown that the patients with the highest homocysteine levels had the greatest risk of developing ischemic heart disease and stroke. In addition, in other retrospective studies, increased levels of homocysteine appear to be related to an increased risk of venous blood clots and pulmonary embolism. In women, increased levels are associated with preeclampsia, fetal growth problems, stillbirths, and delivery complications.

As of this writing, a large number of prospective studies are being conducted to determine if supplementing the diet with folic acid and vitamins B6 and B12 will decrease homocysteine levels and, more importantly, decrease the risk of atherosclerosis complications.

Many physicians now recommend a minimum supplementation of 400 mcg of folate, 3–10 mg of vitamin B6, and 10–100 cg of vitamin B12 for a general risk reduction.

Homocysteine Studies Collaboration. "Homocysteine and Risk of Ischemic Heart Disease and Stroke: A Meta-Analysis." *Journal of the American Medical Association* 288, no. 16 (2002): 2,015–2,022.

Ray, J. G. "Meta-Analysis of Hyperhomocysteinemia as a Risk Factor for Venous Thromboembolic Disease." *Archives of Internal Medicine* 158, no. 19 (October 26, 1998): 2,101–2,106.

Vermeulen, E. G., C. D. Stehouwer, J. W. Twisk, et al. "Effect of Homocysteine-Lowering Treatment with Folic Acid Plus Vitamin B6 on Progression of Subclinical Atherosclerosis: A Randomized, Placebo-Controlled Trial." *Lancet* 355, no. 9,203 (2000): 517–522.

homocystinuria A hereditary disorder that affects the metabolizing of methionine, an amino acid. Newborns with homocystinuria may appear to have mild developmental delays or FAILURE TO THRIVE. As the condition progresses further, the patient may resemble a person with MARFAN'S SYNDROME because of the characteristic tall and slender build with disproportionately long legs and long, thin fingers.

Homocystinuria can lead to blood clots that are dangerous because they can travel to the brain and cause a stroke. The condition may also lead to poor vision and even to double vision.

Diagnosis and Treatment

If physicians suspect that a patient has Marfan's syndrome, they should also screen for homocystinuria. X-rays will show that the patient with homocystinuria has OSTEOPOROSIS. An examination by an ophthalmologist (eye doctor) will usually show that the patient has both a dislocated lens (typically, the lens is dislocated downward rather than upward, as is seen in Marfan's syndrome) and nearsightedness. Children with homocystinuria may have glaucoma, cataracts, and retinal detachment, all eye diseases that are abnormal among children.

Laboratory tests of the blood and urine will show elevated levels of homocystine and methionine in patients who have homocystinuria. If a liver biopsy and enzyme assay are performed, they will show the lack of cystathionine beta synthase, an enzyme. A biopsy of the skin will show the absence of cystathionine beta synthase and folate-related enzyme levels in fibroblasts among patients with homocystinuria. These enzymes can also be measured in blood cells.

If homocystinuria is diagnosed, there is no cure for this condition. Despite this, many patients respond well to high doses of pyridoxine (vitamin B6). If the patient is an infant or young child, a low methionine diet may help to prevent the child from becoming mentally retarded and from developing other aspects of the disease as it progresses. Some states screen newborn infants for homocystinuria so that they can be treated promptly if the condition is present.

hormone replacement therapy (HRT) Typically refers to the combined use of estrogen and progesterone in women who are estrogen deficient and who still have an intact uterus. In women without a uterus who have had natural or surgical MENOPAUSE, only estrogen is required, and this replacement therapy is referred to as estrogen replacement therapy (ERT). Hormone replacement therapy may also refer to any use of one or more hormones to replace an existing deficiency.

In the late twentieth century, many physicians routinely placed postmenopausal women on either HRT or ERT when they experienced any symptoms of menopause, most notably HOT FLASHES. Sometimes even when women experienced few or no menopausal symptoms, physicians placed women on hormones because it was believed that such treatment would be beneficial to women's health. However, studies released in the early twenty-first century revealed that HRT was riskier than was previously known and that it carried an increased risk for women developing breast cancer, heart disease, and other illnesses. As a result, many physicians began limiting the use of HRT, and many women also voluntarily chose to stop taking the drugs.

One of the key studies that revealed health risks of hormone therapy, the Women's Health Initiative, was ended early in 2002 because of its findings. In this study, researchers followed more than 16,000 women taking estrogen/progestin combination (Prempro) combination therapy for five years. The researchers found that the women taking hormone therapy faced a significantly greater risk of developing breast cancer as well as an increased risk for developing a stroke and heart attack. The women experienced a lower than expected rate of colorectal cancer and fewer fractures, but these apparent protective factors were insufficient to justify the higher risks of developing other diseases.

Some women have continued with HRT because it rids them of distressing menopausal symptoms such as hot flashes, vaginal dryness, and insomnia. An analysis of 21 double-blind, randomized, placebo-controlled clinical studies of 2,511 women showed that hormone replacement therapy decreased hot flashes in women by 77 percent compared with placebo.

In both the Women's Health Initiative and the Heart and Estrogen/Progestin Replacement (HERS) study, hormones were not found to offer either primary or secondary protection against coronary artery disease. Thus, in 2004, most physicians will consider the use of HRT in menopausal women for unremitting vasomotor symptoms only. They will also use the lowest possible dosages for the shortest possible period of time. Both osteoporosis and coronary heart disease can be prevented and treated with multiple other agents with fewer adverse effects than HRT.

Some women have chosen to try "natural" remedies, such as supplements of vitamin E, soy, black cohosh, and other options for their menopausal symptoms. Women should also discuss such supplements and medications with their physicians in advance to ensure they would experience no adverse effects from combining such drugs with other medications that they already take.

See also ESTRADIOL; ESTROGEN; ESTROGEN REPLACEMENT THERAPY; HORMONES.

Grady, D., et al. "Cardiovascular Disease Outcomes During 6.8 Years of Hormone Therapy: Heart and Estrogen/Progestin Replacement Study Follow-up (HERS II)." *Journal of the American Medical Association* 288, no. 1 (2002): 49–57.

Grodstein, Francine, Thomas B. Clarkson, and JoAnn E. Manson, M.D. "Understanding the Divergent Data on Postmenopausal Hormone Therapy." *New England Journal of Medicine* 348, no. 7 (February 13, 2003): 645–650.

McKane, W. Roland, et al. "Mechanism of Renal Calcium Conservation with Estrogen Replacement Therapy in Women in Early Menopause—A Clinical Research Center Study." *Journal of Clinical Endocrinology & Metabolism* 80, no. 12 (1995): 3,458–3,464.

Writing Group for the Women's Health Initiative Investigators. "Risks and Benefits of Estrogen Plus Progestin in Healthy Postmenopausal Women." *Journal of the American Medical Association* 288, no. 3 (July 17, 2002): 321–333.

hormone resistance The inability of the body to use properly some or all of the hormones that are naturally produced by the body. This resistance may be partial or complete. The essential feature of Type 2 diabetes is resistance to the effects of insulin secreted by the pancreas. Patients with Type 2 diabetes have structurally normal insulin receptors and near-normal numbers of receptors, yet these receptors do not function properly.

In some syndromes, patients have abnormal receptors or sometimes make none at all. In FAMILIAL HYPERCHOLESTEROLEMIA, patients lack the receptors to bind and thus to metabolize low-density lipoproteins (LDL).

Most hormonal systems exist in a balance in which the number and activity of receptors can adjust to the amount and activity of the hormone that is available.

See also HORMONES.

hormones   Substances secreted by the endocrine glands that send chemical messages through the bloodstream, usually causing an action. Some examples of hormones are thyroxine (produced by the thyroid gland); adrenaline, aldosterone, and cortisol (produced by the adrenal gland); insulin (produced by the beta cells in the pancreas); testosterone (produced by the testicles); and estrogen (produced by the ovaries).

Typically, these hormones exert their effects at places distant from where they are produced. For example, one endocrine effect is that insulin goes from the pancreas to affect muscles and cells throughout the body. Hormones can also exert paracrine effects. For example, insulin produced in the beta cells of the pancreas also has effects on the adjacent alpha and delta cells. The word *endocrine* implies a secretion into the blood and movement of the secretion to another area. In contrast, *paracrine* refers to secreting directly into the surrounding cells or tissue without going into the systemic circulation—it is a local effect.

When the body produces an inadequate amount or none of the needed hormone, supplements can often be taken. For example, people with Type 1 diabetes are lacking in insulin, and they can take supplemental insulin. Individuals who are hypothyroid can take supplemental thyroid drugs, such as levothyroxine.

Some women who are menopausal take ESTROGEN REPLACEMENT THERAPY (ERT), although the

risks and benefits should be carefully considered beforehand. Men who are low in testosterone may consider testosterone replacement therapy. Individuals who are low in parathyroid hormone usually take both supplemental calcium and CALCITRIOL.

According to the National Center for Health Statistics, the number of hormones prescribed in the United States increased by 25 percent from 1997–2000. This may be due in large part to an aging population that is more likely to need hormones to treat diabetes, hypothyroidism, and declining levels of testosterone or estrogen. However, because of concern over hormone replacement therapy for women, increases of hormone prescriptions may flatten out despite the aging population.

See also ALDOSTERONE; CORTISOL; ESTROGEN; GROWTH HORMONE; INSULIN; LEVOTHYROXINE; TESTOSTERONE.

hot flashes   A generic description of a symptom complex that includes a sudden onset with a sensation of increased body temperature (generalized or focal) at times associated with sweating, facial flushing/blushing, and a generalized sense of discomfort and/or anxiety. Hot flashes may last for seconds and rarely last longer than a few minutes.

The hot flash is also known as a hot flush or as vasomotor instability and may have its onset in the perimenopausal period or in MENOPAUSE. Experts believe that it represents true thermoregulatory dysfunction. The areas of the brain that control heat regulation are actually located in the hypothalamus near an area that contains a large number of nerves containing gonadotropin-releasing hormone (GNRH).

Interestingly, hot flashes are not seen in women with TURNER SYNDROME who have never been treated with estrogens. Some experts hypothesize that the cause of the hot flashes may be decreased central opioid activity.

Women who have undergone the complete surgical removal of their ovaries also experience hot flashes. These hot flashes are often more severe than those among women who are experiencing the hot flashes of menopause. This occurs because natural menopause involves a steady decline in estrogen, while the surgical removal of the ovaries causes a sudden shutdown of estrogen production.

Hot flashes are often experienced in the evening, causing difficulties with sleep, although they may occur at any time. Hot flashes may be minor and tolerable, or they may be extreme, waking women from a deep sleep and finding themselves bathed in sweat and with a rapid heartbeat. Chills sometimes follow hot flashes, and the woman who had thrown off all her bed covers will suddenly need extra blankets. This can be a difficult experience not only for the woman but also for anyone sharing her bed.

Diagnosis and Treatment

Hot flashes are usually diagnosed based on the woman's report of her signs and symptoms. If menopause is suspected, measurement of both her FOLLICLE-STIMULATING HORMONE (FSH) and ESTRADIOL levels may be helpful.

Women seeking medical assistance from their physicians to overcome their hot flashes will usually be informed about hormone replacement therapy (HRT) medications, which are a combination of estrogen and progesterone, and estrogen replacement therapy (ERT), which is the administration of estrogen only. ERT is generally prescribed only for women who have undergone complete hysterectomies (removal of both the uterus and the ovaries), because estrogen may increase the risk for uterine cancer as well as ovarian cancer. Fortunately, very small doses of estrogens will usually treat and/or prevent hot flashes.

If estrogen supplementation alone does not help or the patient is unable to tolerate estrogens, other drugs may provide relief. Clonidine, a drug used mainly to lower blood pressure, can decrease hot flashes by as much as 80 percent. However, clonidine can cause low blood pressure (with dizziness and light-headedness), dry mouth, and sleepiness or sedation.

The antidepressant drugs Effexor and Effexor-XR (venlafaxine), Paxil and Paxil-CR (paroxetine), and Prozac (fluoxetine) have been shown to decrease hot flash activity significantly. Another medication, Neurontin (gabapentin), has been shown to decrease hot flashes by 45 percent in a 12-week trial. The data is much more limited for nonprescription supplements.

Until about 2002, many doctors routinely prescribed both HRT and ERT to menopausal woman. However, major clinical studies have shown that the risks of some diseases, such as breast cancer, myocardial infarction (heart attack), and stroke may be increased in women taking these medications. Some doctors also believe that taking HRT or ERT for a certain period of time, such as several years, is acceptable but that they should not be taken for the rest of a woman's life.

Some women take supplements to deal with their hot flashes, such as vitamin E, black cohosh, soy products, and other remedies whose manufacturers purport that their products can help to manage menopausal symptoms. However, women who are considering taking any supplements should first discuss this issue with their physicians, despite the fact that some of these supplements are not prescription drugs. The reason for this is that some alternative medications may not work well with the other drugs that a woman takes. Consequently, supplements may either weaken the other medications or boost their effect. Either action can be problematic to an individual.

Some women prefer to avoid taking ERT, HRT, or supplements altogether. They may be comforted to know that the hot flashes of menopause generally abate over time as the body adjusts and usually end altogether within about two to five years.

See also ESTROGEN REPLACEMENT THERAPY; HORMONE REPLACEMENT THERAPY.

human growth hormone   See GROWTH HORMONE.

hypercalcemia   Excessively high levels of calcium in the bloodstream. Most experts define hypercalcemia as blood calcium levels that are greater than 10.5 mg/dl (8.5–10.5 mg/dl is the normal range). Blood levels greater than 12.0 mg/dl may represent a medical emergency requiring immediate medical treatment.

Because symptoms are not usually apparent unless hypercalcemia is severe and has also caused prolonged damage, the condition is often not suspected by physicians. Instead, it is often detected serendipitously when a patient has a blood profile drawn for a routine physical examination or for other purposes. This eventuality has become less common, however, as Medicare and many managed care organizations will no longer pay for routine profiles and screening.

Many laboratories now measure blood levels of ionized calcium. This is a far more accurate measurement than the total serum calcium level. Total calcium levels and ionized calcium levels are best measured in the early morning when the patient has fasted, with no food or drink other than water for the prior 10–12 hours.

Laboratory errors commonly occur. This is why, in the case of a person who was not previously diagnosed with hypercalcemia, it is crucial to repeat the test two or even three times and also to confirm an elevated total blood calcium level with an ionized calcium level. Using the ionized calcium level as the gold standard removes the issue of a falsely elevated calcium level due to increased or abnormal binding proteins. When total calcium is assayed, it measures calcium bound to proteins, mainly albumin and globulins. Thus, if the patient has abnormal levels of these proteins, he or she may also appear to have an abnormal calcium level.

A less common form of hypercalcemia is known as FAMILIAL HYPOCALCIURIC HYPERCALCEMIA (FHH). This condition can sometimes be mistaken for primary hyperparathyroidism. In this syndrome, the patient's body does not sense calcium levels properly, which results in higher-than-normal calcium levels in the blood but also in low levels of calcium in the urine. Patients suffer no ill effects and do not require any treatment. As the name implies, familial hypocalciuric hypercalcemia runs in families. Once one person in a family is found with it, others should also be screened to avoid being misdiagnosed with another illness at a later date.

Signs and Symptoms

Most people with hypercalcemia are asymptomatic. Thus, most cases of hypercalcemia are found by chance. If the calcium level rises sufficiently, however, it can cause symptoms such as increased urination during the day (polyuria) or at night (nocturia). Hypercalcemia is also associated with such symptoms as constipation, vague abdominal pain (on rare occasions, due to PANCREATITIS), muscle weakness, lethargy, fatigue, and a variety of other nonspecific symptoms that often lead patients to seek the counsel of their physicians. At its most severe, hypercalcemia may cause cognitive problems and even coma.

When hypercalcemia persists for a long period of time, depending upon its cause, it may lead to the development of kidney stones (known as nephrolithiasis/urolithiasis) and/or to OSTEOPOROSIS. Hypercalcemia due to primary hyperparathyroidism leads to bone loss because the excess parathyroid hormone in the blood stimulates the extraction of calcium from the bone into the bloodstream, which is then lost into the urine because it overwhelms the kidneys' ability to conserve this calcium.

Osteoporosis is an asymptomatic disease of bone loss until there is a bone fracture. With longstanding hypercalcemia caused by primary hyperparathyroidism (excessive levels of parathyroid hormone), a patient may develop multiple vertebral fractures with pain and with kyphosis or dowager's hump. Rarely, a deposit of calcium in the eye (band keratopathy) or tongue fasciculations (tiny involuntary muscle contractions that cause the muscle to quiver) can also be noted in patients with hypercalcemia.

Causes of Hypercalcemia

Primary hyperparathyroidism is the most common medical ailment leading to elevated blood calcium levels. This diagnosis represents the cause of about 70–90 percent of hypercalcemia in outpatients and 20–30 percent among hospitalized patients. Primary hyperparathyroidism has a prevalence of about one in every 2,000–3,000 people.

Medical students are taught the phrase, "stones, moans, bones, and groans" to describe the key elements of hyperparathyroidism. This refers to kidney stones (stones) and the pain that they cause (moans), the osteoporosis (bones), and the potential FRACTURES (groans) that may occur.

The most common type of hyperparathyroidism itself is caused by a single benign growth of one of the parathyroid glands, a parathyroid adenoma. However, the disease can also be caused by hyperplasia (a benign growth of all four of the parathyroid glands) and, rarely, by a parathyroid carcinoma.

Many types of CANCER can cause hypercalcemia, and as many as half of all hospitalized patients with hypercalcemia have cancer. (Hyperparathyroidism and cancer together account for about 90 percent of all causes of hypercalcemia.) When a cancerous tumor is identified as the cause of hypercalcemia, it is classified as either a humoral hypercalcemia of malignancy (HHM) or as a non-HHM case.

Many diseases in which the body forms granulomas can lead to hypercalcemia. A granuloma refers to a specific clustering of white blood cell monocytes that have gone into various body tissues and have become tissue macrophages. This may occur in diseases such as tuberculosis, sarcoidosis, and histoplasmosis.

Other medical problems can sometimes cause hypercalcemia. Hyperthyroidism (overactive thyroid) from any cause can lead to mild hypercalcemia as can simple immobilization (bed rest), although this is typically seen only in young patients (such as an adolescent with paraplegia due to a car crash). Inflammatory diseases may also sometimes cause hypercalcemia. Even silicone implants may sometimes induce the condition.

Rare causes of hypercalcemia include ADDISON'S DISEASE, PHEOCHROMOCYTOMA, PAGET'S DISEASE, sarcoidosis, and rhabdomyolysis.

Sometimes medications that are taken for other medical problems can lead to the development of hypercalcemia. For example, drugs such as thiazide diuretics (hydrochlorothiazide) and lithium may cause mild cases of the condition. Excessive doses of theophylline, taken for asthma, can also lead to hypercalcemia, as can the use of tamoxifen, which is given to women with breast cancer and bone metastases. Retinoic acid given to cancer patients may also lead to the condition.

There are other causes of hypercalcemia. For example, an ingestion of excessive calcium and/or VITAMIN D can also lead to this condition. Years ago, before more potent drugs such as the histamine 2-blockers and proton pump inhibitors were available to patients with heartburn, dyspepsia, and ulcers, these medical problems were often treated with large doses of calcium-containing antacids. Many of these patients subsequently developed what was known as MILK-ALKALI SYNDROME with hypercalcemia. Now this syndrome is not seen frequently, although it can occur among patients who chronically use calcium-containing antacids. (Such patients should consult with a gastroenterologist to find out the underlying cause of their digestive disorder.)

Individuals who take very high levels of other vitamins, such as vitamin A, may also induce hypercalcemia.

Treatment of Hypercalcemia

Typically, the treatment of hypercalcemia is aimed at the underlying cause, once it has been identified. However, if the hypercalcemia is severe and has led to DEHYDRATION and mental status changes in the patient, then hospitalization and immediate treatment is usually needed. Hospitalized patients with hypercalcemia are usually given intravenous fluids in the form of normal saline (0.9 percent sodium chloride solution, which is basically salt water). They are also often given a loop diuretic such as furosemide (Lasix) and an intravenous BISPHOSPHONATE medication, usually pamidronate (Aredia).

Patients with hypercalcemia may also be given steroid medications, such as prednisone. CALCITONIN may also be added to the therapy if the other medications fail or if the patient has pain that is secondary to a fracture. Calcitonin will decrease the patient's blood calcium levels. Often physicians treat patients with a combination of medications.

Once the patient has stabilized from an emergency condition, doctors seek to identify and treat the underlying cause of the hypercalcemia. Surgical removal of a parathyroid adenoma may be necessary as would be treatment of the underlying cancer or medical therapy for causal conditions such as sarcoidosis.

See also CALCIUM ABSORPTION; CALCIUM BALANCE; HYPERPARATHYROIDISM; HYPOCALCEMIA.

Bilezikian, John P. "Management of Hypercalcemia." *Journal of Clinical Endocrinology & Metabolism* 77, no. 6 (1993): 1,445–1,449.

Sanders, Leonard, R., M.D. "Hypercalcemia," in *Endocrine Secrets*, 3d ed. Philadelphia, Pa.: Hanley & Belfus, Inc., 2002, 66–71.

hypercholesterolemia See CHOLESTEROL; FAMILIAL HYPERCHOLESTEROLEMIA.

hyperglycemia   Abnormally high levels of blood sugar (glucose). Hyperglycemia is a hallmark feature of diabetes, although an individual can be temporarily hyperglycemic and yet not have diabetes. It is also possible for a person with diabetes to develop HYPOGLYCEMIA. A normal fasting blood glucose level is defined as less than 100 mg/dl.

The key symptoms of hyperglycemia (and diabetes) are as follows:

• Increased urination
• Increased thirst
• Unexplained weight loss
• Blurred vision

Individuals with one or more of these symptoms should see their physicians for an evaluation.

See also DIABETES MELLITUS; GESTATIONAL DIABETES; TYPE 1 DIABETES; TYPE 2 DIABETES.

hyperlipidemia   Excessive levels of blood fats, particularly low-density lipoprotein (LDL) cholesterol (bad cholesterol) and trigylcerides. This is a dangerous condition that can lead to serious medical consequences, such as a stroke or heart attack. Patients with DIABETES MELLITUS have an increased risk for developing hyperlipidemia. Patients with hyperlipidemia may experience ERECTILE DYSFUNCTION. Some elderly patients with HYPOTHYROIDISM present with hyperlipidemia.

Physicians usually make recommendations for dietary changes to patients with hyperlipidemia. If the patient is obese, weight loss is recommended to improve the condition. The doctor may also prescribe medications to lower CHOLESTEROL levels.

See also APOLIPOPROTEINS; FAMILIAL COMBINED HYPERLIPIDEMIA: FAMILIAL HYPERCHOLESTEROLEMIA: FAMILIAL HYPERTRIGLYCERIDEMIA.

hypernatremia   Excessively high levels of sodium in the blood or above 145 millimoles per liter in an adult. High blood levels of sodium may result from a severe lack of water compared with the sodium in the body, which is the cause of most cases of hypernatremia. Those who face the greatest risk of experiencing hypernatremia are infants, elderly people, and some severely ill hospitalized patients.

Hypernatremia may also be caused by a variety of illnesses, including infections causing diarrhea and vomiting as well as by CUSHING'S SYNDROME, DIABETES INSIPIDUS, HYPERGLYCEMIA, HYPERCALCEMIA, and sometimes the overtreatment of hypokalemia (insufficient potassium). Hypernatremia may also result from the failure of a person to consume sufficient fluids over a given period of time or from an accidental excessive intake of sodium. In addition, some medications can cause hypernatremia, such as lithium, amphotericin B, foscaret, and methoxyflurane.

Signs and Symptoms of Hypernatremia
Babies with hypernatremia usually exhibit some or all of the following indicators:

• Insomnia
• Very high-pitched cry
• Lethargy

Children and adults who are hypernatremic may have muscle weakness and confusion and may lapse into a coma. Elderly individuals may exhibit no apparent signs or symptoms until the hypernatremia becomes severe or is greater than 160 millimoles per liter. Patients may be thirsty; however, thirst is not always present.

Diagnosis and Treatment
Sodium levels in the blood can be measured to determine if the patient is hypernatremic. The treatment depends on the cause. For example, if the hypernatremia stems from a bacterial infection, antibiotics can combat the infection and help to resolve the patient's hypernatremia. Whatever the cause, the hypernatremia itself must also be reversed.

If possible, hypernatremia is reversed orally or with a feeding tube. If that is not possible or feasible, then intravenous fluids are given. The speed of reversal often depends on how quickly the hypernatremia occurred. If it occurred over several hours, it can usually be reversed fairly quickly. In contrast, if the hypernatremia occurred over a longer period or an unknown period, reversal is usually performed more slowly.

One risk that doctors face with a rapid reversal of hypernatremia is cerebral edema, which can risk the life of the patient. Periodic reevaluations of the sodium level in the blood need to be performed as the patient is treated.

Adrogue, Horacio J., M.D., and Nicolaos E. Madias, M.D. "Hypernatremia." *New England Journal of Medicine* 342, no. 20 (May 18, 2000): 1,493–1,499.

hyperoxaluria   The condition in which excessive oxalic acid or oxalate is excreted in the urine. Hyperoxaluria may be caused by a primary genetic defect and overproduction of oxalate or may be an acquired condition, generally due to excessive absorption.

Primary hyperoxaluria is a rare inherited metabolic condition in which enzyme defects lead to severe elevations of oxalate. This form of hyperoxaluria is usually diagnosed in children who are younger than five years old and also have kidney failure. These young children often do not have kidney stones, although older children with the condition will develop kidney stones. Children with primary hyperoxaluria are usually treated by a pediatric endocrinologist.

With primary hyperoxaluria type I, or PHI, the liver generates high levels of oxalic acid that is excreted into the individual's urine. This acid combines with calcium filtered from the bloodstream by the kidneys and subsequently results in the formation of kidney stones. If the disease further progresses to kidney failure, this condition is known as oxalosis. PHI is a hereditary disease that stems from a missing liver enzyme, hepatic enzyme alanine-glyoxylate aminotransferase (AGT), which is a substance that normally rids the urine of excessive levels of oxalate. This defective gene is mapped to chromosome 2q36-37.

There is also a primary hyperoxaluria type II, which is called PHII. This is also a hereditary disease, and it stems from a defective gene in the liver, known as hepatic hydroxypyruvate reductase (HPR). This defective gene is mapped to chromosome 9. PHII is not usually as severe a disease as is

PHI, although some patients with PHII will develop kidney failure.

As the kidney function declines, oxalate can be deposited throughout the body, leading to other complications such as cardiac arrhythmias. If diagnosed early, these children can be treated by forcing fluids, placing them on a low oxalate diet (avoiding chocolate, rhubarb, spinach, and tea), and providing high dosages of vitamin B6 (pyridoxine). Neutral phosphates, magnesium oxides, and potassium citrate can also be used to protect the kidneys. In end-stage cases of kidney failure, kidney and combined kidney-liver transplantations can be undertaken.

A kidney transplant will restore normal kidney function. However, the continued high production of oxalate can act to damage the new kidney. A liver transplant is the only known cure to hyperoxaluria as of this writing.

Patients with hyperoxaluria may also be treated with orthophosphate and pyridoxine therapy. This treatment is especially important in children and adolescents with hyperoxaluria. According to researchers who studied patients with primary hyperoxaluria, who reported on their findings in a 1994 issue of the *New England Journal of Medicine,* "The importance of increasing the doses of orthophosphate during childhood and adolescence was illustrated by the development of new stones or an increase in the size of existing stones during growth spurts in five patients. When the dose was increased, stone formation ceased."

The researchers wrote that early diagnosis and treatment was advantageous to patients. They also said, "Treatment with orthophosphate and pyridoxine before the onset of renal failure reduces calcium oxalate crystallization in the urine and appears to preserve renal function."

Acquired Hyperoxaluria

Some patients have no genetic cause of hyperoxaluria, but the condition occurs due to other causes. For example, it may be caused by a person eating extremely large amounts of substances containing oxalate, such as large quantities of rhubarb, or by ingesting substances that are converted by the body to oxalate, such as massive doses (four grams or more per day) of vitamin C. Acquired hyperoxaluria may also result from a deficiency of thiamine (vitamin B1).

Some patients develop hyperoxaluria as a result of surgery to remove part of their bowel. In addition, patients with chronic digestive diseases (such as Crohn's disease) may also develop hyperoxaluria. In these cases, the condition is known as enteric hyperoxaluria.

Symptoms of Hyperoxaluria

The key symptom of any form of hyperoxaluria is the presence of kidney stones. Kidney stones are extremely painful, and the patient may be initially diagnosed and treated for kidney stones in a hospital emergency room. After a patient is diagnosed with kidney stones, physicians will normally attempt to ascertain the cause of the stones. A 24-hour collection of urine from the patient is obtained, and the amount of excreted oxalate is measured. If the level of urine oxalate is greater than 1.2 millimoles (approximately 100 mg) per 1.73 meters square over 24 hours, then the diagnosis of hyperoxaluria is likely.

Patients with acquired hyperoxaluria are advised to ingest large amounts of fluids, particularly water, and to avoid excessive amounts of the foods that are rich in oxalates. Kidney dialysis is ineffective at ridding the body of the excess levels of oxalate, which is another reason why patients should be treated early on and before kidney function deteriorates.

For further information, contact:

Oxalosis and Hyperoxaluria Foundation
201 East 19th Street
Suite 12E
New York, NY 10003
(800) OHF-8699 (toll-free)
www.ohf.org

Milliner, Dawn S. "The Primary Hyperoxalurias." *NORD Guide to Rare Disorders: The National Organization for Rare Disorders.* Philadelphia, Pa.: Lippincott Williams & Wilkins, 2003.
Milliner, Dawn S., et al. "Results of Long-Term Treatment with Orthophosphate and Pyridoxine in Patients with Primary Hyperoxaluria." *New England Journal of Medicine* 331, no. 23 (December 8, 1994): 1,553–1,558.

hyperparathyroidism   Excessive   levels   of parathyroid hormone, which is produced by the PARATHYROID GLANDS.

Primary hyperparathyroidism refers to the condition in which one or more of the four parathyroid glands located in the neck, near the thyroid gland, produces an excessive amount of parathyroid hormone in an autonomous fashion. This excess parathyroid hormone activity leads to HYPERCALCEMIA.

Secondary hyperparathyroidism is an appropriate physiological response of the parathyroid glands when the body's levels of calcium are low. This is often due to poor nutrition leading to vitamin D deficiency and inadequate calcium absorption from the gut.

Tertiary hyperparathyroidism generally only occurs in patients with kidney failure who have secondary hyperparathyroidism that is physiological and then enters an autonomous phase in which the parathyroids continue to excrete excess parathyroid hormone. This occurs even when the calcium and vitamin D levels are adequate.

The risk for developing hyperparathyroidism increases with age. Among people who are over age 65, about one in every 1,000 men and two or three in every 1,000 women will develop hyperparathyroidism.

Causes of Hyperparathyroidism

In 90 percent or more of the cases, primary hyperparathyroidism is caused by the development of a single parathyroid adenoma. This is a benign growth that functions autonomously on one of the four glands. It continues to secrete excess amounts of parathyroid hormone even when the blood calcium is elevated. The other three parathyroid glands typically respond appropriately, which is to say they atrophy (stop working), making it a bit easier for the experienced surgeon to find the abnormal gland.

In about 10 percent of the cases, parathyroid hyperplasia develops with excess growth of all four glands and excess secretion from all four glands as well. In very rare cases, the excess parathyroid hormone secretion can be due to the development of a parathyroid cancer, typically involving one of the four glands.

In some cases, lithium therapy that is given to patients who are bipolar (manic-depressive) may also induce hyperparathyroidism.

Secondary hyperparathyroidism is caused by a decrease in calcium levels (HYPOCALCEMIA). This may stem from any process that impairs the body's ability to absorb or retain calcium, such as an underlying kidney disease; vitamin D deficiency (as in RICKETS in children or OSTEOMALACIA in adults); malabsorption syndromes due to pancreatitis, ulcerative colitis, Crohn's disease, or other gut problems; or leakage of calcium from the kidneys into the urine (renal hypercalciuria).

Signs and Symptoms

Most patients with primary hyperparathyroidism are asymptomatic. After they are diagnosed and treated, however, some patients in retrospect will realize that they had some symptoms. Individuals vary in how they present with hyperparathyroidism, but some common signs and symptoms of this medical problem include:

- Back pain
- Joint pain
- Fatigue
- Upper abdominal pain
- Muscle weakness
- Increased thirst
- Increased urination
- Itching skin
- Bone pain
- Muscle and tongue fasciculations (tiny involuntary muscle contractions that cause the muscle to quiver)
- Band keratopathy (usually noted only by a special examination by an eye specialist)

Diagnosis and Treatment

Hyperparathyroidism is diagnosed based on the patient's medical history and physical examination as well as on laboratory tests of calcium, phosphorus, parathyroid hormone, and kidney function. Typically, total calcium or ionized calcium levels are elevated, although more frequently normocalcemic hyperparathyroidism can be diagnosed. Increased levels of protein that bind to calcium can falsely elevate the total serum calcium level, but this can be sorted out by measuring the nonbound or ionized calcium.

Serum phosphorus levels are often decreased in patients with primary hyperparathyroidism, while serum alkaline phosphatase levels may be increased. The confirmatory test is measurement of the intact parathyroid hormone level, which is nearly always elevated. Again, though, in very early cases, it may run at the upper limits of the normal level.

Patients with hyperparathyroidism may have reduced BONE DENSITY, especially of the forearm, taken in a DEXA scan. (There is more cortical bone in the forearm, and this bone decreases sooner than the other types of bone do.)

Primary hyperparathyroidism can be mistakenly diagnosed in patients with familial hypercalcemic hypocalciuria. In this condition, patients have elevated calcium levels, normal or high-normal parathyroid hormone levels, but very low excretion of calcium in the urine. This is an inherited defect in which patients' bodies do not properly sense blood calcium levels. They do not develop osteoporosis, kidney stones, myopathy, or any of the complications of hyperparathyroidism and thus do not need treatment, especially parathyroidectomy.

This condition is typically excluded by measuring a 24-hour urine for calcium. The patient collects all urine that is excreted over a 24-hour period, to be evaluated by a laboratory. Normally patients will excrete two to four milligrams per kilogram of calcium in the urine per day. Patients with hyperparathyroidism excrete at least this much and often much more than patients with familial hypercalcemic hypocalciuria, who always excrete much less.

Surgical Treatment

The best therapy for primary hyperparathyroidism is surgery. Indications for surgery include kidney stones, bone loss (especially osteoporosis), severe hypercalciuria, and total calcium levels that are greater than 11 to 12 mg/dl. On occasion, surgery may also be attempted if a patient is suffering with aches and pains and/or cognitive dysfunction that cannot be explained by any other mechanism.

Patients must find a surgeon who has significant experience in parathyroid surgery. Using an experienced surgeon is essential because finding the offending gland may be difficult and distinguishing between a small adenoma and hyperplasia at the time of surgery is often difficult. In addition, the parathyroids' blood supply is limited. Excess damage to the area can lead to permanent hypoparathyroidism, a condition that must be treated with both calcium and vitamin D. Also, the recurrent laryngeal nerves are in this area. Damage to one or both of them can lead to chronic hoarseness or vocal cord paralysis.

In the case of parathyroid hyperplasia, the surgeon will often remove three-and-one-half of the four glands and transplant one-half of one gland into the forearm. Some of the other parathyroid tissue can be frozen and preserved for future use if needed.

In the rare cases of cancer, as much as possible of the cancer should be excised at the time of surgery, as it does not respond well to radiation or chemotherapy. An experienced surgeon will locate the offending adenoma in about 90 percent of the cases.

Preoperative imaging is not necessary, but it is being done more frequently as techniques have improved. As of this writing, the most sensitive imaging seems to be a nuclear medicine scan called a sestamibi subtraction scan. This scan may be particularly advisable in the cases of older and sicker patients, as it may help to localize the surgeon's efforts and also shorten the duration of the operation. In addition, it can lead to very directed and limited small incision surgery under local anesthesia with the use of intraoperative nuclear medicine probes, although this is not standard therapy as of this writing.

Tertiary hyperparathyroidism requires the adjustment of dosages of calcium and vitamin D supplements and often parathyroid surgery as well.

Nonsurgical Therapy

Patients who do not have any indications for surgery can be followed conservatively with close attention paid to blood calcium levels, kidney function, and bone density. Two large trials have attempted to determine which patients will require surgery, and both have failed to achieve that goal.

Some patients will go for many years without any significant signs and symptoms of hyperparathyroidism, while others will progress rapidly. Thus, patients are counseled to use a moderate amount of calcium and salt and to force fluids in order to keep the urine dilute and decrease the risk of developing kidney stones.

Patients who have secondary hyperparathyroidism may be treated with calcium and vitamin D to correct the deficiencies. They may also be treated with cinacalcet (Sensipar, Amgen). Cinacalet is the first drug in a new class of agents called calcimimetics. Cinacalcet sensitizes calcium receptors in the parathyroid glands (the parathyroid glands perceive there is more calcium in the system) and causes direct lowering of parathyroid hormone. It is approved by the Food and Drug Administration (FDA) for the treatment of secondary hyperparathyroidism in patients with chronic kidney disease.

See also CALCIUM BALANCE; PARATHYROID GLANDS.

Dang, Devra K. "Cinacalcet." *Formulary* 39 (2004): 482–489.

Lips, Paul. "Vitamin D Deficiency and Secondary Hypoparathyroidism in the Elderly: Consequences for Bone Loss and Fractures and Therapeutic Implications." *Endocrine Reviews* 22, no. 4 (2001): 477–501.

Marx, Stephen J., M.D. "Hyperparathyroid and Hypoparathyroid Disorders." *New England Journal of Medicine* 343, no. 25 (December 21, 2000): 1,863–1,875.

hyperphosphatemia/hypophosphatemia Abnormally high levels of phosphorus in the blood (hyperphosphatemia) or abnormally low blood levels of phosphorus (hypophosphatemia). Hypophosphatemia is a rare condition that is most commonly seen in patients who suffer from starvation/malnutrition or alcoholism. Because phosphates are ubiquitous in the diets of most Americans, one meal can usually restore levels to normal. In cases of primary hypophosphatemia in which phosphorus is lost in the urine, treatments become more complicated.

Hyperphosphatemia is most often seen in patients with end-stage kidney (renal) disease. It may also be caused by chemotherapy treatment for cancer (tumor lysis syndrome), caused by the destruction of many cancer cells with the subsequent release of phosphorus from inside the cells. Hyperphosphatemia can result in long-term, dangerously decreased levels of calcium in the blood (HYPOCALCEMIA).

Some endocrine diseases associated with hyperphosphatemia include ACROMEGALY, HYPOPARATHYROIDISM, PSEUDOHYPOPARATHYROIDISM, and THYROTOXICOSIS.

Treatment of hyperphosphatemia is aimed at identifying and treating the underlying cause of the problem as well as the resultant symptoms such as hypocalcemia. In patients with end-stage kidney disease (also known as kidney failure), compounds called phosphate binders (which bind the dietary phosphates) are used to treat or to prevent hyperphosphatemia.

Growing children normally have blood phosphorus levels that are higher than those of adults. Pseudohyperphosphatemia does exist and is usually due to excess and/or abnormal protein levels in the blood (as with Waldenström's macroglobulinemia, monoclonal gammopathy, and multiple myeloma). Pseudohyperphosphatemia can also be caused by other blood abnormalities that interfere with the phosphorus assay, such as hyperlipidemia, excess bilirubin (a cause of jaundice), and hemolysis (the destruction of red blood cells).

hyperplasia The term used when more cells of an organ are synthesized than usual. The cells are typically normal, that is, benign or nonmalignant, but may cause problems due to their size or the production of excess hormones. Hyperplasia is different from hypertrophy, in which the number of cells remains the same but each individual cell increases in size.

Hyperplasia is seen in CONGENITAL ADRENAL HYPERPLASIA. This occurs when enzyme abnormalities cause problems with the normal feedback control systems and excessive numbers of adrenal cells are synthesized. The consequences are due to the excessive amounts of hormones that are synthesized.

hypertension See BLOOD PRESSURE/HYPERTENSION.

hyperthyroidism The clinical condition caused by the metabolic effects of excessive levels of thyroid hormones in the blood. This clinical syndrome can range from minimal to severe. It can also be referred to as biochemical hyperthyroidism, in which the hormone levels are elevated but the patient has no symptoms (also known as subclinical hyperthyroidism). It can also be referred to as clinical hyperthyroidism, in which the patient has both abnormal thyroid hormone levels and the typical clinical signs and symptoms of hyperthyroidism.

The most common cause of hyperthyroidism is GRAVES' DISEASE. Other causes are a multinodular goiter, various forms of thyroiditis, toxic or autonomously functioning thyroid nodules, medications, and iodine.

Signs and Symptoms of Hyperthyroidism

Patients with hyperthyroidism usually exhibit some or all of the following signs and symptoms:

- Shortness of breath caused by minimal activity
- Fatigue
- Heat intolerance (patients with hypothyroidism, in contrast, have cold intolerance)
- Hyperactivity
- Increased perspiration (hyperhydrosis)
- Irritability
- Menstrual disturbances (typically oligomenorrhea (infrequent periods) or AMENORRHEA)
- Nervousness
- Heart palpitations/rapid heart rate
- Weight change (usually weight loss, but some patients experience weight gain)
- Sleep disturbances, including nightmares
- Muscle weakness (usually of the proximal muscles)

- Warm, moist, and smooth (velvety) skin
- Presence of a goiter (the thyroid may be small, normal, or large)

Elderly people with hyperthyroidism sometimes will not present with hyperactivity and, instead, will exhibit what is called apathetic hyperthyroidism or thyrotoxicosis. These patients may seem to be depressed and apathetic. They may also lose weight and may experience congestive heart failure. The physician then generally orders laboratory tests, suspecting hypothyroidism, and may be surprised to find hyperthyroidism instead. Administration of antithyroid medication or radioactive iodine can induce a significant improvement and remission of the patient's symptoms.

Diagnosis and Treatment

Hyperthyroidism may be diagnosed by taking a careful medical history and performing a physician examination, especially checking the patient's neck for the presence of a GOITER. Then thyroid function tests are obtained. Usually measurements of thyroid-stimulating hormone (TSH), free T4, and in many instances total T3 blood levels are ordered.

If the diagnosis is in doubt, the physician may order a radioactive iodine uptake test. This test measures the avidity with which the thyroid gland traps iodine to create more thyroid hormones. In most cases of hyperthyroidism, the uptake is increased above normal (usually 15–30 percent at 24 hours). In the various forms of thyroiditis, the radioactive iodine uptake is quite low, usually less than 3 percent and often near zero. The thyroid can be scanned using an isotope known as technetium to ascertain the shape, size, and homogeneity (or lack thereof) of the thyroid gland.

To treat Graves' disease, antithyroid drugs or radioactive iodine are used. For a multinodular goiter or toxic nodule, the best therapy is usually radioactive iodine therapy. For thyroiditis, the symptoms are usually treated with beta-blocker medications and the underlying condition will resolve on its own over time.

If these therapies fail, a THYROIDECTOMY, or removal of the thyroid gland, may be performed. However, it is usually chosen as the last resort.

See also HASHIMOTO'S THYROIDITIS; HYPOTHYROIDISM; THYROID BLOOD TESTS; THYROID-STIMULATING HORMONE.

Miller, K. K., and G. H. Daniels. "Lithium Therapy Can Cause Silent Thyroiditis and Hyperthyroidism." Clinical Endocrinology 55, no. 4 (2001): 501–508.

hypertriglyceridemia   Excessively high levels of triglycerides in the blood, primarily composed of very low-density lipoproteins (VLDL). Patients with hypertriglyceridemia typically have elevated triglyceride levels in the 200–500 mg/dl range. Often there are no physical signs of hypertriglyceridemia. However, if the patient's triglyceride levels increase above 1,000 mg/dl, the retinal blood vessels of the eye may appear as a milky-reddish yellow color. This condition is known as lipemia retinalis.

Hypertriglyceridemia may be a primary or a genetic condition. It is also often seen secondary to other metabolic disorders such as DIABETES MELLITUS (mainly TYPE 2 DIABETES, especially if the diabetes is poorly controlled), HYPOTHYROIDISM, alcohol ingestion, use of estrogens or steroids, and kidney insufficiency or failure. FAMILIAL HYPERTRIGLYCERIDEMIA is an autosomal dominant disorder in which there is both an increased production of VLDL by the liver and a decreased clearance of VLDL. Other rare, familial forms exist, but most are recessive.

Hypertriglyceridemia is often accompanied by low levels of high-density lipoproteins (HDL) or good cholesterol. Triglycerides are mainly synthesized in the liver, and their synthesis is driven by carbohydrate intake and flux through the liver.

The initial therapy for hypertriglyceridemia is diet. In particular, carbohydrates should be limited to decrease the synthesis of new triglycerides. Exercise will also help to decrease triglycerides, as it will increase the production of the enzymes that help to metabolize the triglycerides.

When medications are needed, Hydroxymethylglutaryl (HMG) coenzyme (Co A) reductase inhibitors, or statins, are often first used if the triglyceride levels are lower than 500 mg/dl. These medications lead to an increase in LDL receptors that further leads to a decrease in the cholesterol in the blood. If the patient's triglyceride level is 500 mg/dl or greater, there is an increased risk of developing pancreatitis. Consequently, drugs known as fibric acid derivatives (fibrates) and nicotinic acid may be added to or substituted for statins. In the United States, the fibrates Lopid (gemfibrozil) and Tricor (fenofibrate) may be administered. They will decrease triglyceride levels by 40–60 percent and also increase HDL levels by 10–20 percent. These agents must be used carefully; in patients with renal impairment, they may also be associated with the development of gallstones. When taken with statin medications, they can be associated with myositis and rhabdoymyolysis.

Niacin will lower triglyceride levels by 20–50 percent and increase HDL by 15–40 percent. It can cause upset stomach, increased liver enzymes, increased uric acid (and may precipitate the onset of gout), increased glucose levels (typically only 5–15 mg/dl), and flushing and itching that can be severe but that can usually be prevented by taking a 325 mg aspirin prior to the niacin.

See also CHOLESTEROL.

hypocalcemia A condition resulting from abnormally low levels of calcium in the blood, often due to unusually low levels of parathyroid hormone. Normal total calcium levels are 8.5–10.5 mg/dl for individuals of all ages, and levels below 8.5 are abnormally low.

Patients with chronic problems with hypocalcemia should generally be treated by endocrinologists, who have particular expertise in both normal and abnormal functions of the endocrine glands. Errors of extremes, which means providing either inadequate or excessive therapy, could result in severe medical consequences. When treating patients with hypocalcemia, endocrinologists are unlikely to make such errors.

Hypocalcemia can deteriorate. If left untreated, it can lead to heart arrhythmias and cataracts. It can also lead to a medical emergency known as TETANY, in which the person's calcium levels drop so low that he or she begins experiencing severe muscle cramps and spasms and may also have seizures. If calcium and vitamin D are not administered intravenously to the convulsing person, the patient may die. Fortunately, such severe hypocalcemia is a very rare condition, and death from hypocalcemia is highly unusual. Most people with hypocalcemia experience some identifiable symptoms that precede the development of tetany, such as severe muscle cramps, and thus the majority of patients can be treated well before their condition becomes dangerous.

Risk Factors

Infants born to mothers with DIABETES MELLITUS are at risk for hypocalcemia. Supplemental calcium and vitamin D can be administered to the newborn to resolve the problem, once diagnosed. Individuals who have undergone thyroid or parathyroid surgery within the past 48 hours have the highest risk for developing hypocalcemia. These individuals are experiencing HYPOPARATHYROIDISM, or abnormally low levels of the parathyroid hormone. Hypocalcemia may also occur after a partial (sometimes called a subtotal) thyroidectomy. However, it is more commonly found after a total thyroidectomy or parathyroid surgery, when the entire gland is removed because of cancer or for other medical reasons.

In most postsurgical cases of hypocalcemia, the problem is temporary. Only about 3 percent of people who have undergone thyroid surgery will have a permanent problem with hypocalcemia.

Other individuals may also be at risk for developing hypocalcemia. They include those who:

- Are deficient in magnesium (hypomagnesemia)
- Have severe kidney disease, particularly kidney failure
- Have liver disease
- Have pancreatitis
- Are alcoholic
- Are in an intensive care unit with a severe illness, especially malnutrition

Function of Calcium

Calcium in the blood and bones is carefully regulated by the parathyroid glands, which are endocrine glands embedded in and around the thyroid gland.

The parathyroids control the transfer of calcium among the blood, bone, and other tissues. Dietary calcium may also protect against hypertension, colon cancer, and other medical problems. Vitamin D is also involved in the absorption of calcium.

Signs and Symptoms of Hypocalcemia

The most frequently occurring symptom of hypocalcemia is a feelings of pins and needles (paresthesia), usually experienced in the fingers, toes, and around the mouth.

Other indicators of chronic hypocalcemia include the following:

- Coarse hair
- Very dry skin
- Chronic yeast infections (candida)

Indicators of acute hypocalcemia (requiring emergency medical treatment, which is the intravenous administration of calcium), include:

- Severe muscle cramps
- Numbness
- Irritability
- Low blood pressure (hypotension)
- Mental confusion and psychiatric problems

Diagnosis and Treatment of Hypocalcemia

Several classic physical examination tests may indicate hypocalcemia. For example, if the nerve in the cheekbone is lightly tapped by the physician, the face of the person with hypocalcemia will often react involuntarily with an uncontrollable, sneer-like contortion of the mouth. This particular facial tic is known as CHVOSTEK'S SIGN, named after the doctor who identified the phenomenon.

Another clinical test for hypocalcemia is to inflate a blood pressure cuff on the patient's arm. If the person has hypocalcemia, within several minutes the person's arm will usually spasm and/or cramp uncontrollably (this is called TROUSSEAU'S SIGN).

In addition to checking for clinical signs, such as Chvostek's or Trousseau's signs, the physician should take a complete medical history and order laboratory tests to determine both the patient's calcium and magnesium levels. If these levels are found to be below normal, the patient will require supplemental calcium and may also need high doses of prescribed vitamin D. The severely ill patient will need to receive these supplements intravenously, but the patient whose levels are slightly low will usually improve after taking oral preparations. Some patients need to take vitamin D regularly.

Calcium preparations in the form of calcium carbonate or calcium citrate are available at virtually any pharmacy, supermarket, or health food store. Calcium carbonate is the most popular form of supplemental calcium used in the United States, followed in popularity by calcium citrate. Some individuals take calcium lactate, which can be difficult to find, although it can be ordered from sites on the Internet.

Treatment with calcium may cause minor side effects such as constipation. The addition of magnesium, in about half the dose of the calcium that is taken, may help to rectify cases of constipation. However, the individual's physician should be consulted before a patient adds a magnesium supplement because the supplement could interact with other medicines the patient may be taking. The physician should also determine the dose of any supplemental magnesium.

People who have been diagnosed with hypocalcemia will usually require periodic testing of their blood and urine. The frequency of such testing will be determined by the patient's physician. In some cases, if the underlying problem is corrected, patients who have hypocalcemia may regain a normal blood level of calcium, in which case they would no longer need to take supplemental doses of calcium and vitamin D. In fact, continued supplementation for such people could cause them to develop HYPERCALCEMIA, a dangerously high level of calcium in the blood.

If the hypocalcemia was caused by damage to or a malfunction of the parathyroid glands, the individual usually needs to take supplemental calcium and vitamin D for life. The patient should be tested periodically to verify that his or her blood calcium levels remain in the appropriate range. With aging, most individuals will also need to increase their intake of vitamin D and calcium supplements.

See also HYPERPARATHYROIDISM.

Headley, Carol M. "Hungry Bone Syndrome Following Parathyroidectomy." *ANNA Journal* 25, no. 3 (June 1998): 283–289.

Lepage, R., et al. "Hypocalcemia Induced During Major and Minor Abdominal Surgery in Humans." *Journal of Clinical Endocrinology & Metabolism* 84, no. 8 (1999): 2,654–2,658.

Marx, Stephen J., M.D. "Hyperparathyroid and Hypoparathyroid Disorders." *New England Journal of Medicine* 343, no. 25 (2000): 1,863–1,875.

Petit, William A. Jr., M.D., and Christine Adamec. *The Encyclopedia of Diabetes.* New York: Facts On File, Inc., 2002.

hypoglycemia   Abnormally low levels of blood sugar. Having extremely low levels of blood sugar is known as insulin shock. Physicians determine the presence of hypoglycemia based on the patient's symptoms as well as the chemical analysis of the patient's blood sugar, which is typically defined as a fasting glucose level of less than 55 mg/dl.

Risk Factors

Individuals with DIABETES MELLITUS and ADDISON'S DISEASE are at risk for developing hypoglycemia. If the person with diabetes has a severe bout of hypoglycemia, the condition may devolve into DIABETIC KETOACIDOSIS, a dangerous condition requiring emergency hospitalization and treatment. Hypoglycemia can also occur among individuals with insulin-secreting tumors of the pancreas as well as among patients with liver disease or kidney disease. Some individuals develop hypoglycemia after drinking alcohol. Sometimes the cause of hypoglycemia cannot be determined.

Symptoms of Hypoglycemia

Some key symptoms of hypoglycemia are as follows:

- Cold sweats
- Fatigue
- Confusion
- Headache
- Shakiness
- Hunger
- Rapid heartbeat

Treatment

Hypoglycemia is usually treated by consuming glucose-containing foods or drinks. However, if the individual becomes unconscious, emergency medical treatment is required to avoid coma and even death. The patient will usually be given glucose or glucagon by emergency medical personnel. Once the glucose levels are stabilized, the patient usually normalizes as well.

Advance Preparation for Chronic Hypoglycemic Attacks

People who suffer from chronic hypoglycemia or from conditions that can often lead to hypoglycemia should not skip any meals, because failing to eat regular meals can exacerbate the condition. They should also avoid drinking much or any alcohol.

In addition, patients with chronic attacks of hypoglycemia should also wear medical bracelets or necklaces that state their medical problem and that are easily seen on the person's body. Medical cards are not sufficient because they are usually left in wallets, and emergency personnel may not have access to wallets or have time to search them. People with frequent bouts of hypoglycemia should also keep glucose-containing snacks in their homes and their cars. Some patients may need a glucagon kit for emergency use, which can be prescribed by their doctors.

Patients who exhibit hypoglycemic symptoms while driving should pull off the road as soon as possible and should also consume an item with glucose in it. If they have blood-testing equipment available (as patients with diabetes should have), they should check their blood sugar level 15 minutes after eating the glucose snack. If it is above 70 mg/dl, the person should, in most cases, be able to drive.

See also COMA.

For further information on hypoglycemia, contact the following organizations:

American Diabetes Association
National Service Center
1710 North Beauregard Street
Alexandria, VA 22311
(800) 342-2383 (toll-free)
http://www.diabetes.org

Juvenile Diabetes Research Foundation
    International
120 Wall Street
Ninth Floor
New York, NY 10005
(800) 342-2383 (toll-free)
http://www.jdrf.org

hypogonadism   Abnormally low levels of TESTOS-TERONE in males. An estimated one in 500 males are affected by this condition. Hypogonadism may be either primary or secondary. Primary hypogonadism results from abnormalities in one or both testicles. Secondary hypogonadism is usually caused by a problem with the pituitary gland, which controls the production of testosterone.

Effects of Hypogonadism Depend on When It Occurs

Hypogonadism may occur as early as during fetal development. It may also occur during puberty or after adulthood. The symptoms and signs of hypogonadism vary depending on at what stage in life the hypogonadism occurred. For example, if it occurred before birth and the gonads did not produce enough male hormone, then the child may have genitals that are neither clearly male nor female.

If the condition occurs at or before puberty, the boy will not experience the normal adolescent changes of most adolescent males, such as a deepened voice, increased body hair, and further growth of the penis and testes. Instead, the boy will experience greater-than-normal growth in the arms and legs, and he may also experience GYNECOMASTIA (enlarged breast tissue).

If the fully developed male becomes hypogonadal, he will usually experience problems with ERECTILE DYSFUNCTION (impotence), INFERTILITY, decreased muscle mass, increased fat, gynecomastia, and OSTEOPOROSIS. He may also experience the symptoms that are common among women in menopause, such as HOT FLASHES, mood swings, diminished sexual drive, depression, and fatigue.

Of interest is that in some cases, hypogonadism is purposely induced. For example, men with advanced prostate cancer are often treated with hormone therapy to stop testosterone production, because testosterone makes prostate cancer grow faster. As a result, such men experience all the symptoms and signs of hypogonadism. When they stop taking the hormones, their normal levels of testosterone resume, and the signs and symptoms of hypogonadism disappear.

Causes of Hypogonadism

Hypogonadism has many different causes. In infants and toddlers, the cause may be an undescended testicle, which can be corrected by surgery. KLINEFELTER SYNDROME, a chromosomal disorder, is another cause. Males normally have one X and one Y chromosome, but with Klinefelter syndrome, the individual has two or more X chromosomes as well as the Y chromosome.

Other causes of primary hypogonadism include:

- Hemochromatosis (excessive levels of iron in the blood)
- Damage to the testicles
- Hernia surgery

Causes of secondary hypogonadism include the following:

- Kallmann's syndrome (impaired development of the hypothalamus, which ultimately affects the release of testosterone)
- Disorders of the pituitary gland, such as tumors
- Sarcoidosis
- Mumps orchitis
- Some medications, such as some psychiatric drugs or other medications

Diagnosis and Treatment

In addition to taking a complete medical history and performing a physical examination, particularly of the penis and testicles, the physician will usually order a test of the male's blood levels of testosterone. The physician may also order imaging tests, such as an ultrasound or MAGNETIC RESONANCE IMAGING (MRI) scan. In adult males, the doctor may also order a semen analysis to determine whether the sperm count is within the normal range.

If the hypogonadism did not occur during fetal development, the male with hypogonadism can often be treated with testosterone replacement therapy (TRT). Boys and men on TRT must be carefully monitored, because levels that are too high can cause other health problems, such as prostate disease and infertility. Testosterone can be given in the form of an injection every two weeks, and patients can be trained to self-inject. Patients may also use a testosterone transdermal patch that is placed onto the scrotum or onto another part of the body. Testosterone is also available in the form of a skin gel.

See also HERMAPHRODITISM, KALLMANN'S SYNDROME.

Lange, Paul M., M.D., and Christine Adamec. *Prostate Cancer for Dummies.* New York: Wiley Publishing, 2003.

Nachtigall, Lisa B., M.D., et al. "Adult-Onset Idiopathic Hypogonatatropic Hypogonadism—A Treatable Form of Male Infertility." *New England Journal of Medicine* 336, no. 6 (February 6, 1997): 410–415.

Petak, Steven M., M.D. "American Association of Clinical Endocrinologists Medical Guidelines for Clinical Practice for the Evaluation and Treatment of Hypogonadism in Adult Male Patients—2002 Update." *Endocrine Practice* 8, no. 6 (November/December 2002): 439–456.

Sih, Rahmawati, et al. "Testosterone Replacement in Older Hypogonadal Men: A 12-Month Randomized Controlled Trial." *Journal of Clinical Endocrinology & Metabolism* 82, no. 6 (1997): 1,661–1,667.

Snyder, Peter J., et al. "Effects of Testosterone Replacement in Hypogonadal Men." *Journal of Clinical Endocrinology & Metabolism* 85, no. 8 (2000): 2,670–2,677.

hypogonadotropism Decreased or absent gonadal function (in the ovary or the testes) due to the absence of the gonadal-stimulating pituitary hormones, including FOLLICLE-STIMULATING HORMONE (FSH) and LUTEINIZING HORMONE (LH). This condition is also known as gonadotropin deficiency, KALLMANN'S SYNDROME, or secondary hypogonadism.

Hypogonadotropism is characterized by the lack of pubertal development in adolescence and the absence of secondary sexual indicators, such as pubic hair, underarm (axillary) hair, or facial hair in males. Some patients have an inability to smell (anosmia).

This condition is diagnosed by tests of hormone blood levels as well as the gonadotropin-releasing hormone (GnRH) stimulation test. This latter test measures hormone levels after they are stimulated by injected hormones.

Male patients with hypogonadotropism are treated with intramuscular injections of testosterone. Females are usually treated with female hormones, such as estrogen and progesterone pills. Males and females may also be treated with growth hormone.

See also HYPOGONADISM.

hyponatremia A lower-than-normal concentration of sodium in the bloodstream. It is invariably a problem of water. In other words, too much water is in the system in relationship to the amount of sodium. This is contrary to a common misconception, which is that the hyponatremia results from inadequate sodium or salt intake. Hyponatremia is diagnosed when sodium levels are less than 135 millimoles per liter in an adult. The most common causes of hyponatremia are the use of thiazide diuretic medications for hypertension or loop diuretics that were given to remove excess salt and water from the body.

HYPOTHYROIDISM can sometimes lead to hyponatremia, as patients with hypothyroidism are unable to excrete any excess water in the system. Primary ADRENAL INSUFFICIENCY will also lead to hyponatremia due to the deficiency in mineralocorticoids. In addition, an extreme intake of water can also dilute the serum sodium, causing hyponatremia. The condition can also be seen in the syndrome of inappropriate secretion of antidiuretic hormone (SIADH) and sometimes (very rarely) in abused infants and children. Mentally ill individuals, such as patients with schizophrenia, may also ingest excessive amounts of water, causing hyponatremia.

Symptoms of Hyponatremia

The common symptoms of hyponatremia are malaise, nausea and vomiting, headache, lethargy, muscle cramps, and decreased deep tendon reflexes. If the hyponatremia is not resolved, patients may further worsen to the point of seizures, coma, brain damage, and even death.

Diagnosis and Treatment

Physicians will suspect that a patient may have hyponatremia based on the clinical symptoms and medical history, especially with respect to medications that were recently taken. Hyponatremia is diagnosed by blood testing that reveals a lower-than-normal serum sodium concentration.

To treat hyponatremia, the patient is typically given an intravenous sodium chloride containing solution with a concentration of sodium that is greater than what exists in the individual's bloodstream, even to the point of using very small doses of hypertonic saline (a 3 percent sodium chloride solution). On occasion, a loop diuretic, such as furosemide, may be used. Often free water must be withheld from the patient as well; patients are not allowed to drink as they wish, and water intake is limited to less than 1.0–1.5 or sometimes 0.5 liters per day. If the case is a mild one, patients can be observed only, while water is withheld.

See also HYPERGLYCEMIA.

Adrogue Horacio, J., M.D., and Nicolaos E. Masias, M.D. "Hyponatremia." *New England Journal of Medicine* 342, no. 21 (May 25, 2000): 1,581–1,589.

hypoparathyroidism   A condition in which there is inadequate parathyroid hormone in the bloodstream as well as in the bone, the gut, the kidneys, and other organs. Parathyroid hormone is produced by the parathyroids, which are glands embedded in the neck behind the thyroid gland.

If hypoparathyroidism becomes severe, the patient develops a condition called HYPOCALCEMIA and, in extreme cases, may have seizures. Without treatment after seizures from hypocalcemia, the patient may die. This occurs for several reasons. One is that without adequate parathyroid activity in the bloodstream, the kidneys cannot hold onto needed calcium so excessive calcium is lost via the urine. Some excess calcium may be deposited into the tissues of the kidneys and lead to calcification of the kidneys (nephrocalcinosis) or to the devel-

opment of kidney stones (nephrolithiasis). Thus, ironically hypocalcemia can cause calcification.

Causes of Hypoparathyroidism

The most common cause of this condition is surgery on the thyroid or parathyroid glands or other neck surgery that causes the removal of or damage to the parathyroid glands. In some cases, hypoparathyroidism is caused by the autoimmune destruction of the parathyroid glands. Autoimmune hypoparathyroidism may exist on its own or as a part of a deficiency syndrome involving many organs. In rare cases, hypoparathyroidism results from radioactive iodine treatment given to treat hyperparathyroidism (a condition of excessively high levels of parathyroid hormone).

Rarely, severe deficiencies of magnesium, a condition seen in malnourished patients and alcoholics, can lead to a state of hypoparathyroidism and hypocalcemia (abnormally low blood levels of calcium).

Signs and Symptoms of Hypoparathyroidism

Patients with hypoparathyroidism may experience some or all of the following signs and symptoms:

- Muscle cramps
- Abdominal pain
- Tingling in the feet, hands, and face
- Spasms in the hands or feet

In severe cases, patients may experience seizures or convulsions caused by TETANY, a dangerous condition of extremely low calcium blood levels.

Diagnosis and Treatment

Physicians diagnose hypoparathyroidism based on the patient's medical history, particularly any past history of any form of neck surgery, as well as the apparent presence of hypocalcemia. Patients with hypocalcemia may respond with a characteristic facial twitch when the cheekbone is tapped (CHVOSTEK'S SIGN). Others may show TROUSSEAU'S SIGN, an arm spasm and cramp that results from a test using a blood pressure cuff.

The doctor will also order laboratory tests of the patient's serum calcium levels. Low levels indicate hypocalcemia. The doctor may also check serum parathyroid hormone levels (which are below normal in the presence of hypoparathyroidism), serum phosphorus levels (which are high with hypoparathyroidism), and serum magnesium levels (which are low with hypoparathyroidism). The physician may also order tests of ionized calcium in the blood and/or calcium excretion in the urine.

To treat hypoparathyroidism, physicians order over-the-counter oral calcium. They also order CALCITRIOL (prescribed vitamin D), often in very high doses. (Vitamin D supplements available in health food stores are not sufficient.) If the patient is very ill, he or she may need to be hospitalized to receive calcium and vitamin D intravenously.

The ENDOCRINOLOGIST must be careful to recommend adequate yet not excessive amounts of calcium and vitamin D to alleviate the patient's symptoms while avoiding the patient from losing a severe amount of calcium via the urine. Often patients do not need to attain normal calcium blood levels, however, which may be too high for these patients and could cause complications of the kidneys, or even kidney failure and death.

See also CALCIUM ABSORPTION; CALCIUM BALANCE.

Abugassa, Salem, et al. "Bone Mineral Density in Patients with Chronic Hypoparathyroidism." *Journal of Clinical Endocrinology & Metabolism* 76, no. 6 (1993): 1,617–1,621.

Marx, Stephen J., M.D. "Hyperparathyroid and Hypoparathyroid Disorders." *New England Journal of Medicine* 343, no. 25 (December 21, 2000): 1,863–1,875.

Stock, John L., et al. "Autosomal Dominant Hypoparathyroidism Associated with Short Stature and Premature Osteoarthritis." *Journal of Clinical Endocrinology & Metabolism* 84, no. 9 (1999): 3,036–3,040.

hypopituitarism Excessively low or insufficient levels of pituitary hormone production. In the most extreme cases, complete PITUITARY FAILURE (panhypopituitarism) occurs, although this condition is rare.

Any one of the six anterior pituitary hormones may become deficient: adrenocorticotropic hormone (ACTH), FOLLICLE-STIMULATING HORMONE (FSH), GROWTH HORMONE (GH), LUTEINIZING HOR-

MONE (LH), PROLACTIN, and THYROID-STIMULATING HORMONE (TSH). The production of the posterior pituitary hormone desmopressin acetate (DDAVP) can also be impeded, although this is certainly less common unless there is significant destruction of the pituitary gland. Typically, the pituitary hormones decline in a specific order. In other words, some of the cells are more susceptible to damage than others. The usual order of decline is LH, FSH, GH, TSH, ACTH, and then prolactin.

Hypopituitarism may result in ADRENAL INSUFFICIENCY, HYPOTHYROIDISM, HYPOGONADISM, and GROWTH HORMONE DEFICIENCY as well as deficiencies of antidiuretic hormone (ADH) and prolactin. Abnormal or unexpected pairings of laboratory test results may indicate hypopituitarism. For example, the patient's levels TSH may be normal but the levels of T3 and T4 are low, which should lead the physician to consider laboratory error, EUTHYROID SICK SYNDROME, or pituitary or hypothalamic dysfunction.

Patients with hypopituitarism should wear medical bracelets describing their condition in the event that it should worsen and they require emergency treatment. Studies performed in the United Kingdom and Sweden indicate that hypopituitarism increases the risk of death by double or more compared with individuals of the same age and gender without the condition. Much of this increased mortality is due to cardiovascular causes.

Causes of Hypopituitarism

Hypopituitarism has many different possible causes. It may be caused by a macroadenoma (a tumor greater than one centimeter in diameter) of the pituitary gland, which damages or destroys the remainder of the pituitary. Sometimes a cyst (Rathke's cleft cyst) or tumor (craniopharyngioma) in the hypothalamus may cause hypopituitarism. This medical problem may also be a complication of irradiation of the pituitary in the course of the patient receiving treatment for tumors of the pituitary or from radiation of nearby tissue in the nose, throat, or brain.

Rarely, hypopituitarism is caused by pituitary apoplexy, which results from severe bleeding (hemorrhage) and subsequent enlargement of the pituitary gland. POSTPARTUM PITUITARY NECROSIS

(Sheehan's syndrome), which is caused by severe bleeding after childbirth, may also result in hypopituitarism. In addition, some rare diseases may cause the condition. These diseases include hemochromatosis (an iron overload disease), sarcoidosis (one of several granulomatous conditions that may damage the pituitary), and genetic disorders such as KALLMANN'S SYNDROME. A direct injury to the pituitary, such as an injury caused by a car crash, may also result in hypopituitarism.

Diagnosis and Treatment

The diagnosis of hypopituitarism may be difficult, because the patient's symptoms may mimic hypothyroidism or other disorders, which must be ruled out. With hypopituitarism, patients have a secondary form of hypothyroidism—growth hormone deficiency—and thus often have a milder form of symptoms.

Because the etiology is secondary—that is, the patients' bodies no longer make TSH but their thyroid gland is still intact—the thyroid still makes some thyroid hormone. In contrast, in patients who have a primary thyroid problem in which the thyroid gland is completely destroyed, their bodies make no thyroid hormones at all, and their symptoms are much worse.

If a patient's hypopituitarism is caused by a tumor that can be surgically removed, the condition may reverse itself completely after surgery. If the cause is not treatable, if tissue has been destroyed by radiation or trauma, for example, then treatment involves partial or complete hormone replacement so that the results of the dysfunction can be managed. As a result, such patients who are exhibiting hypothyroid symptoms are treated with supplemental levothyroxine (T4).

Patients with adrenal insufficiency are given glucocorticoids, such as hydrocortisone, prednisone, or cortisone acetate. Men with hypogonadism (insufficient production of testosterone) are treated with supplemental testosterone (transdermal or intramuscular). Women with an insufficient production of estrogen are treated with hormone replacement therapy (transdermal, oral, or intramuscular). Growth hormone replacement in adults is a mildly controversial issue. As of this writing, most growth hormone-deficient adults are not given growth hormone. Nonetheless, growing evidence indicates that treating growth hormone deficiency leads to a better quality of life.

If hypopituitarism is not treated, patients may experience a loss in bone density due to hypogonadism and a greater-than-normal risk of developing osteoporosis.

See also PITUITARY GLAND.

Mulinda, James R., M.D. "Hypopituitarism (Panhypopituitarism)," Available online. URL: http://www.emedicine.com/med/topic1137.htm. Downloaded on January 15, 2004.

Schmidt, Diane N., M.D., and Kathleen Wallace, M.D. "How to Diagnose Hypopituitarism." *Postgraduate Medicine* 104, no. 7 (July 1998): 77–87.

Vance, Mary Lee. "Hypopituitarism." *New England Journal of Medicine* 330, no. 23 (June 9, 1994): 1,651–1,662.

hypotension Abnormally low blood pressure readings, which may be found among very ill or elderly individuals or among those with severe HYPERTHYROIDISM, PITUITARY FAILURE, or ADDISON'S DISEASE. Some medications, such as drugs with sedating qualities, some antidepressants, antianxiety medications, heart medicines, and other medications can cause low blood pressure. Some conditions, such as DEHYDRATION (which can be caused by HYPERGLYCEMIA, heart failure, shock, or cardiac arrythmias) can also cause hypotension to occur.

Hypotension can be dangerous because it can impair people so much that they experience severe falls and FRACTURES. Studies have shown that the type of hypotension that occurs after eating a meal (postprandial hypotension) is also a high-risk indicator for falls, especially among patients with DIABETES MELLITUS or those who take three or more medications. In general, chronic hypotension refers to patients who have blood pressure levels below 90/60.

ORTHOSTATIC HYPOTENSION refers to a sudden drop in blood pressure (about 20 mm Hg in the systolic blood pressure) that occurs when a person changes from a lying-down to a sitting-up position or from a sitting-up to a standing position.

Emergency symptoms of hypotension that indicate urgent medical treatment may be needed include the following:

- Chest pain
- Shortness of breath
- A fever over 101 degrees Fahrenheit
- Severe headache
- Severe pain in the upper back region
- Diarrhea and vomiting that lasts more than a day
- The presence of black or maroon-colored stools
- Urine that smells foul
- Fainting

Diagnosis and Treatment

When hypotension is diagnosed, the cause is sought through a medical history and physical examination as well as tests such as a complete blood count (CBC), urinalysis, chest X-rays, and tests for thyroid function. When the doctor has determined the probable cause, a treatment plan can be developed to improve the hypotension. For example, if the hypotension is caused by medications, the doctor may be able to change the medication or reduce the dosage. If Addison's disease is the cause of hypotension, supplemental steroids and intravenous fluids will improve the condition.

See also BLOOD PRESSURE/HYPERTENSION.

hypothalamic-pituitary-adrenal axis (HPA axis)   Refers to the connections and interconnections between the organs of the hypothalamus, pituitary, and the adrenal glands. The HPA axis is also affected by input from both the cerebral cortex and the brain stem.

The HPA axis is activated by stress. Part of the stress response may lead to inflammation by causing the production of cytokines. These further lead to the creation of tumor necrosis factor, interleukin-1 and interleukin-6, and other mediators of inflammation used to protect the body.

All other anterior pituitary hormones have a hypothalamic-pituitary–end organ axis that is the main controller of that end organ's functional status. All three exist in a homeostatic loop to maintain hormone function at the appropriate levels.

Chrousos, George P., M.D. "The Hypothalamic-Pituitary-Adrenal Axis and Immune-Mediated Inflammation." *New England Journal of Medicine* 332, no. 20 (1995): 1,351–1,362.

hypothalamus   The endocrine gland ultimately responsible for directing the release of the anterior pituitary hormones: thyrotropin-releasing hormone (TRH), growth hormone-releasing hormone (GHRH), gonadotropin-releasing hormone (GRH), corticotropin releasing hormone (CRH), and dopamine. Each of these hormones triggers the production of other key hormones needed by the body (see Table).

The hypothalamus also helps to regulate blood pressure, appetite, satiety (a feeling of fullness after eating), libido, and body temperature. Malfunctions of the hypothalamus may range from minor medical problems to life-threatening conditions.

A cyst or tumor in the hypothalamus may cause HYPOPITUITARISM. Excessive release of GHRH, leading to further release of GROWTH HORMONE, causes ACROMEGALY. If the condition occurs before puberty, it is called GIGANTISM because it causes the individual to be much larger in height and size than the average person. The impaired development of the hypothalamus in the fetus leads to KALLMANN'S SYNDROME.

PITUITARY HORMONES THAT CAUSE THE STIMULATION OF OTHER KEY HORMONES

Pituitary Hormone	Effect
TRH	Releases TSH
GHRH	Releases GH
GRH	Releases LH and FSH
CRH	Releases ACTH
Dopamine	Inhibits prolactin

TSH = thyroid-stimulating hormone
GH = growth hormone
LH = luteinizing hormone
FSH = follicle-stimulating hormone
ACTH = adrenocorticotropic hormone

The hypothalamus releases antidiuretic hormone (ADH), also called vasopressin or desmopressin acetate (DDAVP). This hormone is released directly into the posterior pituitary via neurons and if insufficient amounts are released, will cause the development of DIABETES INSIPIDUS.

See also HYPOTHALAMIC-PITUITARY-ADRENAL AXIS.

hypothyroidism The metabolic condition caused by abnormally low levels of thyroid hormone in the bloodstream, usually due to an undersecretion from the thyroid gland. Experts estimate that more than 10 million Americans are affected by this medical problem.

Causes of Hypothyroidism

Hypothyroidism may be mild, moderate, or severe. As with hyperthyroidism, hypothyroidism can be subclassified as biochemical or subclinical (low levels of thyroid hormone activity without any signs or symptoms) or clinical (with typical signs and symptoms).

Some infants are born with CONGENITAL HYPOTHYROIDISM, which must be treated immediately to avoid long-term irreversible developmental delays in physical and intellectual functioning. An estimated one in every 3,000 babies has congenital hypothyroidism. (Newborns are screened for low thyroid levels.) Hypothyroidism is also caused by the surgical removal of the thyroid gland or by its destruction through external radiation or radioactive iodine treatments.

The most common cause of hypothyroidism is HASHIMOTO'S THYROIDITIS, which is an autoimmune disorder that damages the thyroid gland over the course of years. Early on in this syndrome, the thyroid gland may be normal in size. As the disease progresses and thyroid-stimulating hormone (TSH) levels increase, the gland typically enlarges to a GOITER (an abnormally enlarged thyroid gland). Finally, after years of exposure to the destructive antibodies, the thyroid gland may become small or may atrophy.

Another cause of hypothyroidism, although rarely seen in the United States, Canada, and other developed countries, is iodine deficiency.

Medications, such as lithium (used for bipolar illness) can induce hypothyroidism, impairing the synthesis of thyroid hormone. Usually if the lithium is replaced by another drug, the patient's normal thyroid functioning will return. Some drugs have excessively high levels of iodine and can impair thyroid function, such as amiodarone, a cardiac drug. Interferon, commonly used to boost the immune system in patients with hepatitis C, can lead to hypothyroidism. In addition, antithyroid drugs given to treat hyperthyroidism, such as propylthiouracil and methimazole, may induce hypothyroidism in some patients.

Very rarely, diet can induce hypothyroidism, particularly a diet very high in bamboo shoots, cabbage, cassava, and sweet potatoes.

Sometimes the thyroid gland itself continues to function normally, but a malfunction in either the pituitary or the hypothalamus causes the condition of secondary or central hypothyroidism (inadequate stimulation of the thyroid gland by thyroid-stimulating hormone). In these cases, the free T4 level may be low normal or low while the TSH level is normal or low. Thus, if a TSH level is measured first, the physician is more likely to suspect hyperthyroidism than hypothyroidism.

Hypothyroidism May Be Misdiagnosed as Depression

Sometimes hypothyroidism is misdiagnosed as depression, particularly when the signs and symptoms are mild. As a result, all patients diagnosed with possible depression should be screened for hypothyroidism before receiving any antidepressant medications (unless the patient is severely depressed and withholding medications until the blood was tested for thyroid disease would be considered dangerous).

Both hypothyroidism and depression may share the common symptoms of constipation, decreased concentration, decreased libido, depressed mood, diminished interest in activities that formerly appealed to the patient, fatigue, sleep increase, and weight increase. People who are depressed, however, may also have suicidal thoughts. People with hypothyroidism also have cold intolerance, delayed relaxation phase of the deep tendon reflexes, goiter, less and coarser hair, skin changes (thicker, drier, and doughier), and slow heart rate (brady-cardia), features not commonly found among people with depression alone. However, a person with hypothyroidism can also have depression, complicating the diagnosis and treatment. Treating the hypothyroidism is critical because antidepressant medications do not work optimally in an untreated hypothyroid patient.

Signs and Symptoms of Hypothyroidism

There are several common symptoms of hypothyroidism. However, children age five and under who are hypothyroid may have no apparent symptoms (although they will often have decreased growth). Adolescents may have only a few signs and symptoms, such as facial puffiness and fatigue. Doctors should not prescribe thyroid hormone to a patient without checking his or her blood to verify that the thyroid levels are too low. The patient may have another medical problem altogether, and the administration of unnecessary thyroid hormones could create other medical problems, such as iatrogenic HYPERTHYROIDISM.

The general symptoms and signs of hypothyroidism include:

- Fatigue
- Cold intolerance (patients with hypothyroidism get cold faster and the cold bothers them more than others)
- Chronic constipation
- Decreased appetite
- Apparent (or actual) depression
- Muscle cramping and weakness, especially of the proximal muscles
- Anemia
- Reduced sexual libido
- Decreased perspiration
- Paresthesias (pins and needles feelings)
- Carpal and tarsal tunnel syndromes
- Weight increase/difficulty with weight loss
- Sleepiness
- Decreased memory/concentration
- Hoarseness (thickened vocal cords)

- Slowed movements
- Thinning of the outer third of the eyebrows (also known as Queen Ann's eyebrow)
- High cholesterol levels (about 56 percent of patients experience this sign)
- Skin that is cool and dry to the touch
- Puffy face
- Failure to ovulate (ANOVULATION)
- Excessively heavy menses (menorrhagia)
- Enlarged tongue (macroglossia)

If hypothyroidism is severe and continues untreated, the following signs and symptoms may occur:

- HYPOGLYCEMIA (low blood sugar)
- Hypothermia (below-normal body temperature)
- Hypoventilation (below-normal breathing rate)
- HYPONATREMIA (inadequate levels of sodium in the blood)
- Water retention
- Bradycardia (slow heartbeat)
- Depression
- Shock
- MYXEDEMA COMA

Some studies have shown other indicators of hypothyroidism. In a 1997 issue of *The Physician and Sportsmedicine*, the authors reported on the case of a male athlete with knee and shoulder pain who had been diagnosed with tendonitis and fibromyalgia. Routine blood tests showed a highly elevated TSH level. The patient was treated with levothyroxine, and his problems resolved.

Said the authors of this study, "Previous musculoskeletal symptoms and fatigue did not recur. He has since attained personal best race times and has had his best triathlon season." They concluded that "the dramatic improvement and complete resolution of the symptoms with thyroid replacement therapy after failure with other medical treatments suggest that normal tendon healing is impaired in hypothyroidism."

Risk Factors

Women face about 10 times the risk of developing hypothyroidism as men, and the risk is greatest for women who are older than age 40. Nearly 10 percent of all women between the ages of 45 and 64 are hypothyroid. About 12 percent of women over age 60 have elevated levels of TSH, indicating hypothyroidism. About 7 percent of men between the ages of 65 and 74 have hypothyroidism. Women who are menopausal are also at risk for hypothyroidism. Women who already take medications for hypothyroidism may need to increase their dosage of thyroid hormone based on the results of their blood levels.

Thyroid disease (of all types) is often hereditary. As many as 50 percent of patients with thyroid disease inherited the gene for thyroid disorders.

Diagnosis of Hypothyroidism

Physicians assess thyroid status by performing a physical examination and ordering laboratory tests that check TSH levels, levels of free T4, total T3, and antithyroid antibodies (usually antithyroid peroxidase antibody or anti-TPO). Physicians should also take a careful medical history, noting the presence of any past thyroid disease or whether a patient has any first-degree relatives (parents or siblings) who have thyroid disease since thyroid disease runs in families.

In a physical examination, the doctor palpates the neck to check for any unusual enlargement of the thyroid. The doctor will also measure for slow pulse, look for enlarged tongue and a delayed relaxation phase of the deep tendon reflex, and check for edema (fluid retention), especially under the eyes. Blood pressure is usually higher in patients with hypothyroidism and often decreases after the condition is treated.

Based on the 2003 guidelines from the American Academy of Clinical Endocrinologists (AACE), in most laboratories, treatment for hypothyroidism should be considered if the TSH levels are above 3.04 mU/l. In the past, the cutoff for hypothyroidism was at a higher level, or 5.0 mU/l, which did not include many patients with mild hypothyroidism.

Sometimes the diagnosis for hypothyroidism may be missed altogether. For example, hypothyroidism is a common problem among people over age 65. However, doctors may assume that older people are "supposed" to feel tired, lethargic, and constipated and thus may mistakenly attribute the symptoms of hypothyroidism to "normal" aging.

Treatment

In most cases, patients quickly improve with the administration of LEVOTHYROXINE (l-thyroxine), usually in an oral form, such as Synthroid or Levoxyl. In addition, the TSH should be measured about six to eight weeks after any change in either l-thyroxine brand or a change in the prescribed dosage of the medication.

Once patients are stabilized, they should be monitored regularly and should receive at least annual checks of their TSH blood levels. Patients diagnosed with hypothyroidism should also have regular checks of their total cholesterol levels, because studies have shown that hypothyroidism increases the risk of HYPERCHOLESTEROLEMIA (high cholesterol levels in the blood). Once thyroid levels are within the normal range, however, cholesterol levels often drop as well.

Sometimes patients have only slightly elevated TSH levels or have some symptoms of hypothyroidism but also have normal blood levels. Mild thyroid failure may be caused by autoimmune thyroiditis, treatment for GRAVES' DISEASE (a prominent form of hyperthyroidism), lithium carbonate therapy for bipolar disorder (manic depression), radiation to the neck, and iodine and iodine-containing medications.

In such cases, physicians often treat patients with thyroxine supplements. The reason for such treatments is to prevent a progression to overt hypothyroidism, to prevent enlargement of the thyroid gland, to alleviate symptoms, to help with symptoms of depression, to normalize serum lipid levels, and also to normalize the cardiac function of patients.

Hypothyroidism and Pregnancy

About 2.5 percent of all pregnant women are hypothyroid. Hypothyroidism is often associated with an increased risk of obstetrical complications. In addition, pregnant women with positive thyroid antibodies face an increased risk of suffering from miscarriages.

Hypothyroidism can be more difficult to diagnose during pregnancy because the symptoms of weight gain and fatigue are also commonly seen in nearly all pregnant women. In addition, about one-third of pregnant women who are hypothyroid have no symptoms at all, and only one-third have moderate symptoms. Also, the TSH levels in hypothyroid women are often unchanged and continue to lie within the normal range. Instead, the total T4 and total T3 are increased, and the thyroid hormone binding ratio (T3-resin uptake) is decreased.

Risk factors for developing hypothyroidism among pregnant women are as follows:

- The presence of a goiter
- Previous therapy for hyperthyroidism
- The presence of TYPE 1 DIABETES
- A family history of thyroid disease
- The presence of other autoimmune disorders
- HYPERLIPIDEMIA
- Previous experience with high-dose external neck radiation
- Previous postpartum thyroiditis

Untreated hypothyroidism among pregnant women can have serious consequences in addition to miscarriage. Other possible consequences include:

- Gestational hypertension (hypertension that occurs only during pregnancy)
- Preterm delivery
- Anemia
- Fetal complications
- Postpartum hemorrhage

When hypothyroidism is diagnosed among pregnant women, they are generally prescribed levothyroxine. About half of the women who take levothyroxine before their pregnancy will need to take an increased dose of the drug during their pregnancies. Thus, their TSH blood levels should be measured in each trimester during the pregnancy and should then be rechecked again within six to eight weeks after the birth of the child.

Postpartum Thyroiditis

Some women do not become hypothyroid before or during pregnancy, but instead, their hypothyroidism occurs postpartum. The prevalence of postpartum thyroiditis (including both hypothyroidism and hyperthyroidism) is about 8 percent. Of the women who develop postpartum thyroiditis, about 36 percent have hypothyroidism only, 38 percent have hyperthyroidism only, and 26 percent have hyperthyroidism first, which is then followed by hypothyroidism.

The usual course is first to develop hyperthyroidism that can last from one to four months, with the levels returning to the normal range for the following one to two months. After this time, thyroid levels may dip to hypothyroid levels for one to two months before again returning to normal. It is not uncommon for the postpartum hypothyroidism to be permanent. Thus, with the plethora of symptoms that many postpartum women can have, as well as the ups and downs that their thyroid levels may go through after giving birth, the diagnosis of hypothyroidism can be delayed and may sometimes be completely missed by physicians.

Women with the highest risk of developing postpartum thyroiditis include those who:

- Have Type 1 diabetes
- Have a previous history of postpartum hypothyroidism
- Have other autoimmune diseases, such as HASHIMOTO'S THYROIDITIS or Graves' disease

See also THYROID BLOOD TESTS; THYROIDITIS; THYROID-STIMULATING HORMONE.

Arafah, Baha M., M.D. "Increased Need for Thyroxine in Women with Hypothyroidism During Estrogen Therapy." *New England Journal of Medicine* 344, no. 23 (June 7, 2001): 1,743–1,749.

Baskin, H. Jack, M.D., et al. "American Association of Clinical Endocrinologists Medical Guidelines for Clinical Practice for the Evaluation and Treatment of Hyperthyroidism and Hypothyroidism." *Endocrine*

Practice 8, no. 6 (November/December 2002): 457–469.

Daniel K. Cherry, M.S., Catharine W. Burt, and David A. Woodwell. "National Ambulatory Medical Care Survey: 2001 Summary." *Division of Health Care Statistics, Centers for Disease Control and Prevention,* no. 337, August 11, 2003.

Guha, Bhuvana, M.D., Guha Krishnaswamy, M.D., and Alan Peiris, M.D. "The Diagnosis and Management of Hypothyroidism." *Southern Medical Journal* 95, no. 5 (2002): 475–480.

Kamel, Hosam K., M.D. "Hypothyroidism in the Elderly," Available online. URL: http://www.mmhc.com/cg/articles/CG9911/kamel.html. Downloaded on November 10, 2003.

Knopp, William D., M.D., Matthew E. Bohm, M.D., and James C. McCoy, M.D. "Hypothyroidism Presenting as Tendinitis," Available online. URL: http://www.physsportsmed.com/issues/1997/01jan/knopp.htm. Downloaded on January 5, 2004.

Marlash, Cary N., M.D., and Jack H. Oppenheimer, M.D. "The Thyroid Gland," in *Endocrine Pathophysiology.* Madison, Conn.: Fence Creek Publishing, 1998, 37–59.

Toft, Andrew D., M.D. "Subclinical Hypothyroidism." *New England Journal of Medicine* 345, no. 7 (August 16, 2001): 512–516.

impaired glucose tolerance (IGT) A condition in which an individual's blood glucose levels are higher than normal but are not high enough that the person could be diagnosed as having diabetes. Former names of IGT, no longer in use (because they are inaccurate), are *borderline diabetes, subclinical diabetes, chemical diabetes,* and *latent diabetes.* More recently, the condition has become known as PREDIABETES.

Patients may go on to develop Type 2 diabetes. However, some studies have demonstrated that lifestyle changes such as weight loss, increased exercise, and decreased sugar consumption can prevent or delay the onset of diabetes. In one study, published in *The New England Journal of Medicine,* one group of individuals with impaired glucose tolerance made lifestyle changes and subsequently experienced an 11 percent incidence of diabetes. Members of the control group, who made no lifestyle changes, showed a significantly higher incidence of diabetes, 23 percent.

See also HYPERGLYCEMIA.

Davies, M. J., N. T. Raymond, J. L. Day, et al. "Impaired Glucose Tolerance and Fasting Hyperglycemia Have Different Characteristics." *Diabetes Medicine* 17, no. 6 (2000): 433–440.
Tuomilehto, Jaakko, M.D., et al. "Prevention of Type 2 Diabetes Mellitus by Changes in Lifestyle among Subjects with Impaired Glucose Tolerance." *New England Journal of Medicine* 344, no. 18 (2001): 1,343–1,350.

infants Newborn babies and children up to about age two. Even newborns can suffer from endocrine diseases and disorders (although, fortunately, such situations are rare). CONGENITAL HYPOTHYROIDISM is one endocrine disease for which newborns are screened. This disease must be diagnosed and treated as soon as possible to avoid the long-term, serious consequences of major developmental delays in the physical and intellectual functioning of the child.

Infants may also suffer from other endocrine diseases and disorders, such as TYPE 1 DIABETES. This is why newborns are carefully screened by pediatricians when born and also followed up shortly afterward. Sometimes illnesses are not immediately apparent and may be found during a routine checkup of the child by a pediatrician.

infertility The inability to create a pregnancy due to a medical problem. Infertility can be found in men and in women. Primary infertility is defined as the failure to conceive a pregnancy within one year of attempting to do so, which is a problem for 10–20 percent of couples who are actively seeking to have a child. Secondary infertility refers to infertility that occurs to couples who have borne one or more children but are now unable to achieve a pregnancy.

Many different medical reasons cause both males and females to be unable to reproduce. The key reason is age, because fertility nearly always declines with aging, particularly for women. Even women who are as young as 35 years have a significantly reduced ability to attain a pregnancy when compared with younger women. Each passing year increases a woman's risk of having a fertility problem.

Male fertility, in contrast, may continue until the male is elderly, although the odds of fathering a child generally decrease in aging men due to problems such as ERECTILE DYSFUNCTION, TYPE 2 DIABETES, hypertension, and other illnesses.

In a study among women who had sought the services of fertility clinics in 1999, published in 2001 by the Centers for Disease Control and Prevention (CDC) in the United States, researchers found that only 15.9 percent of women ages 41–42 years achieved a pregnancy, compared with 24.4 percent of women ages 38–40 years, and 31.6 percent of women ages 35–37 years. The highest success rate (37.3 percent) occurred among women younger than age 35.

These statistics are a matter of concern because many people in the United States, Canada, and other developed countries purposely delay childbearing as they concentrate on their careers. Many women and men mistakenly believe that women can easily become pregnant in their late 30s or in their 40s and are shocked to learn that they are, instead, at risk for infertility.

Causes and Treatments for
Infertility Among Women

Age is not the only factor affecting fertility. Other potential problems include endometriosis, blocked fallopian tubes, past infections that have scarred the woman's fallopian tubes, and other causes, such as hormonal imbalances: For example, undiagnosed and untreated HYPOTHYROIDISM may impair a woman's fertility. A history of amenorrhea (lack of menstrual periods) or oligomenorrhea (infrequent periods) indicate a potential underlying medical problem that physicians should investigate. The past use of intrauterine devices may also have affected a woman's fertility.

In some women, the problem lies with failed interactions in the hypothalamic-pituitary-ovarian axis, which basically means that biochemical changes that should occur do not occur. According to Dr. Eli Adashi and Dr. Jon Hennebold in their 1999 article for the New England Journal of Medicine, "The operational characteristics of the reproductive axis leave little room for error, which may explain the relatively high incidence of cycling disorders in women. Most of these are thought to be acquired disorders of suprapituitary origin, but some women may be genetically predisposed to them.

"Most genetically determined cycling disorders are of suboptimal [below normal] origin, with the ovary being the most common site of origin."

Some genetic abnormalities that may cause infertility are KALLMANN'S SYNDROME, hypergonadotropic HYPOGONADISM, CONGENITAL ADRENAL HYPERPLASIA, and MCCUNE-ALBRIGHT SYNDROME. Some women may also be resistant to FOLLICLE-STIMULATING HORMONE (FSH), LUTEINIZING HORMONE (LH), or gonadotropin-releasing hormone (GnRH).

Some women may require surgery to open blocked tubes or to correct other structural defects that are preventing a pregnancy from occurring.

In many cases, infertile women are given fertility drugs to cause the ovaries to release one or more eggs. These eggs are then harvested, and a pregnancy is created in an in vitro fertilization (IVF) procedure. Several states (Illinois, Massachusetts, and Rhode Island) have mandated that health insurance companies must cover the entire cost of IVF treatment. Five states (Arkansas, Hawaii, Maryland, Ohio, and West Virginia) require at least partial coverage.

In the other states, patients must pay for the costs of IVF treatments out of their own pockets. In an interesting study of insurance coverage and IVF outcomes, published in a 2002 issue of the New England Journal of Medicine, the pregnancy rate was found to be higher in states that did not require insurance coverage. The reasons for this are unclear but should be considered by legislators making public policy.

Because IVF is costly for most people (at least $11,000 per cycle in 2003), experts are attempting to find ways to bring down costs. According to a 2003 article in the Wall Street Journal, some fertility clinics are retrieving immature eggs even before ovulation occurs and then inducing growth in the laboratory before attempting fertilization with sperm. With this procedure, fertility drugs are not needed as part of treatment and the cost to consumers is lower than with traditional IVF.

As an aside, one problem with in vitro fertilization as well as with intracytoplasmic sperm injection is that the infants conceived in this manner have twice the risk of suffering from major birth defects, according to a 2002 issue of the New England Journal of Medicine.

Causes of Infertility Among Men

There are many causes of infertility among men. One cause is the absence of sperm (azoospermia), a problem experienced by an estimated 8 percent of infertile males, according to Dr. Victor Brugh and his colleagues in their article in a 2003 issue of *Endocrinology and Metabolism Clinics of North America.* Insufficient sperm or sperm that have poor motility (movement) are other common causes of infertility. Some men may also have scarring from sexually transmitted diseases, which impedes their fertility.

According to Dr. Brugh and his colleagues, many infertile men (as many as 20 percent) have an underlying endocrine disorder. Tests of serum testosterone and FSH can identify many abnormalities. Physicians may also test levels of LH, PROLACTIN, and estradiol. When medical problems are identified, they can often be treated. Some males have decreased testosterone-to-estradiol ratios, which can sometimes be remedied with oral aromatase inhibitor medications and thereby improve fertility.

Another common problem is varicocele, which is a dilated spermatic vein that impedes fertility. Varicocele can often be repaired by physicians. Sometimes medications such as nitrofurantoin or spironolactone can cause infertility in men by affecting their sperm count. Heavy marijuana use also impairs fertility.

Procedures such as intracytoplasmic sperm injection (ICSI) have enabled some men to overcome the problem of a low sperm count as long as they produce at least a few sperm. In this procedure, one sole sperm is injected directly into the female egg in an in vitro (outside the body) procedure. The fertilized egg is later implanted into the woman's uterus.

Some men may also suffer from chromosomal abnormalities or immunological problems that prevent them from achieving a pregnancy with their partner. Some men may need minor or more serious surgery to correct structural problems although chromosomal problems cannot be corrected.

In some cases, the cause for infertility cannot be detected or, if detected, cannot be treated with current therapies.

Joint Reasons for Infertility

Sometimes both the man and women have infertility problems, and both problems must be resolved (if possible) before the couple can have a child. For example, the man may have a low sperm count and the woman may also have endometriosis or blocked fallopian tubes. If both infertility problems are successfully corrected, then the odds of achieving a pregnancy are usually increased, although creating a pregnancy is never a certainty, even with a healthy man and woman who have no detectable medical problems.

Unknown Reasons for Infertility

In many cases, doctors can find no cause for the infertility in either the man or the woman, which is an extremely frustrating situation for both individuals and may be very hard for them to accept. Some individuals continue to seek answers for their infertility from other physicians, who also cannot find a specific cause for the infertility. Infertile couples may blame themselves or may blame each other. The situation can become extremely stressful, straining their relationship. In such cases, a skilled and sympathetic counselor may be effective at pointing out the flaws in their thinking and helping them to accept their situation.

If Pregnancy Is Not Possible

Although some couples who are infertile choose to remain childless, other couples decide to adopt a baby or older child and later say they wonder what took them so long to make this decision. They may adopt a child from the United States or from another country. (Interestingly, studies have shown that only about 15 percent of couples who adopt children later have a biological child, contrary to popular rumors that adopting a child somehow makes infertile couples fertile.)

Still other couples or individuals hire a surrogate to carry a child. The pregnancy may be created from a husband's sperm or donor sperm and the surrogate's ovum. Sometimes the embryo is derived from both the sperm of a husband and the ovum of a wife. In other cases, neither partner has a genetic relationship to the baby that the surrogate is carrying. Laws on surrogacy vary drastically from state to state, and some states do not address the issue. Infertile individuals considering surrogacy should be very familiar with their state laws before choosing this option.

See also FEMALE REPRODUCTION; FERTILITY; MALE REPRODUCTION; REPRODUCTIVE ENDOCRINOLOGY.

For further information on resolving infertility, contact the following organizations:

American Fertility Association
666 Fifth Avenue
Suite 278
New York, NY 10103
(888) 917-3777 (toll-free)
http://www.theafa.org

American Society for Reproductive Medicine
1209 Montgomery Highway
Birmingham, AL 35216
(205) 978-5000
http://www.asrm.org

RESOLVE: The National Infertility Association
7910 Woodmont Avenue
Suite 1350
Bethesda, MD 20814
(301) 652-8585
http://www.resolve.org

Adashi, Eli Y., M.D., and Jon D. Ahennebold. "Single-Gene Mutations Resulting in Reproductive Dysfunction in Women." *New England Journal of Medicine* 340, no. 9 (1999): 709–718.

Brugh, Victor M., III, M.D., H. Merrill Matschke, M.D., and Larry I. Lipshultz, M.D. "Male Factor Infertility." *Endocrinology and Metabolism Clinics of North America* 32, no. 3 (2003): 689–707.

Guzick, David S., M.D. "Sperm Morphology, Motility, and Concentration in Fertile and Infertile Men." *New England Journal of Medicine* 345, no. 19 (November 8, 2001): 1,388–1,393.

Hansen, Michele, et al. "The Risk of Major Birth Defects After Intracytoplasmic Sperm Injection and In Vitro Fertilization." *New England Journal of Medicine* 346, no. 10 (March 7, 2002): 725–730.

Jain, Tarun, M.D., Bernard L. Harlow, and Mark D. Hornstein, M.D. "Insurance Coverage and Outcomes of In Vitro Fertilization." *New England Journal of Medicine* 347, no. 9 (August 29, 2002): 661–666.

Marcus, Amy Dockser. "Finding a Cheaper Way to Make a Baby." *Wall Street Journal* (March 6, 2004): D1.

United States Department of Health and Human Services, Atlanta, Georgia, Division of Reproductive Health, National Center for Chronic Disease Prevention and Health Promotion. Centers for Disease Control and Prevention. *1999 Assisted Reproductive Technology Success Rates: National Summary and Fertility Clinic Reports.* December 2001.

insulin   A protein hormone normally produced by the beta cells, specifically in the islets of Langerhans in the pancreas. All individuals with TYPE 1 DIABETES (and some individuals with long-term Type 2 diabetes as well) must inject insulin in order to live. Insulin is secreted into the bloodstream in response to changes in ambient blood glucose levels as well as in response to ingested nutrients, specifically carbohydrates and proteins. In an individual with normal pancreatic physiology, insulin is cosecreted with amylin, while at the same time glucagons and other hormone levels decrease.

The insulin first travels to the liver via the portal vein, where it decreases the amount of glucose that the liver is secreting into the bloodstream. Insulin helps the amino acids that are extracted from dietary proteins assimilate into new proteins. It also helps store the breakdown of ingested fats into triglycerides. Inadequate insulin will lead to increases in blood glucose levels (HYPERGLYCEMIA), and excess insulin will lead to low blood glucose levels (HYPOGLYCEMIA). On very rare occasions, the pancreas can form tumors, called INSULINOMAS, that secrete excess insulin.

Insulin was discovered in 1921 by Dr. Frederick Banting and Mr. Charles Best (a medical student at the time) in Canada. Their breakthrough finding enabled many patients with Type 1 diabetes to lead normal lives rather than dying young, as was the inevitable outcome for patients before then.

Today many different types of insulin preparations are available, including rapid-acting, short-acting, intermediate-acting, long-acting, and very long-acting. In addition, some forms may be combined into one injection. As of this writing, all of the available insulins are recombinant human insulins that are made synthetically. Compared with the previously available beef and pork insulins, they are more pure and begin to work more quickly, but they also do not last quite as long as the previous types.

Although these synthetic forms of insulin are very similar to the endogenous insulin made by the pancreas itself, all patients who have been taking insulin for a significant length of time will develop some antibodies to the insulin, which may decrease its efficacy slightly. Usually these antibodies do not cause clinically significant problems.

As of this writing, insulin is either injected subcutaneously by the patient, using a syringe or pen device, or administered via a catheter attached to an insulin pump. In addition, a variety of inhaled insulin preparations are being studied. These inhalers are similar to but more sophisticated than those currently used to deliver asthma drugs into the lungs.

See also BASAL-BOLUS THERAPY.

insulinoma A tumor, usually benign, of the insulin-secreting cells that lie within the pancreas. About 5–10 percent of all insulinomas are malignant tumors. Insulinomas cause an excessive production of insulin, which can lead to HYPOGLYCEMIA. The hypoglycemia may range from mild to severe. Insulinomas are also called islet cells adenomas. They occur in only about one in 250,000 individuals. People with MULTIPLE ENDOCRINE NEO-PLASIA, Type 1 (MEN 1) have an increased risk for developing insulinomas.

Some key indicators of the presence of an insulinoma are the following symptoms:

- Rapid heart rate
- Sweating
- Headache
- Confusion
- Dizziness
- Loss of consciousness
- Anxiety

Most of these indicators are the signs and symptoms of hypoglycemia. Patients with postprandial (after-eating) hypoglycemia, anxiety, depression, HYPERTHYROIDISM, cardiac irregularities, and other conditions, may show the same symptoms. The key difference is that when these indicators occur only or mainly in the morning prior to eating, hypoglycemia and possibly insulinoma should be suspected.

Because these symptoms may occur with many other conditions, physicians must further investigate with tests. A low blood glucose level and a

INSULIN FORMS AND SPEED AND LENGTH OF ACTION

	When Insulin Begins to Work	PEAK Effect	Typical Length of Effect
Rapid			
Lispro* (Humalog)	15 minutes	1 hour	3–5 hours
Aspart (Novolog)	15 minutes	1 hour	3–5 hours
Short			
Regular* (Humulin and Novolin)	45 minutes	2–3 hours	5–8 hours
Intermediate			
NPH* (Humulin and Novolin)	2–4 hours	4–10 hours	10–16 hours
Lente* (Novolin and Humolin)	3–4 hours	4–12 hours	12–18 hours
Long			
Ultralente (Humulin)	6–8 hours	10–18 hours	16–24 hours
Glargine† (Lantus)	2–4 hours	No peak	20–26 hours

* Also available in pen devices.
† Glargine is an acidic insulin that cannot be combined with other insulins.

Premixed Forms of Insulin

70/30 Insulin* (Humulin and Novolin)	70% NPH/30% Regular
75/25 Insulin* (Humulin)	75% Neutral protamine lispro/25% lispro
50/50 Insulin (Humulin)	50% NPH/50% Regular

* Available in pen devices.
Note: Onset, peak, and length of effects are significantly affected by injection site, activity, smoking, kidney function, and a variety of other factors.

high blood insulin level, as well as a high C-peptide level, can all indicate the possible presence of an insulinoma. If the ratio of insulin to glucose is inappropriate and an insulinoma is suspected, imaging studies may then be undertaken.

Typically, COMPUTERIZED TOMOGRAPHY (CT) or a MAGNETIC RESONANCE IMAGING (MRI) is used to localize the tumor. In some cases, such as when a CT scan or MRI do not show any tumor but the physician is still concerned that one may be present, pancreatic arteriography may also be performed. In this procedure, a small catheter is threaded into the arteries supplying the pancreas, and intravenous contrast is given to image the pancreas carefully, section by section. In some cases, the tumor cannot be localized preoperatively and the surgeon will palpate the pancreas at surgery to locate the tumor.

If a patient is diagnosed with an insulinoma, the treatment is usually surgery. Patients who have multiple tumors may need a partial pancreatectomy. Doctors try to leave at least 15 percent of the pancreas intact so that it can continue to create the pancreatic enzymes needed to digest food. If no tumor is found or if surgery would be dangerous for an individual patient, the physician may order medication such as diazoxide (Acetazolamide) to decrease insulin secretion and, in turn, to reverse hypoglycemia. In some cases, another medication known as octreotide is given to decrease insulin production.

insulin resistance   A condition in which the pancreas produces sufficient insulin but the patient's body is unable to use it. If insulin resistance levels should worsen, the condition will be diagnosed as Type 2 diabetes. Insulin resistance may be a problem for years before the insulin resistance and/or diabetes is actually diagnosed. Insulin resistance does not always proceed to diabetes, although it increases the risk of developing diabetes in future years. The problem of insulin resistance is worsened in large part by both obesity and the lack of sufficient physical activity. Some researchers have also found that prediabetic insulin resistance tends to be much higher among smokers.

Both women and men experience insulin resistance. Women with insulin resistance have a greater risk for developing POLYCYSTIC OVARY SYNDROME (PCOS). It is also important to note that birth control pills may increase insulin resistance. This is especially true for progesterone-only contraceptives.

If a person has a genetic predisposition to developing Type 2 diabetes (that is, if an individual has a parent or sibling who has diabetes) and if he or she already has insulin resistance, some medications may cause diabetes. Some examples of medications that may induce diabetes include:

- Glucocorticoids
- Nicotinic acid/niacin (generally has a small effect)
- Alpha-adrenergic agonists
- Thiazides that cause low potassium levels
- Dilantin (this rarely induces diabetes)
- Pentamidine
- Interferon alpha therapy
- Diazoxide

Diagnosis and Treatment

If a patient has PREDIABETES, which means that oral glucose tolerance tests and other tests show levels that are not high enough to indicate diabetes but are above normal, most physicians will urge the patient to exercise and to lose weight if obesity is a problem. Some physicians will prescribe low doses of medications in an effort to avert the development of diabetes, although studies have not shown this to be efficacious.

See also OBESITY.

Facchini, Francesco S., et al. "Insulin Resistance as a Predictor of Age-Related Diseases." *Journal of Clinical Endocrinology & Metabolism* 86, no. 8 (August 2001): 3,574–3,578.

Matthaei, Stephan, et al. "Pathophysiology and Pharmacological Treatment of Insulin Resistance." *Endocrine Reviews* 21, no. 6 (2000): 585–618.

Petit, William A. Jr., and Christine Adamec. *The Encyclopedia of Diabetes.* New York: Facts On File, Inc., 2002.

insulin resistance syndrome The metabolic syndrome that may exist when a person is resistant to the hormonal effects of insulin. The characteristic components of this syndrome—insulin resistance, diabetes, hypertension, and dyslipidemia—are also known as the deadly quartet. Insulin resistance syndrome is also called metabolic syndrome, metabolic-cardiovascular syndrome, and syndrome X. (A variant form of angina pectoris is also known as syndrome X.)

Insulin resistance syndrome is always modulated by OBESITY. The more obese the person is, the worse the insulin resistance. This is most true of abdominal obesity, specifically visceral abdominal obesity (fat that is within the abdominal cavity as opposed to being purely subcutaneous). An extreme example of such a case would be a person who is at a normal body weight but has increased abdominal fat and insulin resistance. People with this syndrome are also at high risk for developing abnormal clotting in blood vessels that may contribute to atherosclerosis, heart attacks, or stroke.

The national Cholesterol Education Program's Adult Treatment Panel III suggests that any person with three of five risk factors can be clinically diagnosed with insulin resistance syndrome. These factors include:

- Waist circumference of greater than 40 inches in men and greater than 35 inches in women

- Triglyceride levels greater than or equal to 150 mg/dl

- High-density lipoprotein (HDL) levels less than 40 mg/dl in men and less than or equal to 50 in women

- Blood pressure that is greater than or equal to 130/85 mm Hg

- Glucose levels greater than 100 mg/dl

When applying these criteria to a survey of nearly 9,000 adults, the prevalence of insulin resistance syndrome was found to be 22 percent in all adults and as high as 43.5 percent in those ages 60–69 years.

Doctors strongly recommend that patients with insulin resistance syndrome begin a program of proper medical nutrition and exercise, leading to weight loss to decrease their risk of complications.

As of this writing, no single drug is approved to treat all of the components of insulin resistance syndrome. Yet there are plenty of data to suggest that the medication metformin (Glucophage, Glucophage-XR) will indirectly help decrease the insulin resistance. The medication's specific cellular and biochemical actions cause changes that lead to decreased insulin resistance. In addition, two thiazolidinedione drugs, rosiglitazone (Avandia) and pioglitazone (Actos), will decrease insulin resistance directly. These medications directly cause biochemical and cellular changes that decrease the resistance to insulin. Several studies have shown that these drugs will also decrease the risk of developing overt diabetes mellitus. Many pharmaceutical companies are actively working to develop newer versions of these drugs that will treat/prevent diabetes and also slow or prevent atherosclerosis.

Insulin resistance syndrome is to be distinguished from the clinical issue of resistance to insulin. About 80–95 percent of all patients with Type 2 diabetes have at least some insulin resistance and as it increases, they require more therapy in the form of large doses of oral medications or increased dosages of insulin.

The medication's specific cellular and biochemical actions cause changes that lead to decreased insulin resistance. In addition, there is an extremely rare syndrome where patients develop antibodies to insulin and/or to the insulin receptor and require tremendously high doses of insulin (such as thousands of units of insulin per day). Interestingly, they do not die, and sometimes their condition improves. There are so few of such patients that little is known about their natural history.

See also CHOLESTEROL; HYPERLIPIDEMIA; INSULIN RESISTANCE; PREDIABETES.

iodine-induced thyrotoxocosis Extreme output of thyroid hormone caused by an individual ingesting high levels of iodine. This is a rare condition.

See also THYROTOXICOSIS.

Joslin Diabetes Center A prestigious, nonprofit diabetes treatment, research, and educational institution affiliated with Harvard Medical School. The Joslin Diabetes Center specializes in treating patients with diabetes and performing leading-edge research on both diabetes treatment and prevention. It is the largest single organization in the United States devoting its energies and efforts solely to diabetes research and care. The Joslin Diabetes Center provides comprehensive clinic services for patients with diabetes, including endocrinology, ophthalmology, nephrology, pediatric endocrinology, obstetrics, mental health, nutrition, and exercise physiology.

The Joslin Center was originally formed in 1898 by Elliott P. Joslin, M.D., a noted Boston physician and author dedicated to treating diabetes. Today the Joslin Diabetes Center has affiliates throughout the United States.

For more information, contact the Joslin Diabetes Center:

One Joslin Place
Boston, MA 02215
(617) 732-2415
http://www.joslin.harvard.edu

Affiliates to Joslin Diabetes Center are as follows:

California

University of California–Irvine
Gohschalk Medical Plaza
Irvine, CA 92697
(949) 824-8656

Connecticut

Lawrence & Memorial Hospital
14 Clara Drive
Suite 4
Mystic, CT 06355
(860) 245-0565

Lawrence & Memorial Hospital
50 Faire Harbor Place
Suite 2E
New London, CT 06320
(877) JOSLIN-1

New Britain General Hospital
100 Grand Street
New Britain, CT 06050
(888) 4-JOSLIN (toll-free)

Florida

Morton Plant Hospital
455 Pinellas Street
Clearwater, FL 33756
(727) 461-8300

Indiana

Floyd Memorial Hospital & Health Services
1850 State Street
New Albany, IN 47150
(812) 949-5700

St. Mary's Medical Center
3700 Washington Avenue
Evansville, IN 47750
(812) 485-1814

Maryland

North Arundel Hospital
301 Hospital Drive
Glen Burnie, MD 21042
(410) 787-4940

University of Maryland Medical System
22 South Greene Street
N6W100
Baltimore, MD 21201
(410) 328-6584

Massachusetts

Anna Jaques Hospital
25 Highland Avenue
Newburyport, MA 01950
(978) 463-1344

New York

Arnot Health
HCGW
600 Fitch Street
Suites 202-203
Elmira, NY 14905
(607) 737-8107

SUNY Upstate Medical University
90 Presidential Plaza
Syracuse, NY 13202
(315) 464-5726

Pennsylvania

Forbes Regional Hospital
Forbes LifeStyle Center
Professional Office Building 2
2580 Haymaker Road
Suite 403
Monroeville, PA 15146
(412) 858-4474

Western Pennsylvania Hospital
5140 Liberty Avenue
Pittsburgh, PA 15224
(412) 578-1724

South Carolina

Prevecare
234 Seven Farms Drive
Daniels Island
Charleston, SC 29492
(843) 576-3700

Washington

Swedish Medical Center
910 Boylston Avenue
Seattle, WA 98104
(206) 215-2440

West Virginia

St. Mary's Medical Center
2900 First Avenue
Huntington, WV 25702
(304) 526-8363

juvenile diabetes   A term once used to describe what is now called TYPE 1 DIABETES. The name was changed to avoid confusion, because juvenile diabetes is also found in many adults. The disease may be diagnosed in childhood or adolescence, or it may not be diagnosed until early adulthood and sometimes later. It continues on throughout the individual's life, requiring lifelong treatment.

Kallmann's syndrome (KS)   A condition that results from a deficiency of gonadatropin-releasing hormone (GnRH) from the hypothalamus and that is associated with anosmia (loss of the sense of smell). Without the anosmia, the condition is called idiopathic hypogonadatropic hypogonadism.

The GnRH deficiency stems from a congenital defect in neurons in the hypothalamus that lead to a deficiency of GnRH. As a result, the pituitary gland secretes decreased amounts of LUTEINIZING HORMONE (LH) and FOLLICLE-STIMULATING HORMONE (FSH), leading to testosterone deficiency, INFERTILITY, and ERECTILE DYSFUNCTION. About one-third of the cases of KS are inherited, while the remaining cases appear to be caused by genetic mutations. An estimated one in 10,000 males and one in 50,000 females are affected.

Kallmann's syndrome is the most common cause of secondary HYPOGONADISM. The syndrome was named after F. J. Kallmann. In 1944, Kallmann and his colleagues reported in the *American Journal of Mental Deficiency* about families in which many members had delayed or absent puberty (eunuchoidism), anosmia, and color blindness. Kallmann noted that some of the individuals with the syndrome were also developmentally delayed (in the past known as mentally retarded).

Signs and Symptoms

DELAYED PUBERTY is a common feature of this syndrome. Males with Kallmann's syndrome may have an extremely small penis (MICROPENIS) as well as undescended testicles (cryptorchism). On occasion, patients will begin puberty but fail to mature completely.

Boys will also have decreased muscle strength and will not be as aggressive as the average male with normal testosterone levels. Males may have a high-pitched voice and lack facial hair. Underarm (axillary) hair may be scanty. Pubic hair may begin to develop due to the presence of adrenal androgens. Usually the testicles are very small, one to two cubic centimeters. On occasion, they may be as large as 12–15 cubic centimeters if any pubertal development occurred. Patients with Kallmann's syndrome who have normal testes and spermatozoa are referred to as fertile eunuchs. Typically there is no GYNECOMASTIA (breast swelling) due to the low levels of estrogen in men.

Females with Kallmann's syndrome may be deficient in estrogen, causing primary amenorrhea in girls. If untreated, this estrogen deficiency may in the clinical course of the condition cause HOT FLASHES, OSTEOPOROSIS, and painful intercourse (dyspareunia) due to insufficient vaginal lubrication. The vagina may be a darker red than is found in women without KS.

Other abnormalities associated with Kallmann's syndrome are cleft lip or cleft palate and hearing loss. In children who have Kallmann's syndrome, the kidneys may fail to develop (renal agenesis), and some patients may become obese. In severe cases, patients have skeletal abnormalities. Patients may also have congenital heart disease. Most patients with KS are infertile, although fertility may be regained with medical treatment.

Some patients with KS have unusually long arms that are five centimeters or greater than normal (eunuchoidal). This is due to the delayed closure of their growth plates (epiphyses) during puberty. Their height is usually normal for their age despite the lack of pubertal development.

Diagnosis and Treatment

Patients with Kallmann's syndrome are diagnosed based on their signs and symptoms, but obviously, diagnosing the condition is easier if there is any family history of KS. Blood tests of testosterone levels (serum testosterone) will reveal extremely low testosterone levels in males, while serum estradiol will be extremely low in females with KS. A MAGNETIC RESONANCE IMAGING (MRI) scan of the skull will reveal the presence of abnormal olfactory systems, a very common condition among as many as 75 percent of patients with KS.

Other tests that may be performed include a dual-energy X-ray absorptiometry (DEXA) scan to determine if the patient has osteoporosis and an echocardiogram to identify the presence of congenital heart disease.

Patients with KS are usually treated with hormone replacement therapy to restore normal secondary sexual characteristics and fertility and to normalize bone and muscle mass. Males are treated with testosterone replacement and females with estradiol replacement. In women, estrogen is given alone initially, to maximize breast development, and progestational agents are added later. When fertility is desired, GnRH can be used in men and women, although in men, often human chorionic gonadatropin (HCG) is used, followed by FSH.

If other conditions are present (such as osteoporosis, heart disease, and so forth), those medical problems are treated.

See also KLINEFELTER SYNDROME.

Tritos, Nicholas A., M.D. "Kallmann Syndrome and Idiopathic Hypogonadotropic Hypogonadism," Available online. URL: http://www.emedicine.com/med/topic1216.htm Downloaded on December 15, 2003.

Wynbrandt, James, and Mark D. Ludman. *The Encyclopedia of Genetic Disorders and Birth Defects,* 2d ed. New York: Facts On File, Inc., 2000.

Klinefelter syndrome   An extra X chromosome that occurs in about one in 1,000 baby boys. There can be multiple X chromosomes. The greater the number of X chromosomes present, the more the physical abnormalities. Patients with Klinefelter syndrome usually develop HYPOGONADISM and INFERTILITY due to the absence of sperm in the semen (azoospermia) and other health problems.

Dr. Harry Klinefelter first identified the condition in 1942.

Signs and Symptoms

The key feature for virtually all patients with Klinefelter syndrome is small and firm testes. Patients may also have GYNECOMASTIA (enlarged breasts), which is present in 50–75 percent of patients; decreased pubic hair (40–60 percent of patients); and decreased facial hair (60–80 percent). A small penis (MICROPENIS) is present in about 10–25 percent of these patients. Patients with Klinefelter syndrome do not undergo the normal changes of male puberty. Nearly 100 percent are infertile. They also have decreased muscle mass in comparison with their peers. Some males with Klinefelter syndrome are taller than average.

Associated Illnesses

Patients with Klinefelter syndrome have a high risk of developing tumors. Some experts believe that the disease itself may be caused by a tumor. Although breast cancer is rare among men, patients with Klinefelter syndrome have a 20 times greater risk of developing breast cancer than do other men. However, experts say that screening mammography for men with Klinefelter syndrome is not usually recommended since the occurrence of breast cancer is still extremely rare.

Men with Klinefelter syndrome have an increased risk for developing autoimmune disorders, such as rheumatoid arthritis, systemic lupus erythematous, and Sjögren's syndrome. Androgens may be protective against autoimmune disorders. Since men with Klinefelter syndrome have low levels of testosterone, this may be the reason for their greater incidence of autoimmune diseases. Another possible cause may be lymphocyte abnormalities found in these patients.

Patients with Klinefelter syndrome have an increased risk of learning disabilities such as dyslexia and attention deficit disorder. They may also exhibit psychiatric problems such as anxiety disorder, depression, and even psychotic disorders. Boys with Klinefelter syndrome have difficulty with peer groups and are less interested in girls than other boys. Said authors Cynthia Smyth and William Bremner in their 1998 article on

Klinefelter syndrome in *Archives of Internal Medicine,* "The combination of feminine physical features, poor motor coordination, and difficulties in speech and memory probably impairs the attainment of adequate self-esteem, increases anxiety, and promotes insecurity." Testosterone treatment may lead to improvement of the patient's self-esteem.

Because of their androgen deficiency, patients with Klinefelter syndrome are also at an increased risk for developing OSTEOPOROSIS. Testosterone replacement decreases the risk for osteoporosis, especially when it occurs before the male is age 20.

Klinefelter syndrome also increases the risk for endocrine disorders such as DIABETES MELLITUS, although it is usually a mild form of TYPE 2 DIABETES. HYPOTHYROIDISM may be present in some patients.

Varicose veins are common in patients with Klinefelter syndrome. In one study, 20 percent of 104 patients had varicose veins. Patients also experience 10–20 times the risk of venous ulcers and a higher-than-normal risk for pulmonary embolism and deep venous thrombosis.

An estimated 40 percent of patients with Klinefelter syndrome have dental abnormalities, which can be identified with dental X-rays and treated.

Diagnosis and Treatment

Patients with Klinefelter syndrome are diagnosed based upon their medical history as well as on their signs and symptoms. Laboratory tests will also reveal elevated gonadotropin levels and decreased testosterone levels in most patients.

The treatment is usually testosterone replacement therapy. This will not make the man fertile, but it will improve many problems. It will increase the facial and body hair, redistribute body fat, improve sexual desire and ability, improve bone mineral density, and reduce the risk for psychiatric problems. These virilizing changes will usually also improve self-esteem. In general, testosterone replacement therapy is started early in puberty or around age 12 and must continue for the patient's life. Most patients receive testosterone injections, although testosterone creams are also available, as are transdermal skin patches.

See also DELAYED PUBERTY; HERMAPHRODITISM; KALLMAN'S SYNDROME.

Kurzrock, Eric A., et al. "Klinefelter Syndrome and Precocious Puberty: A Harbinger for Tumor." *Urology* 60, no. 3 (2002): 515xiv–515xv.

Smyth, Cynthia M., M.D., and William J. Bremner, M.D. "Klinefelter Syndrome." *Archives of Internal Medicine* 158, no. 12 (June 22, 1998): 1,309–1,314.

levothyroxine A synthetic formulation of thyroid hormone, albeit structurally the same as the molecule made by the thyroid gland, and used primarily to treat individuals with HYPOTHYROIDISM due to all causes (autoimmune hypothyroidism, surgical hypothyroidism, destructive and medication-induced hypothyroidism). Levothyroxine is also called T4 because of the four iodine molecules attached to the tyrosine rings, in contrast to triiodothyronine or T3, in which only three iodine molecules are present.

The usual replacement dosage for a person with no thyroid function is about 2 mcg/kg/day, or about 150 mcg per day in a person weighing 150 pounds (70 kg). The dosage is typically titrated to a thyroid-stimulating hormone (TSH) level of between 0.5 and 2.0 microunits per ml.

The three market leaders of levothyroxine medications in the United States in 2003 were Synthroid, Levoxyl, and generic levothyroxine. These medications had combined sales of over a billion dollars in 2003, and the largest seller was Synthroid, at over $500 million. According to the Centers for Disease Control and Prevention, Synthroid was the seventh most popular of all drugs prescribed to patients during office visits in 2001.

Some patients also take desiccated thyroid hormone extract, which is obtained from pig thyroid glands. Until the late 20th century, this extract was the dominant form of medication for people with hypothyroidism.

Levothyroxine is also used to attempt to suppress thyroid nodules and goiters. The exogenous thyroid hormone that is given increases the levels of hormone in the bloodstream and then decreases the secretion of thyrotropin-releasing hormone (TRH) from the hypothalamus and the secretion of TSH from the pituitary gland. A similar plan is followed with patients who have THYROID CANCER. Levothyroxine is given to the individuals to suppress the secretion of TSH completely with the hopes that if any thyroid cancer cells have been left behind, the lack of TSH will keep them from growing any further.

Lugol's solution A 5 percent iodine and 10 percent potassium iodide solution that is used in three situations, as follows:

1. To block iodine uptake into the thyroid gland transiently in a patient with HYPOTHYROIDISM.
2. To help decrease the blood flow in a thyroid gland just prior to thyroid surgery.
3. To block the thyroid gland during a radiation emergency, blocking radioactive iodine from entering the thyroid gland.

Lugol's solution is also used (in unlabeled uses, that is, not specifically approved for the purpose by the Food and Drug Administration, although doctors may order it) as an expectorant and as a dermatologic treatment to treat Sweet's disease (acute neutrophic dermatosis). It is also sometimes used to treat lymphocutaneous sporotrichosis, a fungal disease.

luteinizing hormone (LH) An important hormone for both men and women, produced by the anterior pituitary. Luteinizing hormone affects the synthesis and release of hormones of the ovaries and the testes, such as estrogen, progesterone, and testosterone. It also affects the synthesis and release of eggs or sperm that are released to create a pregnancy. Luteinizing hormone is also called interstitial cell-stimulating hormone (ICSH).

LH is secreted in a pulsatile fashion. In spite of this, the normal levels in men fall within a fairly narrow range. As with all pituitary hormones, the LH level must be interpreted in the context of the associated testosterone level or semen analysis. In women, marked variations in LH secretion occur throughout the menstrual cycle. Physicians must therefore interpret a woman's LH levels within the context of the specific time of her cycle as well as consider her concomitant estradiol levels.

Luteinizing hormone is involved in a complex FEEDBACK LOOP between the gonad (ovary or testicle), the pituitary gland, and the hypothalamus. For example, during a woman's menstrual cycle, blood LH levels increase, and this, in turn, causes the ovary to produce estradiol. When estradiol levels reach a certain point within the body, the estradiol and the gonadotropin-releasing hormone (GnRH) cause a sharp increase in LH production (the preovulatory surge). This increase causes ovulation to occur. The LH levels reach a certain point, and then they decline.

When women go through menopause, they may experience periodic HOT FLASHES, which are surges of luteinizing hormone in the bloodstream. HORMONE REPLACEMENT THERAPY (HRT) may resolve this symptom, although each woman should discuss with her own gynecologist whether or not to take HRT.

Deficiencies of LH in women of childbearing age or in men may cause INFERTILITY. If estradiol or testosterone levels are low and a concomitant measure of LH is also low, this indicates a possible hypothalamic or pituitary problem. If so, individuals who wish to have children may be treated with hormones, such as luteinizing hormone-releasing hormone (LHRH). Sometimes LH is very low or altogether absent, as in conditions such as hypogonadotropic HYPOGONADISM, KALLMANN'S SYNDROME, or other forms of secondary hypogonadism.

Tumors that secrete excessive amounts of LH are rare. However, inappropriate levels of LH in the blood are seen in a condition called POLYCYSTIC OVARY SYNDROME.

Medical science has enabled doctors to manipulate LH production to the ends of patients. For example, ORAL CONTRACEPTIVES block the LH surge that precedes the release of an egg and thus prevent pregnancy.

See also FOLLICLE-STIMULATING HORMONE.

Griffin, James E., and Ojeda, Sergio R. *Textbook of Endocrine Physiology,* 4th ed. New York: Oxford University Press, 2000.

macrocephaly An unusually large head of a newborn infant. The macrocephaly may be due to an increased brain volume (megencephaly), increased cerebrospinal fluid (hydrocephalus), or bony/vascular enlargement. Large heads are also characteristic of some endocrine disorders. For example, dwarfing syndromes may cause large heads that are disproportionate to the size of the individual's body.

Other causes of macrocephaly include HYPO-PARATHYROIDISM, ADRENAL INSUFFICIENCY, hyperphosphatasia, osteopetrosis (an extremely rare condition inherited by infants that causes dense bones that break easily because of micro-architectural abnormalities), RICKETS, or OSTEOGENESIS IMPERFECTA. Steroid therapy in the mother may also cause macrocephaly in the child that she bears.

See also MICROCEPHALY.

magnetic resonance imaging (MRI) A diagnostic scanning device that uses a magnetic field to form an image of the interior organs being studied. Many physicians use this tool to help with diagnosing a broad array of diseases, ranging from cancer to fractures. It is the imaging test of choice for the PITUITARY GLAND and the HYPOTHALAMUS.

The MRI test is usually painless. On occasion, a nonradioactive element called gadolinium is injected intravenously.

Most scanners are closed, and thus the patient is enclosed in a small chamber that to some patients feels like a tomb. Patients who are claustrophobic have difficulty with undergoing an MRI scan. However, the administration of a drug like diazepam (Valium) about an hour or so beforehand usually calms such fears. Some scanners are open, but these are generally more costly and less preva-

lent, and a patient's health insurance may not provide coverage for the open MRI.

See also COMPUTERIZED TOMOGRAPHY.

male reproduction The ability of a male, with a female, to create a pregnancy and a child. Male reproduction is complex and involves many different factors, such as testosterone production, the durability and presence of sufficient sperm, as well as the health of the sperm. A couple that is unable to create a pregnancy after a year of unprotected intercourse is generally diagnosed with infertility. Initially, whether the cause lies with the female or male or if factors within each person are impairing fertility is usually unknown.

Physicians who are experts in fertility, including obstetricians, urologists, and endocrinologists, can often assist couples in creating a pregnancy, although no doctor can issue a guarantee to any patient. Even healthy individuals with no medical problems sometimes cannot bear children and doctors are unable to determine any underlying cause. This is called unexplained infertility. However, the cause may be a relatively minor problem that is readily resolved. In addition, infertility may also indicate a serious health problem that is present in the male or female, and thus, physicians should investigate it.

Aging decreases male fertility, although it does not end fertility, as it does with females who have undergone menopause. In at least half of all the cases of a couple who are unable to conceive a child together, there is some element of male infertility. In an estimated 30 percent of cases, the infertility is solely caused by a problem with the male. At age 20, there is about a 6 percent rate of male infertility among couples who are unable to conceive, which increases to 64 percent by the ages of 40–44 years.

In a study of 708 infertile couples in England, 28 percent had idiopathic infertility and 24 percent of the cases were caused by male factors. According to Dr. Victor Brugh and his colleagues in their 2003 article on male infertility for *Endocrinology and Metabolism Clinics of North America,* at least 20 percent of infertile men have an underlying endocrine disorder. Laboratory tests of TESTOSTERONE and FOLLICLE-STIMULATING HORMONE (FSH) levels can identify the disorder in nearly all men.

The first analysis, which is nearly always done in a man suspected of infertility, is the semen analysis. After refraining from sexual activities for two to three days, the man masturbates and produces a semen sample. Doctors will then check the semen for the absence of sperm (azoospermia), a problem that about 8 percent of infertile males experience. A sperm count greater than 48 million per milliliter with greater than 63 percent motility is considered a fertile count. For men with low sperm counts, intrauterine insemination of the woman will increase the chance of conceiving.

The physical examination and other tests may reveal other underlying problems. For example, some men (from 19–41 percent of infertile males) have developed varicocele, which is dilated veins that impede fertility, although experts disagree on exactly how they prevent fertility. Repair of the varicocele may improve fertility as well as the quality of the semen.

Some men have disorders producing or secreting hormones, such as gonadatropin-releasing hormone (GRH), luteinizing hormone, or follicle-stimulating hormone. Others have genetic disorders, such as KALLMANN'S SYNDROME, that can be treated with hormonal injections.

Disorders of the pituitary can lead to infertility, such as a tumor in the pituitary gland. Surgery or radiation of the tumor may lead to improved fertility.

Many medications can impair fertility in men, such as calcium channel blockers, beta-blockers, tricyclic antidepressants, tetracycline, nitrofurantoin, and other drugs. In addition, illegal drugs such as cocaine and marijuana are known to decrease sperm production. Alcohol can also impede sufficient sperm production.

Some men have disorders of ejaculation, such as retrograde ejaculation, in which the semen goes the wrong way. This disorder may be treated medically or surgically, depending on the patient.

For couples considering intracytoplasmic sperm injection, genetic studies are performed to check for Y chromosome abnormalities.

See also FEMALE REPRODUCTION; HYPOGONADISM; INFERTILITY.

Brugh, Victor M., III, M.D., H. Merrill Matschke, M.D., and Larry I. Lipshultz, M.D. "Male Factor Infertility." *Endocrinology and Metabolism Clinics of North America* 32, no. 3 (2003): 689–707.
Hull, M. G., et al. "Population Study of Causes, Treatment, and Outcome of Infertility." *British Medical Journal* 291, no. 6510 (1985): 1,693–1,697.

malnutrition   Very serious condition in which an individual's daily caloric intake is so low that if it is not increased soon, he or she will die. The condition may be caused by a disease, such as hepatitis, cirrhosis of the liver, or CANCER. It may also be caused by poverty and/or famine. Malnutrition may sometimes be caused by the inability of an individual (a child or an elderly person) to feed himself when others fail to provide food or purposely withhold it. In some cases, people with eating disorders such as ANOREXIA NERVOSA develop malnutrition and may actually starve themselves to death.

Marfan's syndrome   A genetic disorder that affects the cardiovascular, ocular, and skeletal systems. Marfan's syndrome was named after its discoverer, French pediatrician Bernard-Jean Antonin Marfan, who first identified the syndrome in 1896. This medical condition is very rare. Individuals with Marfan's syndrome should avoid competitive sports because the strain on their hearts from such vigorous activity could be life-threatening. Marfan's syndrome may cause an early death from aneurysm or heart disease. In some cases, HOMOCYSTINURIA may be mistaken for Marfan's syndrome.

Characteristic traits of individuals with Marfan's syndrome may include the following:

- Very long arms, legs, and fingers that are spider-like and disproportionate to the patient's height

- Joints that are hypermobile (can bend beyond the span of most people)
- Spinal curvature (scoliosis)
- Protruding or indented breastbone (pectus carinatum and excavatum)
- Presence of mitral valve prolapse, a serious heart condition that can cause heart arrhythmias, infections of the heart valve, and even death (this condition is treatable if identified)

Treatment

Studies have indicated that replacement of the aortic root in the heart can successfully decrease the risk of heart disease in patients with Marfan's syndrome. Because of the high risk of heart disease in patients with Marfan's, patients with this syndrome should probably have the surgery even before they show any signs of either heart disease or aneurysm.

In a 1999 issue of the *New England Journal of Medicine*, researchers studied the outcomes for 675 patients who had aortic root replacement at 10 surgical centers in the United States and Europe. Most patients (70 percent) were male, and their average age was 34 years. Of the patients, 455 had undergone elective surgery and the others were treated with urgent surgery. The death rate for the patients who had elective surgery was 1.5 percent versus the markedly higher rate of 11.7 mortality for patients who had emergency surgery.

According to the researchers, patients and their families "should understand that cardiovascular complications of Marfan's syndrome can be managed effectively in most cases by moderate restriction of physical activity, β-adrenergic blockade, routine imaging of the aorta, and prophylactic [elective] replacement of the aortic root before the diameter exceeds 5.5 to 6.0 cm."

Gott, Vincent L., M.D., et al. "Replacement of the Aortic Root in Patients with Marfan's Syndrome." *New England Journal of Medicine* 340, no. 17 (April 29, 1999): 1,307–1,313.

Wynbrandt, James, and Mark D. Ludman. *The Encyclopedia of Genetic Disorders and Birth Defects*, 2d ed. New York: Facts On File, Inc., 2000.

maturity onset diabetes of youth (MODY)   A rare genetic form of Type 2 diabetes, generally found in slender African-American adolescents. At least five different genetic subtypes of MODY have been identified as of this writing. MODY accounts for approximately 2–5 percent of all Type 2 diabetes cases. MODY is different from the Type 2 diabetes that is being diagnosed in increasing numbers of children and adolescents due to their obesity and sedentary lifestyles.

MODY is typically inherited as an autosomal dominant condition. The known genetic defects responsible for MODY include abnormalities of glucokinase, the hepatocyte nuclear factor-4 alpha, hepatocyte nuclear factor-1 alpha, insulin promoter factor 1, and the sulfonylurea 1 receptor subunit.

See also ADOLESCENTS; DIABETES MELLITUS.

McCune-Albright syndrome (MAS)   A medical condition, also known as osteitis fibrosa disseminate, that is rare among females and even more rare among males. McCune-Albright syndrome was named after the two physicians (Doctors Donovan James McCune and Fuller Albright) who separately described it in journal articles written in 1936 and 1937. MAS is not inherited, but it is caused by a genetic mutation in the *GNAS1* gene. The cause for this mutation is unknown.

The syndrome is characterized by EARLY PUBERTY and by endocrine diseases such as HYPERTHYROIDISM, short stature, CUSHING'S SYNDROME, PROLACTINOMAS, or ACROMEGALY as well as by skin changes with increased pigment. Most patients with McCune-Albright syndrome also have bone diseases and thus are at an increased risk for developing FRACTURES and deformities of the arms, legs, and skull. As of this writing, MAS cannot be detected or treated before birth.

Precocious Puberty

The key feature among female patients with McCune-Albright syndrome is precocious puberty (early puberty). Small children and even infants have been identified with this medical problem. According to Dr. Boston in his article on MAS, female infants as young as four months have experienced breast development or vaginal bleeding (first menstruation).

Researchers believe that the early puberty characteristic of McCune-Albright syndrome is often caused by estrogens generated by OVARIAN CYSTS. This is difficult to treat because when these cysts are removed, new cysts often develop. In addition, if one cystic ovary is removed, then the other ovary often starts to develop cysts.

Unfortunately, the synthetic drugs used to treat early puberty in other girls and that suppress luteinizing hormone and follicle-stimulating hormone will generally not be effective in girls with McCune-Albright syndrome. Some doctors are trying oral drugs to block the synthesizing of estrogen, including such medications as tesolactone and fadrozole. These medications appear to be effective in some patients with McCune-Albright syndrome, although further studies are needed.

Thyroid Abnormalities

According to the National Institute of Child Health and Human Development in the United States, an estimated half of all girls who have McCune-Albright syndrome have some form of thyroid disease. Many of these patients have GOITERS, THYROID NODULES, or thyroid cysts, although sometimes these abnormalities are not obvious and can be detected only with an ultrasound. THYROID-STIMULATING HORMONE (TSH) blood levels among patients with MAS are often low, indicating hyperthyroidism. Drugs to suppress thyroid synthesis, such as propylthiouracil or methimazone, may be given to treat the hyperthyroidism.

When hyperthyroidism occurs in infants, it may cause a severe FAILURE TO THRIVE and tachycardia. This may result in a heart attack and even death.

Growth Hormone Abnormalities

Some patients with McCune-Albright syndrome have excessive levels of growth hormone secretion. This problem is usually identified when they are young adults and is caused by a pituitary tumor. Such young women have the characteristic features of acromegaly, which include coarse facial features, large hands and feet, and arthritis. Other patients may present with GIGANTISM if the pituitary tumor develops before puberty. Patients may have surgery on the part of the pituitary that secretes growth hormone. The administration of somatostatin, a growth hormone suppressant, is another treatment for acromegaly.

Other Endocrine Disorders

Girls and women with McCune-Albright syndrome may have an excessive production of cortisol (hypercortisolism), which is also known as Cushing's syndrome. Females with this medical problem are obese and also have very sensitive skin. Treatment may involve the removal of the adrenal gland that is causing the problem (ADRENALECTOMY) or administering drugs that block the synthesis of cortisol. Hypercortisolism in infants can cause a lack of appetite and failure to thrive.

Some children with McCune-Albright syndrome have extremely low levels of blood phosphorus, which is due to a loss of phosphorus that is excreted in their urine. This loss of phosphorus may cause bone changes similar to those found in children with RICKETS, a severe pediatric bone disorder. Children with this problem can usually be treated with oral phosphates as well as vitamin D supplements.

Some females with McCune-Albright syndrome have severe bone diseases, while others do not. When bone disease occurs, it is characterized by fibroblast cells that replace normal bone cells. This can cause fractures if the bone displacement occurs in weight-bearing areas such as the upper leg bone (femur). Fibrous dysplasia may also occur in the skull and upper jaw of patients, causing facial deformity. Abnormal bone growth that occurs in the skull may cause blindness or deafness. It is very difficult for physicians to correct these bone deformities, which may require complex surgery.

Liver abnormalities may also occur. Some infants with McCune-Albright syndrome have severe neonatal jaundice.

Skin Changes

Many children and adults with MAS have characteristic café au lait spots, which are easiest to spot in fair-skinned children. These spots are most likely to be seen on the individual's back and cause no medical problems. Adolescents or adults who are troubled by them can usually cover them up completely with makeup.

Diagnosis and Treatment

McCune-Albright syndrome is diagnosed based on signs and symptoms. Laboratory tests will provide further information. Patients are usually tested with a multichemistry panel for liver function, thyroid function, and serum adrenocorticotropic hormone (ACTH) levels. A 24-hour urine collection may be ordered to check for urinary free cortisol. Growth hormone tests may be ordered as well. Imaging tests are also important, such as a pelvic ultrasonography to identify ovarian cysts in females and a bone scan to locate areas of fibrous dysplasia.

Females with MAS are usually treated with testolactone or tamoxifen, while boys are treated with ketoconazole or testolactone and spironolactone. The other manifestations of McCune-Albright syndrome, such as hyperthyroidism, bone diseases, and so forth, are treated as well. Surgery may be needed, such as an adrenalectomy for adrenal tumors.

See also SKIN.

For further information, contact the following organizations:

McCune-Albright Syndrome/Fibrous Dysplasia
    Division
MAGIC Foundation
6645 West North Avenue
Oak Park, IL 60302
(708) 383-0808
http://www.magicfoundation.org

National Arthritis and Musculoskeletal and Skin
    Diseases Information Clearinghouse
1 AMS Circle
Bethesda, MD 20892
(301) 495-4484
http://www.niams.nih.gov

National Institute of Child Health and Human
    Development
P.O. Box 3006
Rockville, MD 20847
(301) 496-5133
http://www.nichd.nih.gov

Boston, Bruce, M.D. "McCune-Albright Syndrome," Available online. URL: http://www.emedicine.com/PED/topic1386.htm. Downloaded on November 30, 2003.

medication interactions   The condition that exists when two or more medications, or a medication and a nutrient, or a medication and a supplement interact directly or indirectly to impair the ability of one or both drugs to provide the appropriate effect. One medication may boost or weaken the action of another drug or change its action in some other way. Some herbal supplements, such as ginkgo biloba, can cause thinning of the blood and should not be taken by patients taking warfarin (Coumadin) or other drugs with similar actions. For this reason, individuals should always report all medications that they take, including any over-the-counter drugs, herbs, or supplements, to their physicians. A medication interaction may cause mild symptoms or may be severe, causing coma and even death.

People who take many medications (including prescribed drugs, over-the-counter drugs, and herbal supplements and vitamins) have a greater risk of experiencing a medication interaction than others. In addition, because they often take three or more medications to manage chronic diseases and may also have slower metabolisms than younger people, elderly people have an increased risk for experiencing a medication interaction. It is critically important that such individuals attempt to fill all prescriptions at a single pharmacy or, if that is not possible, to report all the medications and supplements that they take whenever they do fill a prescription. This will allow the pharmacist to use one of the many computer programs available to assess the possibility of an interaction or adverse effect.

See also ALTERNATIVE MEDICINE; MEDICATIONS.

medications   Drugs that are used to treat medical problems, including prescribed drugs, over-the-counter drugs, and herbal remedies and supplements. Many endocrine diseases and disorders require medications that are hormones. Sometimes supplemental hormones are needed, such as LEVOTHYROXINE for patients with HYPOTHYROIDISM, INSULIN for patients with TYPE 1 DIABETES (and sometimes for patients with long-term TYPE 2 DIABETES), or TESTOSTERONE for males with HYPOGONADISM.

melatonin   A hormone produced by the pineal gland that plays an important role in the sleep cycles of humans. The chemical name for natural melatonin is N-acetyl-5-methoxytryptamine. Melatonin is metabolized in the liver and excreted in the urine. Its precise role in the sleep/wake circadian cycle remains poorly understood, despite studies.

Melatonin secretion in most people starts soon after darkness falls and usually peaks between the hours of 2 and 4 A.M. Melatonin secretion varies by age. Infants who are younger than age three months have very low levels of melatonin secretion. Secretion rises thereafter and generally peaks between the ages of one and three years, dropping gradually after that age.

Many older people have difficulty with sleep disorders. Some may have pineal insufficiency, causing the decreased production of melatonin. In a study reported in a 1995 issue of *Lancet*, researchers found that the elderly subjects had below-normal nocturnal secretions of melatonin. Patients who were given controlled-release melatonin experienced significantly improved sleep over those patients given placebo. The patients given the melatonin did not sleep more hours, but they slept more soundly.

Other Potential Effects of Melatonin

In addition to its effect on sleep cycles, some experts believe that the pineal gland affects puberty through the secretion of melatonin. In medical anecdotal reports, some children whose pineal glands were destroyed by tumors experienced an EARLY PUBERTY. In addition, experts have found that some children with precocious puberty have unusually low levels of melatonin in their blood. Further research is needed to determine if the pineal gland and/or melatonin secretion play a significant role in early puberty.

Some evidence indicates that the release of melatonin by the pineal gland may play a protective role against the development of cancer or in already-existing cancer, although further studies are needed. Sometimes melatonin is used to supplement the effects of chemotherapy in individuals with cancer. Individuals who have undergone a pinealectomy have shown an increased risk for the growth of tumors, while the administration of melatonin improves the condition or even reverses it.

In some patients with advanced cancer, physicians have treated them with large doses of mela-

tonin in concert with radiation therapy or chemotherapy. Some studies have shown improvements in patients with breast cancer and other cancers who took melatonin in addition to the more standard therapies. Further and larger studies are needed to determine the cancer-fighting capabilities of this hormone.

Supplements of Melatonin

Some people who have difficulty sleeping will take supplements of melatonin to improve their sleep quality, although the long-term effect of taking such drugs is unknown. Other individuals have taken melatonin because they must travel long distances and are attempting to stabilize their body rhythms to those of the area where they are traveling and thus avoid jet lag. For example, they may take melatonin to cause themselves to fall asleep at an earlier time than usual but at a time that would be at about right in the area to which they are traveling.

Melatonin supplements at dosages of one to five milligrams have been found to induce melatonin rates in the blood up to 100 times greater than those normally found in patients. Patients should not take any supplements without first checking with their physicians to ensure that the drug is likely to be safe and will not interact with other medications they already take. Problems with purity and quality control have been found in some supplements. So consumers should purchase products manufactured by large companies within their own countries.

See also ELDERLY; PINEAL GLAND.

Brzezinski, Amnon, M.D. "Melatonin in Humans." *New England Journal of Medicine* 336, no. 3 (January 16, 1997): 186–195.

Garfinkel, D., et al. "Improvement of Sleep Quality in Elderly People by Controlled-Release Melatonin." *Lancet* 346, no. 8974 (1995): 541–544.

Kunz, D., et al. "Melatonin in Patients with Reduced REM Sleep Duration: Two Randomized Controlled Trials." *Journal of Clinical Endocrinology & Metabolism* 89, no. 1 (2004): 128–134.

Panzer, A., and M. Vijoen. "The Validity of Melatonin as an Oncostatic Agent." *Journal of Pineal Research* 22, no. 4 (1997): 184–202.

menopause   The stage of life in which women no longer menstruate nor do they release a monthly egg that could be combined with a sperm to produce an embryo. Menopause usually occurs to women in their late 40s or early 50s, although menopause may occur earlier or later. Some experts have defined perimenopause as a stage that precedes menopause for several years, during which time estrogen production is diminished and women are unlikely to become pregnant. Women who have both of their ovaries removed before the normal onset of menopause, because of OVARIAN CANCER, an OVARIAN CYST, or another medical problem, experience an early, surgically induced menopause.

Women who take LEVOTHYROXINE for hypothyroidism may need higher doses if they also take ESTROGEN REPLACEMENT THERAPY (ERT) to counteract the effects of menopause such as HOT FLASHES, vaginal dryness, and mood swings, according to some studies.

Not all women experience signs and symptoms of menopause. For those who do, the signs or symptoms may be short-lived and mild. For other women, the symptoms are very difficult to manage.

Diagnosis and Treatment

Physicians may diagnose women with menopause based on their age and their symptoms. However, it is best to order a blood test of estrogen levels to confirm that menopause has occurred. If the woman is menopausal, she may wish to take HORMONE REPLACEMENT THERAPY (HRT), which is a combination of estrogen and progesterone. Some women take estrogen replacement therapy (ERT) alone, particularly if they no longer have an intact uterus (due to a hysterectomy) and thus do not have to worry about developing uterine cancer.

For further information, contact the following organization:

American Menopause Foundation
350 Fifth Avenue
Suite 2822
New York, NY 10118
(212) 714-2398
www.americanmenopause.org

Arafah, B. M. "Increased Need for Thyroxine in Women with Hypothyroidism During Estrogen Therapy." *New England Journal of Medicine* 344, no. 23 (2001): 1,743–1,749.

menstruation, painful   Difficult menstrual cycle, often accompanied by severe cramping, copious bleeding (menorrhagia)—which is probably the most severe problem, as well as overall achiness, headaches (including migraines), and a general feeling of being out of sorts. Some women have a painful menstruation every month. In such cases, they should consult with a gynecologist to determine if there is a correctable medical cause for the problem. The physician will usually order a blood test for the woman's hormone levels and may order an ultrasound to determine if an ovarian cyst or another condition is present. Some endocrine disorders, such as HASHIMOTO'S THYROITIDIS (a form of hypothyroidism), are associated with painful and heavy menstrual periods.

Some physicians place women with very painful menstrual cycles on birth control pills (ORAL CONTRACEPTIVES) in an attempt to stabilize the cycles. In some cases, women need to see an ENDOCRINOLOGIST to determine if an endocrine disease or disorder rather than a gynecological disorder may be causing their problems.

In the past, some women with severely painful menstrual periods and/or menorrhagia were given hysterectomies despite the lack of cancer or other disease. The removal of the uterus effectively ends all menstruation, permanently. If the ovaries are also removed at the same time, the woman will undergo a sudden onset of MENOPAUSE. More recently, some physicians have turned to less extreme measures, such as endometrial ablation which can be used as an alternative to the hysterectomy.

In one study, reported in a 1996 issue of the *New England Journal of Medicine*, physicians performed an endometrial resection on 95 percent of 525 women with menorrhagia. Of these women, 6 percent experienced surgical complications. Physician follow-ups with questionnaires over the course of five years determined that the majority of the women experienced significant relief. The majority,

80 percent, of the patients did not need further surgery for menstrual problems, and only 9 percent later required a hysterectomy.

O'Connor, Hugh, and Adam Magos, M.D. "Endometrial Resection for the Treatment of Menorrhagia." *New England Journal of Medicine* 335, no. 3 (July 18, 1996): 151–156.

metabolism   The use of energy to perform the overall processing of the body's functions, including digestion, breathing, blood circulation, and so forth. The formal terms for metabolism are basal metabolic rate or resting energy expenditure. Metabolism increases relative to weight from birth until the age of two years old and then gradually declines until puberty. It then increases again until adolescence is complete. Thereafter, metabolism very slowly declines with age, although many variables will affect it.

Basal metabolic rate correlates best with fat-free mass (FFM), and fat-free mass correlates with muscle mass. Thus, the more muscle mass a person has, the higher the basal metabolic rate. Basal metabolic rate can be measured with a technique called calorimetry; unfortunately, this technique is not readily available because it requires expensive complex equipment that is tricky to use accurately. It is often used with patients in intensive care units on ventilators. In addition, there is a significant variation from measurement to measurement with current techniques, leading to a fairly wide normal range. Usually, formulas are used to calculate basal metabolic rate and thus determine the appropriate intake of nutrition.

The rate of metabolism in an individual is affected by many variables. Hormones are key variables, particularly thyroid hormones. Thyroid disease can speed up or slow down a person's metabolism. HYPOTHYROIDISM tends to decrease an individual's metabolism, causing that person to be more sluggish and slow moving. In contrast, HYPERTHYROIDISM generally increases metabolism and causes individuals to have an increased heart rate, more rapid digestion, and so on. However, of importance is that people have varying metabolisms that lie within the normal range. Some highly energetic people do not have thyroid disease or other endocrine disorders, while at the same time, individuals who appear slow moving to others do not necessarily have a metabolic disorder. In addition, some individuals who may appear normal to others do have a metabolic disorder.

In the case of many hormones, although some of the hormone must be present for the person's metabolism to function at a normal level, changes in the levels may not have a dramatic effect on the metabolism. This is referred to as being permissive for normal metabolism. Examples of such hormones are cortisol and growth hormone.

metaiodobenzylguanide scan (MIBG scan)   A test for an endocrine tumor. MIBG is similar in structure to norepinephrines and acts as a precursor for the synthesis of catecholamines. This molecule can be labeled with radioactive iodine (either I-131 or I-123) and used to attempt to locate small pheochromocytomas (adrenal tumors) that have not been found by computed tomography (CT) scans, magnetic resonance imaging (MRI) scans, or other localizing radiological procedures.

The standard rule of thumb for all endocrine tumors is that the physician must first substantiate that the patient has a clinical syndrome consistent with the disorder and also that the appropriate biochemical markers are elevated in the patient's blood or urine. Rarely, if ever, is it appropriate for a physician to attempt to identify a tumor via a scan without first having some biochemical evidence of the presence of a tumor, because there is a high risk of a false-positive result. The presence of a nodule or mass, which is often normal and benign, can cause a false positive.

Before having the MIBG scan, patients need to be taken off any drugs that could affect their catecholamine metabolism, such as beta-blocker medications and tricyclic antidepressants. Patients are given some iodine prior to the test to protect their thyroid glands from damage that could be caused by the radioactive iodine. The scan is usually done as an outpatient test. It can help detect very small tumors and/or the 10 percent of pheochromocytomas that are not adrenal tumors as well as the rare patient who has multiple tumors.

microcephaly   Unusually small head size, usually in a newborn infant. Microcephaly may be an indication of a developmental delay and always implies an abnormally small brain (microencephaly). Severe placental insufficiency due to poorly controlled DIABETES MELLITUS may lead to microcephaly. Organic acidurias such as HOMOCYSTINURIA may also lead to microcephaly.

Standard head circumferences have been developed for children between the ages of birth and 18 years old. Special head curve charts are available for children with NEUROFIBROMATOSIS TYPE 1, achondroplasia, and Williams syndrome.

See also MACROCEPHALY.

micropenis   An unusually small-sized penis, often caused by a genetic disorder. The male infant with a micropenis has a penis that is less than 2.5 centimeters in length and 0.9 cm in diameter. It can be caused by decreased exposure to TESTOSTERONE in the second or third trimesters of pregnancy, insensitivity to androgens, or deficient GROWTH HORMONE or LUTEINIZING HORMONE.

Some infants are candidates for gender reassignment, which means that they are raised as girls. However, this is a highly controversial practice. Many males with Klinefelter syndrome, although not all, have very small penises.

According to Dr. C. R. J. Woodhouse in his 1998 article in *Urology*, some boys with micropenis have this problem due to an isolated growth hormone deficiency, which can be treated with human recombinant growth hormone (HRH). Although this may cause the penis to increase in size, it will still be below the average length in size for males. Another form of treatment in infants and young boys is to administer testosterone or human chorionic gonadatropin (HCG). This treatment may enable the penis to grow to a normal size.

Some physicians have treated boys with micropenis with dihydrotestosterone (DHT) cream that is applied to the penis. This hormone causes both the penis and the prostate gland to increase in size. In one study of 22 children, all of them experienced increased penile growth with DHT treatment, including four boys who had not responded to treatment with other forms of testosterone. The treatment must occur before puberty, as the response after puberty is usually poor.

Studies of the sexual function of men with micropenis indicate they can have normal sex lives. According to Woodhouse, regarding a study of 20 adult males with micropenis, "The most surprising feature of these patients was the firmness with which they were established in the male role and the success that they had in sexual relationships. In the adult group, all were heterosexual, all had erections and orgasms, and 11 of 12 ejaculated." One patient had both a wife and a mistress, and one patient had fathered a child.

See also TESTES/TESTICLES.

Woodhouse, C. R. J. "Sexual Function in Boys Born with Exstrophy, Myelomeningocele, and Micropenis." *Urology* 52, no. 1 (1998): 3–11.

milk-alkali syndrome   The triad of very high blood calcium levels, excess alkali, and kidney insufficiency caused by a combination of an excessive amount of milk and/or alkaline antacids, particularly baking soda (bicarbonate of soda). Patients who are taking vitamin D further aggravate the problem. Milk-alkali syndrome was a common cause of HYPERCALCEMIA prior to the advent of the newer therapies for peptic ulcer disease, especially the use of histamine-2 receptor blockers such as cimetidine (Tagamet) and ranitidine (Zantac).

However, the incidence of milk-alkali syndrome has been increasing as greater numbers of patients use large amounts of calcium carbonate (Tums) supplements to help prevent or treat OSTEOPOROSIS and to decrease blood phosphorus levels among those with severe chronic renal disease. Interestingly, some patients have developed HYPOCALCEMIA when the excess calcium was removed from their diets.

Historically, milk-alkali syndrome first began in 1915 with the introduction of a regimen, by Dr. Sippy, that treated peptic ulcer disease with magnesium carbonate, sodium carbonate, and bismuth subcarbonate. The chronic form of this condition was also called Burnett's syndrome, and the subacute form was known as Cope's syndrome.

Milk-alkali syndrome can cause calcium deposits in the kidneys, which are seen in COMPUTERIZED TOMOGRAPHY (CT) scans, MAGNETIC RESONANCE IMAGING (MRI) scans, X-rays, or ultrasounds of the kidneys. The modern patient who has milk-alkali syndrome typically has no signs or symptoms of this medical problem. However, physicians may suspect the problem based on the patient's history of calcium intake and then the measurement of serum calcium levels as well as other ancillary blood findings. Patients who are heavy users of antacids are at risk for milk-alkali syndrome.

If symptoms do occur, they may include headache, nausea, and weakness. The patient may also have pain in the back or the loins and may experience excessive urination.

Most cases of milk-alkali syndrome are reversible when the patient stops drinking high levels of milk and/or consuming many antacids. In severe cases (which are rare), the kidney is damaged and the patient may experience kidney failure and may require dialysis or a kidney transplant.

See also CALCIUM BALANCE; VITAMIN D.

mineralocorticoids   See ALDOSTERONE.

multiple endocrine neoplasia (MEN)   A rare and serious hereditary disorder of cancer of the endocrine glands. MEN is further subdivided into MEN 1 and MEN 2.

MEN 1

MEN 1 involves multiple tumors that may occur in one or more endocrine glands. This medical problem is a hereditary disorder that occurs in an estimated three to 20 people of every 100,000 individuals. It can present at any age and affects males and females in equal numbers. MEN 1 is also known as multiple endocrine adenomatosis or Wermer's syndrome.

Researchers report that often MEN 1 affects the parathyroid glands in the neck first, causing all four parathyroid glands to become overactive and to secrete excessive levels of parathyroid hormone. This HYPERPARATHYROIDISM then causes high levels

of calcium in the bloodstream (HYPERCALCEMIA), which can then cause kidney stones and renal (kidney) damage. Hyperparathyroidism may also cause constipation, bone pain, muscle pain, fatigue, indigestion, and weakness.

Patients with MEN 1 may also have abdominal pain, nausea and vomiting, vision problems, loss of coordination, lack of appetite, weight loss, and hypotension (low blood pressure). Women may experience infertility and amenorrhea and may also fail to lactate, making it impossible to breast-feed their babies. Men may have decreased libido and a loss of facial or body hair.

If MEN 1 is suspected by the physician, tests are performed on the endocrine glands to evaluate their function. A magnetic resonance imaging (MRI) scan may show a pancreatic tumor. A fasting blood sugar test may be low, while serum glucagon may be high. In evaluating the parathyroid glands, the serum parathyroid hormone and serum calcium levels are elevated if MEN 1 is present. A scan of the head may show that a pituitary tumor is present. Physicians may also check for hormone levels of cortisol, adrenocorticotropic hormone (ACTH), luteinizing hormone, and follicle-stimulating hormone.

If hyperparathyroidism is diagnosed, the usual treatment is to remove three of the four parathyroid glands and part of the fourth gland. (A portion of the fourth parathyroid gland is left in place so that it can continue to generate some parathyroid hormone.)

MEN 2

With MEN 2, patients develop thyroid cancer (medullary carcinoma of the thyroid) as well as cancer of the adrenal glands (pheochromocytoma). MEN 2 is caused by a mutation in the *RET* gene. The incidence is unknown. The cancers do not always appear at the same time. MEN 2 is also known as Sipple's syndrome.

The following symptoms are common with MEN 2:

- Chest pain
- Abdominal pain
- Weight loss
- Coughing blood

- Increased thirst
- Severe headache
- Back pain
- Increased urination

Since these symptoms are common to other disorders, the physician must perform diagnostic testing. For example, an adrenal biopsy may reveal a pheochromocytoma, while an MRI of the abdomen may show a mass in the adrenal glands. Thyroid scans may show nodules, as may an ultrasound of the thyroid gland. Laboratory tests will show elevations of urine catecholamines and urine metanephrine. Patients with MEN 2 also have elevated levels of calcitonin and serum calcium but decreased levels of serum phosphorus.

Patients with MEN 2 need surgery to remove the existing tumors and should be carefully followed up by their doctors. Thyroid tumors are removed with a total excision of the thyroid gland, and patients must take thyroid replacement hormone for the rest of their lives. The thyroid tumors found in MEN 2 are unusually aggressive, which is why the entire gland must be removed to attempt to prevent any spreading of the cancer.

Brandi, Maria Luisa, et al. "Guidelines for Diagnosis and Therapy of MEN Type 1 and Type 2." *Journal of Clinical Endocrinology and Metabolism* 86, no. 12 (2001): 5,658–5,671.

myxedema coma The metabolic syndrome of very severe HYPOTHYROIDISM with associated hypothermia (low body temperature) and other associated organ system dysfunction or failure. It is a rare syndrome with a significant mortality rate (one out of three people die), although this rate has been declining over time due to better diagnosis and supportive care.

Patients typically have long-standing hypothyroidism and have stopped taking their thyroid hormone. Some patients have never been diagnosed with hypothyroidism and thus were never treated for it. Myxedema coma is most common in elderly women and has been seen in all types of hypothyroidism. The crisis can be precipitated by an illness such as pneumonia, influenza, myocardial infarction, urinary tract infection, significant cold exposure, or exposure to narcotics.

These patients are often seen in a hospital emergency department with mental status changes (severe cases are referred to as myxedema madness), low body temperature, slow heart rate (bradycardia), low blood sodium level (HYPONATREMIA), hypoventilation, and low blood sugar (HYPOGLYCEMIA).

If the diagnosis of myxedema coma is suspected, the emergency room physicians will begin therapy before confirmatory laboratory results have been returned. Therapy includes gentle warming, appropriate intravenous fluids (with attention to sodium, glucose, and fluid volume), artificial ventilation if needed, and intravenous levothyroxine and/or triiodothyronine. In addition, if an underlying or precipitating medical illness has not been identified, the physician must still search for one and begin appropriate therapy.

The most common form of underlying hypothyroidism is primary hypothyroidism; the thyroid-stimulating hormone (TSH) is elevated and the free T4 is low. If the TSH is normal or low, the physician must suspect secondary or tertiary hypothyroidism due to pituitary or hypothalamic disease. In these cases, patients must also be tested for CORTISOL deficiency (ADDISON'S DISEASE) and begun on therapy with intravenous glucocorticoids until the testing determines that this hormone is not required.

The term *myxedema megacolon* refers to the severe dilation that can occur in the colon, especially in the cecum, and that can mimic a mechanical bowel obstruction. It usually resolves slowly with the use of thyroid hormones, intravenous fluids and nutrients, and bowel rest (avoidance of solid and liquid food). If the dilation in the cecum exceeds 15 centimeters, surgery may be needed, although in many cases, the colon can be decompressed via a tube placed under radiologic guidance.

The term pretibial myxedema refers to a brawny, nonpitting swelling of the ankles and lower shins. It is nontender, brownish orange in color, and may be plaque-like. It is only seen in patients with GRAVES' DISEASE. The name refers to the appearance of the skin under the microscope, which is similar to what is seen in the skin of patients with severe hypothyroidism.

See also COMA; ELDERLY; HASHIMOTO'S THYROIDITIS.

National Institutes of Health (NIH)   A large federal organization in the United States that oversees such organizations as the National Center for Health Statistics, the Centers for Disease Control and Prevention (CDC), the National Institute of Diabetes and Digestive and Kidney Diseases (NIDDK), the National Institute of Mental Health, and others.

For further information, contact the NIH at:

National Institutes of Health
9000 Rockville Pike
Bethesda, MD 20892
(301) 496-4357

neurofibromatosis type 1 (NF-1)   A serious genetic disorder that is linked to chromosome 17 and affects an estimated one in 3,000 individuals. NF-1 is also known as von Recklinghausen's NF, and it accounts for 85 percent of all NF cases. It is inherited in an autosomal dominant pattern. Those who inherit NF-1 are at risk for all possible complications of the disorder, but variable degrees of disease are seen.

NF-1 patients have about a 6 percent increased risk for developing optic gliomas and outer central nervous system tumors. They are also at an increased risk of noncentral nervous system tumors, such as neurofibrosarcoma and PHEOCHRO-MOCYTOMA (a tumor of the adrenal gland).

Patients with NF-1 also have an increased risk of cognitive dysfunction, learning disabilities, seizures, MACROCEPHALY (a large head), and abnormal results on MAGNETIC RESONANCE IMAGING (MRI) scans of the brain.

Signs and Symptoms

NF-1 patients have neurofibromas and café au lait spots (CALS). According to the National Institutes of Health (NIH), in order to make the diagnosis of NF-1, the patient must have at least two of the following signs and symptoms:

- Six or more CALS (greater than five millimeters in prepubertal individuals and greater than 14 millimeters in postpubertal individuals)
- Two or more neurofibromas of any type or a plexiform neurofibroma
- Axillary (underarm) or inguinal (pelvic) freckling
- An optic glioma
- Two or more hamartomas of the iris (Lisch nodules)
- A distinctive body lesion, such as sphenoid dysplasia with or without pseudoarthrosis
- A first-degree relative (parent or sibling) with NF-1

The café au lait spots present in NF-1 are hyperpigmented skin lesions that usually appear after the patient is age one and that increase in size and number during childhood. Some people without NF-1 may also develop CALS, and one of every four people without NF-1 will have one to three CALS. These CALS fade as a person ages, making the diagnosis more difficult to make later in life.

A Multisystem Disease

Neurofibromatosis is a multisystem disease that affects the endocrine glands, the skin, the central nervous system, and the skeleton. Adults with neurofibromatosis have an increased risk of developing tumors, and some experts have estimated that about 10 percent of adults with this illness will develop pheochromocytomas. The presence of multiple café au lait spots along the anterior axillary line, located at the edge of the armpit, is associated with a greater risk of pheochromocytoma, which means that these individuals should be screened for the presence of pheochromocytomas.

Most children and adults with neurofibromatosis do not require medical attention except for follow-ups for the development of abnormalities that usually occur and for treatment of those medical problems.

Children and NF-1

Children with NF-1 have an increased risk of short stature. In one study of 569 children with NF-1, 213 children were greater than two standard deviations shorter than normal, which means that they were statistically far below the normal height for their age. Scoliosis (a curved spine) occurs in about 15 percent of patients with NF-1. In one large study of children and young adults with neurofibromatosis type 1, about half (48 percent) of the 10-year-old patients had neurofibromas while 84 percent of the 20 year old adults had neurofibromas.

Children with EARLY PUBERTY (precocious puberty) are at risk for developing neurofibromatosis, although some patients with neurofibromatosis may have a DELAYED PUBERTY.

Neurofibromatosis Type 2

There is also a neurofibromatosis type 2. It is characterized by problems with hearing loss and balance—and it may lead to tumors and palsies. The most common symptom of neurofibromatosis type 2 is hearing loss, which may be gradual or sudden. Patients may also experience weakness in the arms and legs caused by tumors in the brain stem or spinal cord. An estimated one in 37,000 individuals have neurofibromatosis type 2. The treatment involves routine hearing tests to evaluate the patient as well as surgery for any tumors that are present.

For further information on neurofibromatosis, contact the following organizations:

National Neurofibromatosis Foundation
95 Pine Street
16th Floor
New York, NY 10005
(212) 344-6633 or (800) 323-7938 (toll-free)
http://www.nf.org

Neurofibromatosis, Inc.
9320 Annaplis Road
Suite 300
Lanham, MD 20706
(301) 918-4600 or (800) 942-6825 (toll-free)
http://www.nfinc.org

Carmi, Doron, M.D., et al. "Growth, Puberty, and Endocrine Functions in Patients with Sporadic or Familial Neurofibromatosis Type 1: A Longitudinal Study." *Pediatrics* 103, no. 6 (June 1999): 1,257–1,262.

Crossen, Margon H., M.D., et al. "Endocrinologic Disorders and Optic Pathway Gliomas in Children with Neurofibromatosis Type 1." *Pediatrics* 100, no. 4 (October 1997): 667–670.

DeBella, Kimberly, Jacek Szudek, and Jan Marshall Friedman, M.D. "Use of the National Institutes of Health Criteria for Diagnosis of Neurofibromatosis 1 in Children." *Pediatrics* 105, no. 3 (March 2000): 608–614.

Short, M. Priscilla, M.D. "Neurofibromatosis Type I," in *NORD Guide to Rare Disorders: The National Organization for Rare Disorders.* Philadelphia, Pa.: Lippincott Williams & Wilkins, 2003.

———."Neurofibromatosis Type 2," in *NORD Guide to Rare Disorders: The National Organization for Rare Disorders.* Philadelphia, Pa.: Lippincott Williams & Wilkins, 2003.

Szudek, J., P. Birch, and J. M. Friedman. "Growth in North American White Children with Neurofibromatosis I (NF 1)." *Journal of Medical Genetics* 37, no. 12 (2000): 933–938.

obesity   Excessive body weight. Obesity is usually measured by body mass index (BMI), which is a person's weight in kilograms divided by his or her height in meters squared, or the weight in pounds divided by height in inches multiplied by 703. Most people prefer to simply look up their BMI status in tables that incorporate these calculations, and individuals need know only their height and weight to find their BMI on the table. An optimal weight is a BMI between 21 and 24.9. A BMI of 25–29.9 constitutes overweight, while obesity is defined as 30 or greater.

High BMIs correlate with a greater risk for illnesses, such as diabetes, heart disease, and hypertension. In addition, some studies have shown that obese individuals have a greater risk of dying from cancer, particularly colon cancer, esophageal cancer, liver cancer, PANCREATIC CANCER, and kidney cancer. Some researchers maintain that obesity is the second-leading cause of deaths that could have been avoided, after smoking.

Individuals who are at risk for INSULIN RESISTANCE have the most urgency for resolving their obesity in order to avoid the consequences of diabetes, hypertension, and other serious illnesses. Diet and exercise are both recommended. As of this writing, a combination of pharmacotherapy and counseling appears to be most efficacious for sustained weight loss, although many people struggle with a lifelong tendency toward obesity.

BMI is a better marker of obesity than are waist measurements or waist-to-hip ratio measurements. Yet some organizations continue to rely upon obesity measurements other than BMI. The National Cholesterol Education Program uses a waist measurement of 40 inches or greater in men or 35 inches or greater in women as a marker for metabolic syndrome. These waist measurements also correlate with a significantly increased risk of the development of TYPE 2 DIABETES, high blood pressure, and coronary artery disease.

Statistical Data on Obese Individuals

According to statistics provided by the National Center for Health Statistics in 2003, nearly 31 percent of all Americans are obese, including 34 percent of women and 27.7 percent of men. African Americans have the highest risk of becoming obese, and 40.4 percent of all African Americans are obese, including 28.9 percent of the men and 50.4 percent of the women. Mexican-American women also have a high percentage of obesity.

In considering a state-by-state look at individuals who are obese, as reported in a 2003 issue of *Morbidity and Mortality Weekly Report* (MMWR), researchers have found that the largest percentage of obese individuals in 2001 were in the following states or territories: Mississippi (27.1 percent), Michigan (25.8 percent), and the Virgin Islands (25.5 percent) (see Table 1).

Increasing numbers of individuals are also severely obese, with a BMI of 40 or greater. Most severely obese individuals weigh at least 100 pounds above the normal weight for their height.

Obesity also has a high economic cost. According to a study published in a 2004 issue of *Obesity Research*, the annual medical expenses incurred as a result of obesity in the United States were $75 billion in 2003, and about half of these costs were borne by Medicare and Medicaid government programs. Furthermore, an estimated 3–7 percent of all health costs are attributable to high weight and obesity, as described by Dr. George Bray in his 2003 article in *Endocrinology and Metabolism Clinics of North America*. The direct costs of obesity were calculated at about $52 billion in

1995, a figure that is probably greatly elevated in 2004, as of this writing.

The number of severely obese adults has increased dramatically in the United States. For example, in a study reported in the *Archives of Internal Medicine,* researchers found that the numbers of people who were severely obese, with a BMI of 40 or greater, had quadrupled from 1986, when about one in 200 adults in the United States were severely obese, to one in 50 by the year 2000.

Abdominal Obesity Is Dangerous

A significant number of individuals who are obese carry much of their weight in the abdominal area. Simply put, they are apple-shaped, with most of their weight apparent around their waist. In contrast, pear-shaped individuals carry their fat primarily around their hips. Studies have shown that abdominal obesity raises the risk of the development of diseases such as DIABETES MELLITUS, hypertension, and coronary artery disease.

Causes of Obesity

Individuals become obese when the total calories (energy) that they take in as food are significantly more, over an extended time, than the total calories they expend. Rarely, illnesses may increase the risk for obesity, such as PRADER-WILLI SYNDROME, which causes patients to have an uncontrollably ravenous appetite. Contrary to popular belief, most endocrine disorders, such as HYPOTHYROIDISM, do not cause obesity, although when such diseases are resolved, the individual may lose a few pounds.

Complex hormonal factors may be at work causing obesity, but they are yet to be discovered. As a result, the only way for most obese people to lose weight is to eat less and exercise more, as unsatisfying as that solution may sound. Unfortunately, many people actively seek the one diet that "works," as evidenced by the continued presence of diet books on best-selling book lists.

Genetic Causes of Obesity

Evidence indicates that some individuals may have a genetic predisposition to being overweight or even to being obese. Researchers have found a genetic link between both Type 2 diabetes and obesity on chromosome 18p11, a connection described in a 2001 issue of *Diabetes.*

Scientists have begun studying genetic risks for the development of obesity in great depth. According to authors Coleen Damcott, Paul Sack, and Alan Shuldiner in their 2003 article on the genetics of obesity in *Endocrinology and Metabolism Clinics of North America,* "There is compelling evidence from family, twin, and adoption studies supporting an important genetic component to obesity. These and other studies estimated that genetics influences 40% to 75% of variation in BMI; however, the genetics of obesity are not simple and rarely follow Mendelian patterns." Instead, say the authors, mutations in several different genes may lead to obesity. For example, mutations in the genes coding for leptin and other substances have been demonstrated to cause obesity in humans.

Studies have linked markers, on a wide variety of chromosomes, to obese individuals as well as to mice. Future research may hold the key to determining which individuals are most genetically susceptible to obesity and may also lead to a method to manipulate these genes.

Some of the obesity-related gene mutations that have been identified to date, according to the Centers for Disease Control and Prevention (CDC), include the following:

- *LEP* (leptin)
- *LEPR* (leptin receptor)
- *POMC1* (pro-opiomelanocortin)
- *SIM1* (human homologue of drosophila single-minded 1)
- *PC1* (prohormone convertase 1)
- *MC4R* (melanocortin-4 receptor)

The presence of a genetic predisposition to obesity does not mean that such individuals are somehow doomed to be fat. Genetic predispositions only indicate greater likelihood of an event occurring, and some individuals with obese parents will be of average weight themselves or even slender. In addition, it is currently nearly impossible for most people to know if they carry a genetic mutation for obesity since such tests are very expensive and complex.

People who are obese, with or without the presence of a genetic propensity, need to work with their doctor on a program of weight loss to reduce their weight as well as their health risks and thus extend their lives.

Medications

In some cases, medications for illnesses other than obesity may cause temporary or chronic increases in weight, although such increases do not usually result in obesity. Some examples of medications that may cause a significant weight gain include GLUCOCORTICOIDS, antidepressants, antipsychotic drugs, and lithium. Sometimes physicians can change or reduce the dosage of the medications to reduce the weight gain. Other times patients need to exercise more frequently and pay close attention to limiting the number of calories they consume.

Television Watching

Some behaviors have been found to be linked with obesity. For example, a study reported in a 2003 issue of the *Journal of the American Medical Association* found that prolonged television watching was significantly linked to both a greater risk of obesity and the presence of Type 2 diabetes. The study considered about 50,000 women in the Nurses' Health Study from 1992–98 who were not obese when the study began. The study also considered about 68,000 women over the same period who did not have diabetes when the study began.

The researchers also looked at other sedentary activities, such as reading, playing board games, sewing, driving a car, and so forth. They still found that prolonged television watching resulted in a lower metabolic rate and a higher risk of obesity and diabetes than the other activities. The researchers said that their study suggested that 30 percent of the cases of patients with obesity and 43 percent of the cases of patients with Type 2 diabetes could be prevented if patients watched less than 10 hours a week of television and walked briskly for 30 minutes or more per day.

Depression and Obesity

Severe obesity is often linked to depression, and researchers have found that a significant weight loss can improve the depression problem. Whether obesity causes depression or depression causes obesity is not clear. However, resolving the obesity often does help alleviate depression.

In a study reported in a 2003 issue of the *Archives of Internal Medicine*, 487 subjects were observed. The researchers found that depression, as measured by the Beck Depression Inventory (BDI), was more commonly found among patients who were young, were female, and had a poor body image. The scores on the BDI improved significantly with weight loss, particularly among women who were severely obese. This may mean that bariatric surgery, also known as gastric bypass surgery, may be indicated in some individuals who are severely obese, although physicians must take each patient's individual health risks into account.

Children and Obesity

Many adolescents and younger children also have a weight problem, and some are obese or even severely obese. The problem of overweight among children has increased dramatically since 1971–1974, when only about 4 percent of children ages 6–11 years old were obese. By 1999–2000, the percentage had increased to 15.3 percent of the children in that age group (see Table 2). Part of the problem may be that children and adolescents take part in fewer physically demanding activities and spend more time watching television than in past years.

Sometimes obesity in young adulthood can be predicted based on parental obesity when children were growing up. In a study reported in a 1997 issue of the *New England Journal of Medicine*, researchers observed 854 young adults, including 135 who were obese. The researchers studied the subjects' childhood obesity and the obesity of their parents when the subjects were children, based on medical records. Their findings state, "Parental obesity more than doubles the risk of adult obesity among both obese and non-obese children under 10 years of age." Clearly, obese parents should have two motivations for weight loss: their own health and the future health of their children.

Resolving Obesity

Researchers fervently disagree about what diets are the safest and best for most people as well as what

TABLE 1: PREVALENCE OF OBESITY* IN ADULTS ≥ AGED 20 YEARS, 1991, 2000, AND 2001 AND BY SEX, 2001— UNITED STATES, BEHAVIORAL RISK FACTOR SURVEILLANCE SYSTEM

| | Both sexes | | | | | | (%) | Men | | Women | |
| | 2001 | | 2000 | | 1991 | | Difference | 2001 | | 2001 | |
State or Territory	%	95% CI* (±)	%	95% CI (±)	%	95% CI (±)	1991–2001	%	95% CI (±)	%	95% CI (±)
Alabama	24.9	2.0	24.5	2.2	14.4	1.9	72.8	24.9	2.	24.9	2.4
Alaska	22.9	2.2	21.5	2.5	13.6	2.6	68.3	20.0	3.	26.3	3.3
Arizona	19.3	2.0	20.1	3.1	11.8	1.9	63.7	20.5	3.	18.0	2.5
Arkansas	23.0	1.8	23.7	1.8	13.5	2.2	70.1	23.5	2.	22.6	2.2
California	22.6	1.6	20.5	1.6	10.8	1.3	109.1	21.5	2.	23.7	2.4
Colorado	15.5	1.8	14.4	1.8	8.9	1.5	75.1	15.8	2.	15.1	2.4
Connecticut	18.2	1.2	17.9	1.4	11.4	1.7	59.8	19.1	1.	17.3	1.4
Delaware	21.4	1.8	17.2	1.8	15.7	2.2	36.4	21.6	2.	21.1	2.4
District of Columbia	20.2	2.4	21.9	2.4	16.2	2.4	24.9	16.3	3.	23.8	3.1
Florida	19.2	1.4	18.9	1.4	10.6	1.5	80.6	19.3	2.	19.2	1.8
Georgia	23.1	1.6	21.9	1.6	9.8	1.5	136.0	22.4	2.	23.8	2.0
Hawaii	18.3	1.8	16.0	1.4	10.5	1.6	74.1	19.9	2.	16.7	2.2
Idaho	21.0	1.4	19.5	1.4	12.3	1.7	71.1	21.9	2.	20.2	1.8
Illinois	21.7	1.6	22.2	1.6	13.6	1.7	59.9	20.8	2.	22.6	2.0
Indiana	25.1	1.6	22.2	1.8	15.7	1.7	59.6	25.5	2.	24.8	2.0
Iowa	23.4	1.6	22.0	1.6	15.0	2.1	55.7	24.7	2.	22.0	2.2
Kansas	22.2	1.4	21.3	1.4	—	—	—	23.9	2.	20.5	1.8
Kentucky	24.8	1.6	23.5	1.6	13.7	1.8	81.0	26.1	2.	23.6	1.8
Louisiana	25.0	1.4	24.2	1.4	16.5	2.4	51.9	25.6	2.	24.4	1.8
Maine	20.0	1.8	20.7	2.0	12.8	2.3	56.5	20.7	2.	19.3	2.4
Maryland	20.4	1.6	20.8	1.6	11.9	1.9	71.6	19.8	2.	21.0	2.2
Massachusetts	17.1	1.0	16.9	1.0	9.3	1.7	83.9	18.1	1.	16.1	1.2
Michigan	25.8	1.6	23.0	2.0	16.3	1.7	58.2	26.2	2.	25.5	2.0
Minnesota	20.4	1.4	17.8	1.6	11.3	1.2	80.1	21.0	2.	19.7	2.0
Mississippi	27.1	2.0	25.3	2.2	16.2	2.2	67.1	26.1	2.	28.0	2.4
Missouri	23.8	1.8	22.5	1.8	12.6	1.8	88.6	25.8	2.	21.8	2.2
Montana	19.2	1.8	16.4	1.8	10.1	1.9	89.7	20.3	2.	18.2	2.4
Nebraska	21.2	1.6	21.4	1.8	13.8	2.1	53.5	22.8	2.	19.6	2.0
Nevada	19.9	2.7	18.3	2.5	—	—	—	22.7	4.	16.8	3.1
New Hampshire	19.9	1.4	18.5	2.2	10.9	1.8	83.2	21.9	2.	17.9	1.8
New Jersey	20.0	1.4	19.0	1.6	10.4	1.8	91.9	19.7	2.	20.3	2.0
New Mexico	20.3	1.6	19.6	1.6	8.5	1.9	140.2	21.5	2.	19.1	2.0
New York	20.8	1.6	17.9	1.6	13.8	1.8	51.2	21.2	2.	20.5	2.2
North Carolina	23.1	1.8	22.0	1.8	13.9	1.9	66.1	22.8	2.	23.3	2.2
North Dakota	20.6	1.8	20.9	2.2	13.7	1.8	50.5	22.0	2.	19.2	2.4
Ohio	22.8	1.8	22.1	2.2	16.2	2.4	40.7	23.2	2.	22.4	2.2
Oklahoma	23.2	1.6	19.9	1.6	12.5	1.8	86.3	25.2	2.	21.1	2.0
Oregon	21.6	1.8	22.0	1.6	12.0	1.2	80.8	20.1	2.	23.0	2.5
Pennsylvania	22.6	1.6	21.7	1.6	15.1	1.6	49.8	22.2	2.	23.0	2.2
Rhode Island	18.1	1.6	17.5	1.4	10.2	1.6	78.1	18.2	2.	18.0	2.0
South Carolina	23.0	1.8	22.7	1.8	14.5	1.9	58.7	23.4	2.	22.7	2.4
South Dakota	21.6	1.4	20.3	1.4	13.1	1.8	64.4	24.1	2.	19.0	1.6
Tennessee	24.2	2.0	23.1	1.8	13.2	1.5	83.9	25.2	3.	23.3	2.2
Texas	25.2	1.4	23.5	1.4	13.0	2.0	93.3	25.5	2.	24.9	1.8
Utah	19.9	1.8	19.7	2.0	10.5	1.6	88.8	20.7	2.	19.0	2.4
Vermont	18.1	1.4	18.4	1.4	10.7	1.7	69.3	19.2	2.	17.0	1.6
Virginia	21.4	1.8	18.7	2.0	10.7	1.7	100.6	22.2	2.	20.6	2.4
Washington	19.9	1.4	19.1	1.6	11.0	1.5	81.6	21.4	2.	18.4	1.8
West Virginia	25.3	1.8	23.7	2.0	15.6	1.7	61.8	25.6	2.	25.0	2.4
Wisconsin	22.7	1.8	20.3	1.8	13.1	2.0	73.9	22.9	2.	22.5	2.2
Wyoming	19.9	1.6	18.4	1.8	—	—	—	20.6	2.	19.3	2.2
Guam	21.9	3.3	—	—	—	—	—	21.2	4.	22.8	4.5
Puerto Rico	22.9	1.8	22.8	1.8	—	—	—	23.9	2.	22.0	2.2
Virgin Islands	25.5	2.4	—	—	—	—	—	20.7	3.	29.5	3.1

Summary					
	Both sexes			Men	Women
	2001	2000	1991	2001	2001
No. of states/territories	54	52	48	54	54
Median	21.6	20.8	12.9	21.9	21.1
Range	15.5–27.1	14.4–25.3	8.5–16.5	15.8–26.2	15. 1–29.5
Mean	21.7	20.5	12.7	22.1	21.3

* Obesity is defined as having a body mass index > 30.0 and < 99.8 kg/m2.
Source: "State-Specific Prevalence of Selected Chronic Disease-Related Characteristics—Behavioral Risk Factor Surveillance System, 2001."
  Morbidity and Mortality Weekly Report 2, no. SS-8 (August 22, 2003), 19.

**TABLE 2: OVERWEIGHT AND OBESITY BY AGE,
UNITED STATES: 1960–2000**

	Children, 6–11 Years	Adolescents, 12–19 Years	Adults, 20–74 Years	
	Overweight		Overweight	Obese
Year	Percent	Percent	Percent	Percent
1960–62	—*	—	44.8	13.3
1963–65	4.2	—	—	—
1966–70	—	4.6	—	—
1971–74	4.0	6.1	47.7	14.6
1976–80	6.5	5.0	47.4	15.1
1988–94	11.3	10.5	56.0	23.3
1999–2000	15.3	15.5	64.5	30.9

* — Data not available.
Source: V. M. Fried, et al. *Chartbook on Trends in the Health of Americans. Health, United States, 2003.* Hyattsville, Md.: National Center for
  Health Statistics, 2003.

physical activities are best. As of this writing, the public is currently enamored of the concept that changes in the ratios of fats, carbohydrates, and proteins in the diet will lead to more rapid, effective, or permanent weight loss. Unfortunately, there is no data to demonstrate that this is true. Two studies have shown that over six months, a diet high in fat was slightly more effective than a balanced diet. However, after 12 months, there was no difference in weight loss. The group on the high-fat diet also had a 40 percent dropout rate, which is to say, 40 percent of the subjects were unable to adhere to the diet over a long term.

Most researchers agree, however, that people who wish to lose weight should eat less and exercise more, particularly walking more frequently. Despite following such advice, many obese people find losing weight to be extremely difficult, which may be due to a combination of a genetic predisposition to obesity as well as hormones, such as GHRELIN, that actively work to keep an individual at a given weight.

Behavioral therapy can be helpful and may lead to about a 8–10 percent weight loss in one year. When added to low calorie diets or medications, it will enhance weight loss. Unfortunately, most of these losses are maintained for only six to 12 months. To date, few people have been able to show good maintenance of weight loss over a three- to five-year period.

Some physicians prescribe diet pills (anorectic agents, or drugs to increase satiety or the feeling of fullness) to obese individuals. Pharmaceutical companies are actively testing many formulations in the hopes of developing a safe and effective antiobesity drug. As of this writing, the most commonly used drugs are phentermine (Adipex-P, Ionamin) and sibutramine (Meridia). These drugs are adjunctive to proper nutrition and exercise.

Phentermine will increase noradrenaline in the hypothalamus and decrease appetite. It can increase blood pressure slightly, disrupt sleep, and increase nervousness and tremulousness. Sibutramine increases the concentrations of noradrenaline, serotonin, and dopamine in the hypothalamus, where there are nerves that increase satiety. This drug can raise blood pressure slightly and cause palpitations, dry mouth, and headache.

The antiseizure drug topiramate (Topamax) has been shown to be effective at helping some individuals lose weight. One trial, using 96–256 milligrams of topiramate in 1,289 patients, including 290 patients with BMIs greater than 35, led to weight losses of 8–13 percent of total body weight. In a second study, doses of 96–192 milligrams per day led to a 5–6 kilogram weight loss as well as lower systolic and diastolic blood pressure and improvement in fat distribution. Common adverse effects include paresthesias (pins and needles), dry mouth, fatigue, and impaired concentration.

Surgery

In extreme cases of obesity, physicians may recommend gastric bypass surgery.

See also BLOOD PRESSURE/HYPERTENSION; EATING DISORDERS; GASTRIC SURGERY FOR WEIGHT LOSS.

Bray, George, A., M.D. "Risks of Obesity." *Endocrinology and Metabolism Clinics of North America* 32, no. 4 (2003): 787–804.

Calle, Eugenia E., et al. "Overweight, Obesity and Mortality from Cancer in a Prospectively Studied Cohort of U.S. Adults." *New England Journal of Medicine* 348, no. 17 (April 24, 2003): 1,625–1,638.

Damcott, Coleen M., Paul Sack, M.D., and Alan R. Shuldiner, M.D. "The Genetics of Obesity." *Endocrinology and Metabolism Clinics of North America* 32, no. 4 (2003): 761–786.

Dixon, John B., Maureen E. Dixon, and Paul E. O'Brien, M.D. "Depression in Association with Severe Obesity." *Archives of Internal Medicine* 163, no. 17 (September 22, 2003): 2,058–2,065.

Faroq, I. Sadaf, M.D., et al. "Clinical Spectrum of Obesity and Mutations in the Melanocortin 4 Receptor Gene." *New England Journal of Medicine* 348, no. 12 (March 20, 2003): 1,085–1,095.

Finkelstein, Eric A., Ian C. Fiebelkorn, and Guijing Wang. "State-Level Estimates of Annual Medical Expenditures Attributable to Obesity." *Obesity Research* 12 (2004): 18–24.

Hu, Frank B., M.D. "Television Watching and Other Sedentary Behaviors in Relation to Risk of Obesity and Type 2 Diabetes Mellitus in Women." *Journal of the American Medical Association* 289, no. 14 (April 9, 2003): 1,785–1,791.

Mokdad, Ali H., et al. "Prevalence of Obesity, Diabetes, and Obesity-Related Health Risk Factors, 2001." *Journal of the American Medical Association* 289, no. 1 (January 1, 2003): 76–79.

Reaven, Gerald M., M.D. "Importance of Identifying the Overweight Patient Who Will Benefit the Most by Losing Weight." *Annals of Internal Medicine* 138, no. 5 (2003): 420–423.

Samaha, Frederick F., M.D., et al. "A Low-Carbohydrate as Compared with a Low-Fat Diet in Severe Obesity." *New England Journal of Medicine* 348, no. 21 (May 22, 2003): 2,074–2,081.

Sturm, Roland. "Increases in Clinically Severe Obesity in the United States, 1986–2000." *Archives in Internal Medicine* 163, no. 18 (October 13, 2003): 2,146–2,148.

Thearle, Marie, M.D., and Aronne, Louis J., M.D. "Obesity and Pharmacologic Therapy." *Endocrinology and Metabolism Clinics of North America* 32, no. 4 (2003): 1,005–1,024.

Whitaker, Robert C., M.D., et al. "Predicting Obesity in Young Adulthood from Childhood and Parental Obesity." *New England Journal of Medicine* 337, no. 13 (September 25, 1997): 869–873.

oral contraceptives Prescribed pills with female hormones that are taken by women on a regular basis in order to prevent a pregnancy from occurring. Also known as birth control pills or "the Pill." The first clinical trials of birth control pills occurred in the 1950s. Oral contraceptives contain estrogen and progestin, with the exception of the minipill, which is a low dose of estrogen only. There are also subdermal forms of contraceptives that physicians can surgically insert under the patient's skin, usually in the arm, for continuous action for about five years. Currently, progestin levonorgestrel (Norplant) is the subdermal contraceptive used in the United States.

Sometimes oral contraceptives are prescribed for other purposes as well, such as to control HIRSUTISM (extreme hairiness in women). Some women also take the drugs to improve difficult menstrual periods or to control the symptoms of POLYCYSTIC OVARY SYNDROME. In one study, reported in a 2002 issue of *Contraception,* researchers reported that about 25 percent of women of all reproductive ages in the United States rely upon birth control bills to prevent pregnancy.

Most types of birth control pills fool the woman's body into thinking that she is already pregnant by blocking the luteinizing hormone surge that comes before ovulation. Thus an egg that could create a pregnancy is not released. (The minipill, an exception, does not work this way.) Oral contraceptives are highly effective when used properly. However, some drugs, such as some antibiotics, can counteract the birth control effect. Thus women taking antibiotics should use alternative methods of birth control to avoid a pregnancy.

Adverse Events Associated with Birth Control Pills

Before birth control pills are prescribed, doctors take a complete medical history to ensure that they are likely to be safe for the patient. Women who are at risk for stroke or heart attack should use alternative means of contraception. Women with well-controlled diabetes can usually take oral contraceptives if they are otherwise healthy. Female smokers should avoid birth control pills because of the increased risk for heart attack.

Past studies have indicated that women who take oral contraceptives may have an increased risk for developing breast cancer. However, the results from the Women's Contraception and Reproductive Experiences (CARE) study, released in 2002, found no association between the past or current use of oral contraceptives and breast cancer among the 4,575 female subjects who had developed breast cancer and the 4,682 controls. The women were ages 35–64 years, a group at a high risk of developing breast cancer.

Controversial Issues

Controversies surround birth control pills, such as whether they should be give to minor children and, if so, under what conditions, such as without their parents' knowledge and consent. State laws differ on the rights of minors to have contraceptives without their parents' permission or awareness.

The antiprogestin mifepristone, also known as RU486 or the morning after pill, is not technically an oral contraceptive because it does not prevent a pregnancy. Instead, it terminates a pregnancy that has already occurred, although the woman taking the drug would not know whether she was actually pregnant because it would be too soon for a pregnancy test to be valid.

Davidson, Nancy E., M.D., and Kathy J. Helzlsouer, M.D. "Good News About Oral Contraceptives." *New England Journal of Medicine* 346, no. 26 (June 27, 2002): 2,078–2,079.

Lidegaard O., B. Edstrom, and S. Kreiner. "Oral Contraceptives and Venous Thromboembolism: A Five-Year National Case-Control Study." *Contraception* 65, no. 3 (March 2002): 187–196.

Marks, Lara V. *Sexual Chemistry: A History of the Contraceptive Pill.* New Haven, Conn.: Yale University Press, 2001.

oral glucose tolerance test (OGTT)   A diagnostic test for DIABETES MELLITUS, either TYPE 1 DIABETES or TYPE 2 DIABETES.

After fasting for eight to 14 hours, the patient's blood is drawn and plasma glucose levels are measured. Blood levels are taken again about one and two hours later after the individual has ingested 75 g of glucose that is provided. Normal fasting plasma glucose is defined as less than 100 mg/dl, and 100–125 mg/dl is categorized as impaired fasting glucose, while greater than or equal to 126 mg/dl is indicative of diabetes. A one-hour level that is less than 140 mg/dl is normal, and higher levels are consistent with impaired glucose tolerance or diabetes. Two-hour glucose levels less than 140 mg/dl are normal. Levels of 140–199 mg/dl are consistent with impaired glucose tolerance, and greater than 200 mg/dl is consistent with the diagnosis of diabetes.

An alternative test to the OGTT is the fasting plasma glucose (FPG) test. The AMERICAN DIABETES ASSOCIATION recommends the FPG test over the OGTT because it is easier, faster, and also less expensive than the OGTT. However, most other institutions tend to disagree. More frequently, the OGTT is used to determine whether a patient has euglycemia (normal glucose levels), impaired glucose tolerance (PREDIABETES), or overt diabetes mellitus.

The percentage of patients with impaired glucose tolerance increases with age and obesity. One large study in the United States, the National Health and Nutrition Examination Survey II (NHANES II), estimated that 11 percent of patients aged 20–74 years have impaired glucose tolerance and 6 percent have Type 2 diabetes.

Results of the OGTT may be helpful in large populations to predict cardiovascular risk. In a study of 25,000 patients followed for seven years, researchers demonstrated that the value of the two-hour glucose correlated with cardiovascular mortality risk, while the fasting glucose level did not provide this predictive information. This was also demonstrated in two large epidemiological studies: and the Framingham study Diabetes Epidemiology: Collaborative Analysis of Diagnostic Criteria in Europe (DECODE).

The OGTT is also used for the diagnosis of gestational diabetes (diabetes that occurs due to pregnancy). First, a 50 g one-hour test is used as a screen. If the one-hour level is greater than or equal to 140 mg/dl, the two-hour test is then done to confirm the initial results. The diagnosis of gestational diabetes is made if a pregnant woman's glucose level exceeds any two of the following three levels:

- Fasting glucose greater than 95 mg/dl
- One-hour glucose level greater than 180 mg/dl
- Two-hour level greater than 155 mg/dl

In the past, a three-hour test was used. Although they use different criteria for diagnosis, both the American Diabetes Association and the World Health Organization now employ the two-hour test.

See also INSULIN RESISTANCE SYNDROME.

The DECODE Study Group on behalf of the European Diabetes Epidemiology Group, "Glucose Tolerance and Mortality: Comparison of WHO and American Diabetes Association Diagnostic Criteria." *Lancet* 354, no. 9,179 (August 21, 1999): 617–621.

orthostatic hypotension   An abnormal decrease in blood pressure that occurs when a person moves from the lying to the seated or standing position. Typically, orthostatic hypotension is defined as a drop in blood pressure by greater than 20/10 mm Hg. Any cause of hypotension in general can cause orthostatic hypotension. Endocrine causes of orthostatic hypotension include autonomic neuropathy due to DIABETES MELLITUS, pituitary failure, HYPOTHYROIDISM, and ADDISON'S DISEASE.

If the cause is autonomic neuropathy, the treatment is multifaceted. Usually the patient is allowed to ingest large amounts of salt, while medications that may exacerbate the condition are adjusted or discontinued. Compressive stockings are prescribed to patients to help push more blood from the legs back into the abdomen and chest cavity. If this fails, medications are added.

As of this writing, the only drug formally approved by the Food and Drug Administration (FDA) for orthostatic hypotension is midodrine (Proamatine), which is an alpha receptor agonist. It is usually administered three times per day in divided doses. The major worrisome side effect is supine hypertension, which is blood pressure that is excessively high when the patient is lying down.

Sometimes the endocrinologist must accept some supine hypertension in order to allow the standing blood pressure to be enough for the patient to stand without being light-headed or fainting. Often the mineralocorticoid drug fludrocortisone (Florinef) is given. Initially, it helps the patient to retain some salt and water. Chronically, though, it causes vasoconstriction, which is contraction of the smooth muscles in the blood vessels in the lower extremities, and forces more blood toward the chest cavity, raising blood pressure.

See also BLOOD PRESSURE/HYPERTENSION; HYPOTENSION.

osteoblasts   Cells within the body that are responsible for the creation of new bone. Osteoblasts work in concert with OSTEOCLASTS (which break down bone), and this mutual work leads to bone remodeling. Some buildup and teardown of bone is normal and healthy. When the processes go awry and there is either too much bone (as with osteopetrosis) or not enough bone (such as with OSTEOPENIA/OSTEOPORO-SIS), patients experience medical problems. Osteoblasts appear to derive from so-called mesenchymal stem cells, which may also develop into muscle, fat, and cartilage cells, depending on how they are stimulated.

Osteoblasts help to synthesize new collagen and other proteins that can later be calcified. Some of the osteoblasts remain behind in the new bone and are called osteocytes. They may be needed by the body in the future for further bone remodeling.

These cells can be affected by many hormones and other cells, including parathyroid hormone, vitamin D (calcitriol), thyroid hormones, growth hormone, insulin-like growth factor, TESTOSTERONE, and estrogen. TERIPARATIDE (Forteo), a recombinant parathyroid drug, is the only medication approved by the Food and Drug Administration (FDA), as of this writing, that will directly stimulate osteoblastic activity and subsequently lead to the formation of new bone. Osteoblastic activity can also be monitored by measurements of a simple blood test called the bone specific alkaline phosphatase (BSAP).

See also ESTROGEN; VITAMIN D.

osteoclasts   Cells in the bone that are responsible for bone breakdown. In concert with OSTEOBLASTS (which build up bone), osteoclasts control bone turnover and remodeling. BISPHOSPHONATES, such as alendronate and risedronate directly affect osteoclasts, decreasing their activity. Thus, these drugs are used by physicians to counter the destruction of bone caused by diseases such as OSTEOPOROSIS or osteopenia.

Physicians can monitor the activity of osteoclasts using simple urinary tests. These tests measure the amounts of protein fragments in the urine called N-telopeptides (NTX) and deoxypyridinolinium cross-links (DpD). Endocrinologists will often measure the activity of osteoclasts for three to six months after starting a patient on bisphosphonates to determine three things:

1. Whether the patient is actually taking the medication.
2. Whether the patient is taking the medicine properly (the medication should be taken on

an empty stomach because it is very poorly absorbed when taken with any food or liquid except water).
3. Whether the medication is working adequately to decrease the activity of osteoclasts in the patient's skeleton. This decrease in osteoclastic activity decreases bone loss and is coupled to osteoblastic activity that leads to bone remodeling and the formation of new bones.

Although osteoporosis causes increased osteoclastic activity, this increased activity also can be detected in cases of HYPERPARATHYROIDISM and PAGET'S DISEASE. In contrast, osteoclast activity is unusually low in a rare condition called osteopetrosis.

Osteoclasts actually come from blood cells called monocytes and can be synthesized in the bone marrow and the spleen before traveling to the bone itself. They can also be affected by parathyroid hormone, prostaglandins, vitamin D (calcitriol), and steroids.

Osteoclasts live only about three to four weeks before they undergo apoptosis, which is genetically preprogrammed cell death. Estrogens may exert some of their beneficial effects on bone by inducing this apoptosis earlier in the life of these cells, thus giving them a shorter time to cause bone breakdown.

See also ESTROGEN.

osteogenesis imperfecta (OI)   A group of four hereditary diseases (type I through type IV), primarily found in infants and small children (and occasionally, in adolescents and adults), which causes patients to have very fragile bones that are prone to developing deformities and fractures. Type II is the most severe form of the disorder. Most patients with this form will die while still in infancy. Type I, the most common form of OI, is also the mildest. Osteogenesis imperfecta is also known as brittle bone disease or osteopsathyrosis.

An estimated one in 10,000 people in the world and one in 20,000 children born in the United States have osteogenesis imperfecta. According to the National Institutes of Health Osteoporosis and Related Bone Diseases National Resource Center, about 20,000–50,000 people in the United States have OI. As a result, it qualifies as an orphan disease, or a disease with less than 200,000 cases, and, thus, one that is less likely for pharmaceutical and other research resources to be expended upon the disease, because so few individuals suffer from the problem in comparison to other diseases.

Some parents of children with osteogenesis imperfecta have been unfairly charged with child abuse and neglect due to the seemingly abnormal frequency of broken bones that can occur in affected children. Furthering this problem is the fact that abused children and children with OI actually share some common traits, such as fractures of the ribs, fractures at various stages of healing, and fractures that cannot be explained.

In most cases (about 75 percent), osteogenesis imperfecta is caused by a mutation in the *COL1A1* or *COL1A2* genes, which are genes that create proteins needed to create collagen. However, over 200 different gene mutations have been associated with OI and OI-like syndromes. Collagen is an important substance in the connective tissues, especially in the bones. It is first synthesized as osteoid, before it calcifies to make mature, healthy bone.

Signs and Symptoms

Individuals with all forms of osteogenesis imperfecta experience, at a minimum, osteopenia, which is a lesser form of bone loss than osteoporosis. As a result, they also often suffer from numerous bone fractures due to their fragile bones. They may also experience easy bruising. Many have a short stature. Some patients have brittle opalescent teeth that wear very quickly (dentinogenesis imperfecta), hearing loss (which may require a cochlear implant), curvature of the spine (scoliosis), loose joints, and a bluish or grayish tint to the part of the eye that is normally white (the sclera).

Adults with type I OI have premature osteoporosis or accelerated osteoporosis after the loss of estrogen secretion at menopause. Some children will require wheelchairs and may develop hearing loss due to defects in the middle ear bones that conduct sound waves.

Children with short stature may be treated with recombinant growth hormone. Adults with type I OI present at an earlier age than those with other types.

Women especially may see a rapid progression of the condition after pregnancy and breast-feeding. The hypermobility of the hands, wrists, and feet may require orthopedic surgical intervention.

Diagnosis and Treatment

Physicians may suspect OI based on frequent fractures. If parents know or suspect that a child has OI, they should advise the child's doctor. This way, the child can be tested and evaluated, and the doctor will not mistakenly report the family for possible child abuse.

Physicians may also test for OI if other family members have been diagnosed with the condition. There is no cure for OI. Fractures should be treated quickly, and patients may need mobility aids, such as braces, wheelchairs, and other devices, particularly when OI is severe. Many physicians recommend swimming as a good source of exercise for patients with OI. If patients can walk, walking is another good exercise. Physical therapy may also help some patients.

Some clinical studies are examining the use of pamidronate for individuals with OI. Bone marrow transplants are being investigated for use in children who have severe osteogenesis imperfecta.

In a study reported in a 2000 issue of the *Journal of Clinical Endocrinology & Metabolism*, researchers in Canada investigated the effects of pamidronate treatment on severely ill children younger than age three. The study size was very small (nine subjects) because few children have severe OI. According to the researchers, "Pamidronate treatment in severely affected OI patients under 3 yrs. of age is safe, increases BMD [bone mineral density], and decreases fracture rate."

See also BONE DISEASES; FRACTURES; OSTEOMALACIA; OSTEOPENIA; OSTEOPOROSIS.

For further information, contact the following organizations:

National Institutes of Health
Osteoporosis and Related Bone Diseases—National
    Resource Center
2 AMS Circle
Bethesda, MD 20892
(202) 223-0344 or (800) 624-BONE (toll-free)
http://www.osteo.org

Osteogenesis Imperfecta Foundation
804 West Diamond Avenue
Suite 210
Gaithersburg, MD 20878
(301) 947-0083
http://www.oif.org

Clark, Robin E., and Judith Freeman Clark with Christine Adamec. *The Encyclopedia of Child Abuse,* 2d ed. New York: Facts On File, Inc., 2001.

Plotkin, Horacio, et al. "Pamidronate Treatment of Severe Osteogenesis Imperfecta in Children Under 3 Years of Age." *Journal of Clinical Endocrinology & Metabolism* 85, no. 5 (2000): 1,846–1,850.

osteomalacia   The bone disorder usually characterized by inadequate mineralization of newly formed bone (the osteoid). In children in whom the growth plates at the ends of the bones (epiphyses) have not sealed, it is called rickets. On bone X-rays, the radiologist cannot differentiate between OSTEOPOROSIS and osteomalacia since both appear as decreased mineralization of bone.

Types and Causes of Osteomalacia

Osteomalacia may be due to an inherited defect (X-linked hypophosphatemic rickets or vitamin D-resistant rickets). It may also be acquired, typically due to a vitamin or mineral deficiency.

The most common form of osteomalacia is caused by calcium and/or vitamin D deficiency. This can be due to malnutrition, failure to absorb nutrients (as in chronic pancreatitis, inflammatory bowel disease), or to medications (GLUCOCORTICOIDS, BISPHOSPHONATES, anticonvulsants, aluminum-containing antacids, and cholestyramine (Questran)).

In institutionalized adults, significant vitamin D deficiency may occur in as many as 50 percent of those tested. These patients, as well as the home-dwelling elderly and any patients with chronic illnesses, may not obtain adequate sunlight, thus leading to the deficiency.

Osteomalacia can also be induced by medication given to treat PAGET'S DISEASE when it is administered for excessively long periods of time or in excessive doses. The medication prescribed is usually a bisphosphonate such as alendronate (Fosamax) or risedronate (Actonel).

Rarely, osteomalacia is caused by a tumor (oncogenic osteomalacia), which is often benign. Removal of the tumor usually resolves the problem. Serum phosphorus levels will return to normal, sometimes within hours or days after the surgery is performed. Some experts believe that these tumors secrete an as-yet undiscovered hormone that causes the loss of excessive phosphorus in the urine. However, the skeletal changes may take months to improve.

The tumors that cause oncogenic osteomalacia may be small and hard for physicians to identify. Thus, these patients may live for years with weakness, bone pain, and/or fractures. Blood tests typically show low phosphorus levels. When a tumor cannot be found, some of these patients improve with phosphorus and vitamin D supplementation. In general, the tumors are more likely to occur in the head and neck and can be sought through COMPUTERIZED TOMOGRAPHY (CT) or MAGNETIC RESONANCE IMAGING (MRI) scans.

Hypophosphatasia is a rare form of osteomalacia that can present in childhood or in a milder form in adults. Adults may have recurrent stress fractures, hip pain, or pseudofractures (abnormalities seen on X-ray that appear to be fractures). These patients also have low alkaline phosphatase levels, with normal or high levels of phosphorus and calcium. There is no known medical therapy for hypophosphatasia as of this writing.

Signs and Symptoms

Patients with osteomalacia have an increased risk for experiencing bone fractures. In addition to showing an increased risk for fracture, patients with osteomalacia often have proximal muscle weakness (shoulder and hip muscles). This weakness makes walking up stairs or lifting objects over the head more difficult. It also causes muscle aches and pains, tender shins and wrists, and at times, neuropathy (problems with the nervous system).

Diagnosis and Treatment

When osteomalacia is suspected, an appropriate evaluation would include measurement of blood calcium, phosphorus, alkaline phosphorus, and kidney and liver tests. In addition, parathyroid hormone is often measured, as patients with osteomalacia often have secondary hyperparathyroidism, with low-normal or frankly low blood calcium levels and elevated parathyroid hormone levels. This increased parathyroid hormone acts at the bone to remove calcium, exacerbating the loss of bone strength, but also to maintain the blood calcium level as close to normal as possible.

A 24-hour urine measurement for calcium (the best biological marker for calcium absorption) will confirm the diagnosis if it is low. The normal range is two to four mg of calcium/kg body weight.

See also FRACTURES; OSTEOGENESESIS IMPERFECTA; OSTEOPENIA; VITAMIN D RESISTANCE.

Carpenter, Thomas O., M.D. "Oncogenic Osteomalacia—A Complex Dance of Factors." *New England Journal of Medicine* 348, no. 17 (April 24, 2003): 1,705–1,708.

Dwivedi, Rohit, M.D., and Michael J. Econs, M.D. "X-Linked Hypophosphatemic Rickets," in *NORD Guide to Rare Disorders: The National Organization for Rare Disorders.* Philadelphia, Pa.: Lippincott Williams & Wilkins, 2003.

osteopenia   The term that defines bone mass that is less than normal but not low enough to meet the definition for OSTEOPOROSIS. Technically, osteopenia is defined as a T-score of 1.0 to 2.49 standard deviations below the peak bone mass that is seen in 25- to 30-year-old patients. Osteopenia is also the correct term for physicians to apply when looking at traditional X-rays: if the bones look thin, they are termed osteopenic. The bone density on the X-ray could be low enough to be consistent with osteoporosis, but the appearance of thin bones could also be due to OSTEOMALACIA or even a problem with the X-ray technique.

Any suspicion of osteopenia, osteoporosis, or osteomalacia should be confirmed by a dual energy X-ray absorptiometry scan (DEXA SCAN) or by a quantitative COMPUTERIZED TOMOGRAPHY (CT) scan.

See also BONE DISEASES; BONE MASS MEASUREMENT; OSTEOGENESIS IMPERFECTA.

osteoporosis   Severe degenerative bone loss. Osteoporosis is a common problem among older individuals, particularly females, although some older men are also at risk for this medical problem. At least 20 million women and men in the United States have osteoporosis. In addition, the National Osteoporosis Foundation estimates that 44 million people (including 30 million women) are estimated to have low bone mass.

When osteoporosis occurs due to aging, it is called primary osteoporosis. However, when medical conditions are contributing to osteoporosis, it is called secondary osteoporosis. Some of the secondary causes include endocrine disorders such as HYPERPARATHYROIDISM, CUSHING'S SYNDROME, DIABETES MELLITUS, VITAMIN D DEFICIENCY, and HYPERTHYROIDISM. Some genetic disorders, like MARFAN'S SYNDROME, TURNER SYNDROME and KLINEFELTER SYNDROME, can also lead to the development of osteoporosis. Certain digestive diseases, such as inflammatory bowel disease, celiac diseases, and primary biliary cirrhosis, can also cause osteoporosis due to decreased absorption of calcium and vitamin D.

Other secondary causes of osteoporosis include the use of a variety of drugs, including glucocorticoids, antiseizure medications such as diphenylhydantoin (Dilantin) and medications such as cyclosporine (Neoral, Sandimmune), and excessive doses of levothyroxine (Synthroid, Levoxyl). In addition, significant liver and kidney disease as well as a variety of malignancies can also lead to osteoporosis.

Risk Factors

Small-boned and elderly (age 65 and older) Caucasian women whose ancestors came from western Europe have the greatest risk of developing osteoporosis, although any woman (or any man) may develop osteoporosis. In general, Caucasians and Hispanics have the highest risk of developing osteoporosis in their senior years: 10 percent each, compared with a risk of 7 percent for African Americans of the same age.

Other risk factors for developing osteoporosis include:

- A family history of osteoporosis
- Eating disorders such as ANOREXIA NERVOSA or bulimia
- Diets low in calcium
- Cigarette smoking
- Heavy alcohol consumption
- Presence of inflammatory bowel disease
- Inactive lifestyle
- Thyroid disease
- Medications such as antiseizure drugs, blood thinners, and corticosteroids

A study of 14,824 men and women in the Norfolk branch of the European Prospective Investigation into Cancer (EPIC-Norfolk) trial showed a linear relationship between the quantitative calculation of heel density by ultrasound and the risk of hip and other fractures.

Signs and Symptoms of Osteoporosis

Osteoporosis often causes no symptoms in the early stages, when it is more readily treatable. At later stages, patients with osteoporosis are at risk for developing fractures. Often the first indicator of osteoporosis is, sadly, a bone fracture. However, if physicians know that there is a family history of osteoporosis, they may screen a women younger than age 65 in an attempt to treat this medical problem before it becomes severe and before fractures occur.

A loss in height of an inch or greater is another possible indicator of osteoporosis.

Diagnosis and Treatment

If the physician suspects osteoporosis, he or she will first obtain a medical history and physical examination to elicit information on the aforementioned risk factors as well as look for the signs and symptoms of secondary causes. If there is suspicion of a secondary cause of osteoporosis, appropriate blood and urine tests will be ordered as well as X-rays. The doctor will then usually order a dual-energy X-ray absorptiometry (DEXA) scan. This test is used to measure bone density.

All patients diagnosed with osteoporosis should be taking sufficient amounts of calcium and vitamin D, 1,000–1,500 mg/day of calcium and 400–800 IU of vitamin D, in divided doses. They should also exercise regularly, a minimum of three hours per week. The best form of exercise is walking.

Other drugs that are prescribed for osteoporosis include:

- Alendronate (Fosamax)
- Risedronate (Actonel)
- Raloxifene (Evista)
- Calcitonin (Miacalcin)
- Recombinant parathyroid hormone or TERIPARATIDE (Forteo)

Alendronate decreases clinical vertebral fractures by 45–55 percent and hip fractures by up to 50 percent. Risedronate has decreased vertebral fractures by 40–70 percent and hip fractures by 30 percent. These studies cannot be compared with each other as they included different groups of women treated for different lengths of time. Both the daily and weekly preparations of these medications appear to be equally effective. Only risedronate is approved by the Food and Drug Administration (FDA) for the prevention and treatment of glucocorticoid-induced osteoporosis as of this writing.

Raloxifene has been demonstrated to decrease vertebral fractures by 30–50 percent. Calcitonin has shown a 33 percent decrease.

In the Women's Health Initiative study, in which the study subjects used hormone replacement therapy, clinical fractures were reduced by 34 percent (vertebral and hip) and 24 percent (all fractures). However, the increased risk, albeit quite small, of breast cancer, heart attack, and stroke make hormone replacement therapy less favored, given the other available medication options.

Teriparatide in a 20 mcg dose has been shown to decrease vertebral fractures by 65 percent and nonvertebral fractures by 53 percent. It is the only FDA-approved agent that will directly increase bone density by up to 15 percent in the spine and by 3–5 percent in the hip in 18 months, the largest increases that are seen with any agent. Teriparatide can cause mild headaches and nausea as well as mild HYPERCALCEMIA, typically not clinically significant.

Other treatments under investigation to treat osteoporosis are vitamin D metabolites and sodium fluoride. Some patients may also improve with supplemental magnesium, which should be taken only under the direction of a physician because high levels of magnesium can be toxic to the body.

Researchers in some studies have used growth hormone and insulin-like growth factor 1 (IGF-1) to enhance and maintain bone mass. Although study results with growth hormone have not been significant, IGF-1 appears to be a more promising agent to combat osteoporosis. Other future potential agents to treat osteoporosis are strontium ranelate, which has been effective in clinical studies, and also medications in the statin drug series, such as lovastatin.

Patients whose osteoporosis causes them pain may obtain some relief with anti-inflammatory medications and other painkilling drugs. Calcitonin appears to have some analgesic effects. Both the subcutaneous and nasal forms have been used for two to 12 weeks after an acute fracture to decrease pain.

In 2004, researchers reported on their findings of treating postmenopausal osteoporosis with strontium ranelate. Both study groups received calcium and vitamin D, and one group received two g of strontium per day. The group that received the strontium had "significant and sustained reductions in the risk of vertebral fractures," according to the researchers, who reported on their findings on the New England Journal of Medicine.

See also BISPHOSPHONATES; DEXA SCAN; OSTEOPENIA.

For more information on osteoporosis, contact:

National Institutes of Health
Osteoporosis and Related Bone Diseases—National
  Resource Center
1232 22nd Street NW
Suite 500
Washington, DC 20037-1292
(202) 223-0344 or (800) 624-BONE (toll-free)
http://www.osteo.org

National Osteoporosis Foundation
1232 22nd Street NW
Washington, DC 20037
(202) 223-2226
http://www.nof.org

Eastell, Richard, M.D. "Treatment of Postmenopausal Osteoporosis." New England Journal of Medicine 338, no. 1 (March 12, 1998): 736–746.

Gallagher, J. C., et al. "Combination Treatment with Estrogen and Calcitriol in the Prevention of Age-Related Bone Loss." Journal of Clinical Endocrinology & Metabolism 86, no. 8 (2001): 3,618–3,628.

Khaw, Kay-Tee, et al. "Prediction of Total and Hip Fracture Risk in Men and Women by Quantitative Ultrasound of the Calcaneus: EPIC-Norfolk Prospective Population Study." Lancet 363, no. 9,404 (January 17, 2004): 197–200.

Meunier, Pierre, J., M.D., et al. "The Effects of Strontium Ranelate on the Risk of Vertebral Fracture in Women with Postmenopausal Osteoporosis." New England Journal of Medicine 350, no. 5 (January 29, 2004): 459–468.

Ringe, J. D., H. Faber, and A. Dorst. "Alendronate Treatment of Established Primary Osteoporosis in Men: Results of a 2-Year Prospective Study." Journal of Clinical Endocrinology & Metabolism 86, no. 11 (2001): 5,252–5,255.

Rubin, Mishaela R., M.D., and John P. Bilezikian, M.D. "New Anabolic Therapies in Osteoporosis." Endocrinology and Metabolism Clinics of North America 32, no. 1 (2003): 285–307.

Stein, Emily, M.D., and Elizabeth Shane, M.D. "Secondary Osteoporosis." Endocrinology and Metabolism Clinics of North America 32 (2003): 115–134.

ovarian androgen overproduction   Excessive production of male hormones (androgens) by the ovary, particularly TESTOSTERONE. The condition is also known as ovarian hyperandrogenism. This medical problem may be caused by an ovarian tumor or a metabolic disorder that leads to increased production of androgens in normal tissues. It may also be caused by other disorders, such as POLYCYSTIC OVARY SYNDROME (PCOS), CUSHING'S DISEASE, or CONGENITAL ADRENAL HYPERPLASIA.

Symptoms of Ovarian Androgen Overproduction

The key symptoms of this disorder are as follows:

- Hirsutism (body hair similar to patterns found among men, such as on the chest and face)
- Oily skin
- Acne
- Decreased breast size in comparison with past breast size
- Increased muscle mass without exercising
- Amenorrhea (absence of menstrual periods)
- Balding or thinning hair

Diagnosis and Treatment

If physicians suspect ovarian androgen overproduction, they order tests to measure the levels of total and free testosterone and possibly androstenedione. Other tests are also ordered to determine if the adrenal glands are overproducing androgens. These tests include measures of adrenocorticotropic hormone (ACTH), 17-hydroxyprogesterone, and DHEA-S (dehydroepiandrosterone). The treatment depends on the cause of the overproduction. If it is an ovarian or adrenal tumor, removal of the tumor should correct the problem.

If there is a benign cause and the ovary is felt to be the culprit, ORAL CONTRACEPTIVES can be used to decrease the stimulation of the ovaries by the pituitary hormones FOLLICLE-STIMULATING HORMONE (FSH) and LUTEINIZING HORMONE (LH). If INSULIN RESISTANCE SYNDROME is the cause, then metformin (Glucophage, Glucophage-XR) can be used, although it is not currently approved by the Food and Drug Administration (FDA) for this purpose. If the adrenal gland is causing the ovarian androgen overproduction, small doses of GLUCOCORTICOIDS can be used, such as dexamethasone (Decadron). In low doses, dexamethasone will decrease the adrenal glands' production of the androgens but still allow the needed amounts of cortisol to be produced.

ovarian cancer A malignant tumor of an ovary. About 20,000 cases of ovarian cancer were diagnosed in the year 2000, with a high of 2,646 cases in California and a low of 37 cases in Alaska (see table). Ovarian cancer appears to be on the increase. The American Cancer Society estimated that about 25,580 women were diagnosed with ovarian cancer in 2004. Ovarian cancer represents about 6 percent of all cancer deaths in women. The National Cancer Institute reports that an estimated one in every 57 women in the United States will be diagnosed with ovarian cancer.

The five-year survival rate for ovarian cancer in the United States is 52 percent (which means that 48 percent will die before five years have passed). However, if the disease is treated in the early stages, when cancer is still localized to only the ovary, the five-year survival rate is much higher: 95 percent. Unfortunately, many cases are not identified in the early stages because most women have few or no symptoms at that point. Some preliminary research on tests that may be able to detect ovarian cancer in the early stages is promising and, if efficacious, will be a welcome breakthrough for many women and their families.

Risk Factors

Some women have a greater risk of developing ovarian cancer than others. Some women carry a rare genetic risk for developing ovarian cancer that can be detected as a *BRCA1* or *BRCA2* mutation. In such cases, some women have their ovaries removed, before any cancer develops, to reduce the risk of developing cancer later on.

Other risk factors are as follows:

- A first-degree relative (sister, mother, or daughter) who has had ovarian cancer; the risk is greater still if two or more first-degree relatives have been diagnosed with ovarian cancer
- Childlessness; the risk declines with the number of children that a woman has borne
- Age; women over age 50 have a greater risk of developing ovarian cancer, and the risk increases further for women over age 60
- A previous history of cancer; women who have previously had breast cancer or colon cancer have an increased risk for developing ovarian cancer
- Race; Caucasian women have the greatest risk for developing ovarian cancer although the reason why is unknown

Protective Factors Against Developing Ovarian Cancer

Some studies have shown that some women have a *decreased* risk for developing ovarian cancer, including those women who have had their uterus (but not their ovaries) removed or women who have had a tubal ligation to prevent future pregnancies. Some studies have also found that using oral contraceptives (birth control pills) decreases the risk for a woman later developing ovarian cancer, although other studies have not found this decreased risk. Interestingly, some studies have shown that women who breast-fed their babies had a lower risk of developing ovarian cancer than women who never breast-fed.

Symptoms of Ovarian Cancer

Most women have no symptoms, which is why ovarian cancer has such a high mortality rate. In general, if symptoms do occur, they appear in the later stages of cancer, although any woman should see a physician if she has the following symptoms:

- Generalized abdominal pain or discomfort (pressure, gas, bloated feeling)
- Early satiety (feeling full after eating very little food)
- Weight gain or loss with no apparent cause
- Unusual bleeding from the vagina (for example, in a postmenopausal women who is no longer menstruating)
- Poor appetite
- Diarrhea or constipation
- Frequent urination

The above symptoms are vague and could be caused by many other medical problems. This is why women who experience such symptoms should really see their physicians. Ruling out a serious problem is best.

Diagnosing Ovarian Cancer

Many women have annual checkups with their gynecologist, which is a good idea. The doctor will perform a pelvic examination to check the woman's ovaries, uterus, vagina, bladder, and rec-tum. Sometimes the doctor may find cause for suspicion during a pelvic examination although he or she is unable to diagnose ovarian cancer. In that case, the doctor will order an internal ULTRASOUND test. If any tumors are present, they should show up on the ultrasound. Some doctors may order a COMPUTERIZED TOMOGRAPHY (CT) test to check for possible ovarian cancer.

If a tumor is identified, the physician will take a biopsy, which is a sample of tissue that will be checked by a pathologist for cancer cells. The biopsy is obtained through a small incision in the belly called a laparotomy. This procedure is performed under anesthesia and causes the woman no pain other than the minor pain involved with inserting an intravenous line through which anesthesia can be administered.

By using the biopsy and other tests, the doctor will stage the cancer, which means that he or she will determine how advanced the tumor is and whether it has spread beyond the ovary. These findings will help determine what treatment is recommended. If the tumor is contained within the ovary, it may be curable by surgical excision of the ovary. If the tumor has metastasized (spread) to other organs, the tumor will be treatable but not curable.

Treating Ovarian Cancer

Most women undergo surgery to treat ovarian cancer. Usually both ovaries, the uterus, the cervix, and the fallopian tubes will be removed. This surgery will render the woman unable to have children. Preserving some eggs before the procedure may be possible, should the woman opt for a surrogate mother to carry a baby at some later point. However, most women who have ovarian cancer are worried about surviving, and reproduction is not a major issue to them. In some cases, particularly if the woman is young and the cancer is localized and low grade, the doctor may remove only the cancerous ovary so that the woman may be able to become pregnant later on.

Some women with ovarian cancer may be treated with radiation therapy, which irradiates the area that has been stricken with cancer in an attempt to kill the cancer cells. Radiation therapy may cause some side effects, such as nausea and vomiting, as well as fatigue and diarrhea.

CANCER OF THE OVARY. INVASIVE CANCER INCIDENCE COUNTS BY U.S. CENSUS REGION AND DIVISION, STATE AND METROPOLITAN AREA AND RACE, UNITED STATES, 2000 (NOT ALL STATES REPORTED DATA.)

	All Races	Caucasian	African American		All Races	Caucasian	African American
Northeast				Georgia	526	410	104
New England				Atlanta	175	120	48
Connecticut	311	293	*	Maryland	390	294	66
Maine				North Carolina	661	547	101
Massachusetts	625	586	*	South Carolina	284	213	63
New Hampshire	101	99	*	West Virginia	188	182	*
Rhode Island	96	92	*				
Vermont	45	44	*	East South Central			
				Alabama	364	302	56
Middle Atlantic				Kentucky	366	342	23
New Jersey	851	754	64				
New York	1,665	1,412	167	West South Central			
Pennsylvania	1,314	1,214	62	Louisiana	316	237	68
Midwest				**West**			
East North Central				Mountain			
Illinois	1,015	898	75	Arizona	380	352	*
Indiana	519	495	20	Colorado	345	334	*
Michigan	860	780	66	Idaho	105	104	*
Detroit	364	299	57	Montana	83	82	*
Ohio	935	848	60	Nevada	154	145	*
Wisconsin	428	411	*	New Mexico	128	111	*
				Utah	144	143	*
West North Central				Wyoming	53	53	*
Iowa	300	292	*				
Kansas	225	220	*	Pacific			
Minnesota	412	381	*	Alaska	37	29	*
Missouri	477	435	37	California	2,646	2,284	115
Nebraska	154	145	*	San Francisco-Oakland	344	261	28
North Dakota	57	57	*	San Jose-Monterey	157	127	*
				Los Angeles	753	604	58
South				Hawaii	84	24	*
South Atlantic				Oregon	306	292	*
District of Columbia	52	17	32	Washington	556	529	*
Florida	1,630	1,497	98	Seattle-Puget Sound	401	380	*

*Counts not given if fewer than 16 cases in a category
Source: U.S. Cancer Statistics Working Group. *United States Cancer Statistics: 2000 Incidence.* Department of Health and Human Services, Centers for Disease Control and Prevention and National Cancer Institute, 2003.

If the cancer is an advanced one, the patient may also be treated with chemotherapy. Chemotherapy refers to cancer-killing drugs. Most chemotherapy used to treat ovarian cancer are administered intravenously. Chemotherapy also usually has side effects, most notably nausea and vomiting.

Women may opt to join a clinical trial on ovarian cancer, which would provide the opportunity to be a part of a study that is testing treatments or medications not available to the general public.

After treatment for ovarian cancer, women should see their physicians at least every three months for two years or longer, depending on the doctor's recommendations. With this follow-up schedule, the doctor may be able to detect any recurrences of disease and provide immediate treatment.

Many women may find it helpful to join a support group composed of other women who have or have had ovarian cancer. Although their spouses and family members can sympathize and try to help women diagnosed with ovarian cancer, they cannot truly know what the experience is like. The woman's physician should be able to recommend support groups in the local area.

See also CANCER.

For further information, contact the following organizations:

Gilda Radner Familial Ovarian Cancer Registry
Rosewell Park Cancer Institute
Elm and Carlton Streets
Buffalo, NY 14263
(716) 845-4503 or (800) 682-7426 (toll-free)
http://www.ovariancancer.com

National Ovarian Cancer Coalition, Inc.
500 NE Spanish River Boulevard
Suite 8
Boca Raton, FL 33431
(561) 393-0005 or (888) OVARIAN (toll-free)
http://www.ovarian.org

Altman, Robert, and Michael J. Sarg. *The Cancer Dictionary.* New York, N.Y.: Facts On File, Inc., 2000.
Knopf, Kevin, and Elise Kohn. "Ovarian Cancer." In *Bethesda Handbook of Clinical Oncology.* Philadelphia, Pa.: Lippincott Williams & Wilkins, 2001.
Modan, Baruch, M.D., et al. "Parity, Oral Contraceptives, and the Risk of Ovarian Cancer Among Carriers and Noncarriers of BRCA1 or BRCA2 Mutation." *New England Journal of Medicine* 345, no. 4 (July 26, 2001): 235–240.
Rebbeck, Timothy R., et al. "Prophylactic Oophorectomy in Carriers of BRCA1 or BRCA2 Mutations." *New England Journal of Medicine* 346, no. 2 (May 23, 2002): 1,616–1,622.

ovarian cyst   Fluid-filled and usually noncancerous growth that occurs on an ovary. Many cysts cause no symptoms, while others are painful. When cysts are large and painful, physicians (usually gynecologists) may remove such cysts and may biopsy surrounding ovarian tissue to rule out the presence of CANCER. The presence of an ovarian cyst may impair a woman's fertility. Ovarian cysts can be detected upon a pelvic examination and confirmed by pelvic and/or vaginal ultrasound. As the technology improves, the diagnostic criteria for ovarian cysts continue to be refined. In one study, up to 23 percent of women volunteers who were considered "normal" and had not been previously diagnosed with any cysts prior to the study met the criteria for polycystic ovaries, or 10 or more cysts at least two to eight millimeters in diameter.

See also OVARY.

ovarian failure, premature   The cessation of the function of the ovary before it would normally occur, or in a woman's 30s or early 40s. This does not include cases in which the ovary was removed because of an ovarian cyst, ovarian cancer, or for other medical conditions. Premature ovarian failure will cause infertility because eggs will no longer be produced.

See also OVARY.

ovary   A female reproductive organ located within the abdominal/pelvic cavity. Normal females have two ovaries. The ovary is the female counterpart to the male testis (also known as the testicle). The ovary releases eggs in a process called ovulation.

One of these eggs may be combined with male sperm to create a human embryo. In a normal premenopausal adult woman, the monthly ovulation process continues unless it is interrupted by ORAL CONTRACEPTIVES, natural or surgically induced MENOPAUSE, or illness.

The ovaries also produce female hormones, including ESTRADIOL and progesterone. These hormones, particularly estradiol, are responsible for female sexual characteristics, such as breast development, the pattern of body hair, fat distribution, and other key aspects of female sexuality. In addition, the ovaries are linked to the woman's monthly menstrual cycle. The normal operation of the ovaries is also tied to the normal operation of other endocrine organs, such as the HYPOTHALAMUS, PITUITARY, and the ADRENAL GLANDS.

If the ovaries malfunction, women may experience problems with infertility. Some women develop OVARIAN CYSTS or OVARIAN CANCER. Others experience ovarian failure, such as with TURNER SYNDROME. POLYCYSTIC OVARY SYNDROME is another example of an ovarian disorder, and it is likely to be induced by INSULIN RESISTANCE SYNDROME. Other disorders may also lead to ovarian malfunctions; for example, the EARLY PUBERTY that is characteristic of MCCUNE-ALBRIGHT SYNDROME is often caused by estrogens generated by ovarian cysts.

Paget's disease   A bone disease primarily characterized by an enlarged and abnormal bone structure and caused by an overproduction of poor-quality bone. First described by Sir James Paget in 1877 (he called the disease *osteitis deformans*), Paget's disease causes joint dysfunction in most patients and may also cause bone pain. When the disease occurs in children or adolescents, it is called juvenile Paget's disease, hyperostosis corticalis deformans juvenilis, or hereditary hyperphosphatasia. Some experts believe that the great composer Ludwig van Beethoven suffered from Paget's disease, causing his hearing loss.

Paget's disease most commonly affects the hip, spine, pelvis, skull, tibia (a leg bone), and humerus (an arm bone). Some experts believe that a virus may cause Paget's disease, although no virus has been isolated to date.

Phases of the Disease

In the early phases of Paget's disease, bone resorption (loss) mediated by overactive OSTEOCLASTS is a key feature. This is followed by a phase in which both the osteoblasts and osteoclasts become overactive. The next phase is one of bone remodeling and sclerosis. At that point, because of the extreme bone changes, physicians may mistakenly believe that the patient has advanced cancer rather than Paget's disease. Making the diagnosis even more difficult, it is also possible for an individual to have Paget's disease and bone cancer at the same time.

A Rare Complication

One rare complication of Paget's disease, occurring in about 1 percent of all patients with the disease, is the development of a malignant bone sarcoma. These tumors are fast growing, and few patients survive for longer than a year. The pelvis, humerus, femur, and tibia are the most common sites for these sarcomas. The patient with a malignant bone sarcoma generally experiences increased bone pain and/or tissue swelling in the area. No treatment is available for this complication.

Risk Factors

The risk for developing Paget's disease increases with age. The disease is found in about 3 percent of all individuals in Europe and North America who are older than age 55. Men are more likely to have Paget's disease than women, in a three-to-two ratio. The disease is more common in people in eastern and northern Europe and in places where Europeans have migrated to, such as to the United States, Australia, and New Zealand. Conversely, the disease is rare in Scandinavia, Asia, and Africa. Racial differences also occur. Caucasians are much more likely to have Paget's disease than African Americans.

The disease also appears to have genetic factors. Certain studies have shown that the risk of a first-degree relative (parent or child) having Paget's disease is seven times greater than it is among individuals who do not have first-degree relatives with the disease. Other studies have demonstrated that the risk for developing Paget's disease, up to the age of 90 years, is 9 percent for people with a first-degree relative, compared with only a 2 percent risk for the general population.

Signs and Symptoms of Paget's Disease

Although some patients have pain with Paget's disease, many do not. In fact, most patients have no signs or symptoms. The disease is often discovered accidentally when X-rays are taken for another purpose and the radiologist notes the characteristic skeletal abnormalities of Paget's disease. Patients with Paget's disease also have an elevated alkaline phosphatase blood level. Sometimes a test for alkaline phosphatase levels is ordered for another purpose and thus the disease is discovered.

Paget's disease may cause difficulty with walking and gait abnormalities because of the bone remodeling that has occurred in the spine, a common site for Paget's disease. Often osteoarthritis is present along with Paget's disease, making the diagnosis more difficult. Some doctors will assume that the problem is solely one of osteoarthritis rather than a combination of both osteoarthritis and Paget's disease.

Paget's disease may also cause a hearing loss by compressing the eighth cranial nerve or affecting the middle ear ossicles. A survey of 958 patients with Paget's disease revealed that 37 percent had some hearing loss, and 31 percent had bowed limbs. Other cranial nerve problems, leading to facial drooping and eye movement disorders, may also be seen with Paget's disease.

If the base of the skull is affected, hydrocephalus may occur (the disruption of the normal flow of cerebrospinal fluid in the brain), necessitating a shunt procedure to prevent coma and/or death in the patient. Fortunately, this complication is rare. In severe cases of Paget's disease, congestive heart failure may also occur due to the large amount of blood diverted to the hypermetabolic bones.

If pain does occur with Paget's disease, it is usually described as a dull and aching pain that is often worse at night.

Other disorders often associated with Paget's disease include the following:

- Arthritis
- Fractures
- HYPERPARATHYROIDISM
- OSTEOPOROSIS
- Thyroid disease
- Kidney stones

Diagnosis and Treatment

Physicians who suspect that a patient may have Paget's disease should order imaging tests and radionuclide studies, although even simple X-rays may show indications of the disease in the intermediate-to-later stages.

Patients with Paget's disease can be treated with BISPHOSPHANATE drugs such as etidronate (Didronel), alendronate (Fosamax), risedronate (Actonel), tiludronate (Skelid), and pamidronate (Aredia). These are all oral medications, except for pamidronate, which must be administered intravenously. These drugs can often suppress the disease process for years. Medications such as salmon calcitonin (including Calcimar and Miacalcin) are also sometimes used to treat patients with Paget's disease. Salmon calcitonin can be administered either intramuscularly or subcutaneously in an injection. It is also available as a nasal spray (Miacalcin), although the nasal spray is generally not as effective as are the injections.

If patients with Paget's disease have bone pain, it is usually treated with acetaminophen (Tylenol) or with one among many different brands of nonsteroidal anti-inflammatory medications (NSAIDs). Nonarthritis pain in the joint is usually responsive to a bisphosphonate medication.

See also CALCIUM BALANCE, OSTEOBLASTS.

For further information on Paget's disease, contact the following organization:

Paget Foundation for Paget's Disease of Bone and
    Related Disorders
120 Wall Street
Suite 1602
New York, NY 10005
(800) 23-PAGET (toll-free) or (212) 509-5335
http://www.paget.org

Delmas, Pierre D., M.D., and Pierre J. Meunier, M.D. "The Management of Paget's Disease of Bone." *New England Journal of Medicine* 336, no. 8 (February 20, 1997): 558–566.

Duncan, William E., M.D. "Paget's Disease of the Bone," in *Endocrine Secrets*. Philadelphia, Pa.: Hanley & Belfus, Inc., 2002.

Gold, D. T., et al. "Paget's Disease of Bone and Quality of Life." *Journal of Bone Mineral Research* 11, no. 12 (1996): 1,897–1,904.

Leach, Robin J., Frederick R. Singer, and G. David Roodman. "The Genetics of Paget's Disease of the Bone." *Journal of Clinical Endocrinology & Metabolism* 86, no. 1 (2001): 24–28.

Siris, E. S. "Epidemiological Aspects of Paget's Disease: Family History and Relationship to Other Medical Conditions." *Seminars in Arthritis and Rheumatism* 23, no. 4 (1994): 222–225.

Whyte, Michael P., M.D., et al. "Oseoprotegerin Deficiency and Juvenile Paget's Disease." *New England Journal of Medicine* 347, no. 3 (July 15, 2002): 175–184.

pancreas   A gland, about six inches in length, that performs several essential functions. The pancreas has both endocrine and exocrine functions.

Endocrine Functions

For its endocrine functions, the pancreas secretes insulin from the beta cells in the islets of Langerhans. These insulin-rich beta cells make up about 50–60 percent of the pancreas.

INSULIN is a hormone that helps the body appropriately assimilate carbohydrates (sugar) so it may be stored as glycogen in the liver and muscle. It also helps to transfer fat (as fatty acids) into triglycerides and store energy, and it allows amino acids to be incorporated into protein. Without insulin, the disease known as DIABETES MELLITUS occurs. With a complete lack of insulin, individuals present with TYPE 1 DIABETES. Prior to the discovery of insulin in 1921, there was a 100 percent fatality rate among all patients with Type 1 diabetes.

The pancreas also secretes glucagon from the alpha cells (which make up about 25 percent of the pancreas). Glucagon helps release glucose from the liver when the pancreas and brain perceive that the ambient glucose level is too low. In addition, the pancreas secretes amylin, a peptide hormone that is cosecreted with insulin and helps slow the emptying of the stomach (thereby smoothing out delivery of nutrients to the bloodstream).

Amylin also decreases the amount of glucagons secreted in response to eating a meal, decreasing the rise in glucose after a meal. By acting directly on the brain, amylin helps to increase satiety (the feeling of fullness) and decrease appetite. Several amylin-like injectable products are in development for use in the treatment of diabetes.

The pancreas also secretes pancreatic polypeptide (from F cells), vasoactive intestinal polypeptide (from neurons in the gastrointestinal tract), and somatostatin and gastrin (from D cells).

Exocrine Function

In its role as an exocrine gland, the pancreas excretes a number of enzymes into the duodenum, via two ducts, in response to ingested meals. Any obstruction of these ducts or the small ducts within the pancreas, especially by gallstones and/or "sludge" from the bile, will lead to PANCREATITIS. These enzymes include lipases, pancreatipase, amylase, trypsins, and others. Most of these enzymes are stored in an inactive form to prevent the pancreas from digesting itself.

When the pancreas malfunctions, as with diabetes mellitus and pancreatitis, the results are serious. PANCREATIC CANCER is nearly always fatal unless diagnosed in the early stages.

pancreatic cancer   A dangerous and usually fatal form of cancer. According to the American Cancer Society, an estimated 31,860 new cases were expected in the United States in 2004. An estimated 31,270 people were expected to die of pancreatic cancer in 2004, including 15,440 men and 15,830 women. Pancreatic cancer represents about two percent of all cancer cases in both men and women.

The five-year survival rate for pancreatic cancer is low. Only about 5 percent of patients with pancreatic cancer will survive for five years; this means 95 percent of patients with pancreatic cancer die before five years have passed.

Despite the dismal outlook with pancreatic cancer as of this writing, researchers are actively seeking information on causes and possible treatments.

Risk Factors for Developing Pancreatic Cancer

Although any individual can develop pancreatic cancer, the risk will vary depending on the following factors:

- Age: the risk increases with age and is highest among people ages 60 and older
- Smoking: people who smoke have a two to three times greater risk of developing pancreatic cancer than nonsmokers

- Diabetes: patients with diabetes have an increased risk
- Race: African Americans have a greater risk of developing pancreatic cancer than Asians, Hispanics, or Caucasians
- Family history: the risk triples if a parent or sibling had pancreatic cancer, and the risk is also increased if a parent or sibling had colon cancer or ovarian cancer

Signs and Symptoms of Pancreatic Cancer

Although signs and symptoms often do not present until the disease is advanced, some indicators of pancreatic cancer should be checked. Patients with these signs and symptoms may have another illness, such as hepatitis that should also be assessed by a physician.

The most common indicators of pancreatic cancer are as follows:

- Yellow skin and eyes (caused by jaundice)
- Dark-colored urine (also caused by jaundice)
- Nausea and vomiting
- Appetite loss
- Unintended weight loss
- Pain in the upper abdomen or the upper back
- Fluid buildup in the abdomen (ascites)

Diagnosis and Treatment

If the physician suspects the presence of pancreatic cancer, he or she performs a physical examination, checking for the presence of jaundice (pronounced yellowing of the skin and eyes caused by a problem with the liver or pancreas). The doctor will also check the abdomen in the area of the pancreas to see if there is pain or an abnormal buildup of fluid. Laboratory tests will show if there is an elevated rate of bilirubin, indicating jaundice that may be caused by a blockage in the pancreatic duct or bile duct due to a tumor. Further information will be provided with a COMPUTERIZED TOMOGRAPHY (CT) scan and ultrasound procedures. A gastroenterologist may perform an endoscopic retrograde cholan-giopancreatography (ERCP), a test in which an endoscope is passed through the patient's mouth and into the stomach and the small intestine. The doctor inserts a catheter through the endoscope to inspect the bile ducts and pancreatic ducts.

The doctor may also perform a biopsy to check for cancer. The biopsy can be achieved during the ERCP or during abdominal surgery. It may also be performed using an internal ultrasound called an endoscopic ultrasound (EUS).

Other options include surgery, radiation therapy, or chemotherapy. Gemcitabine (Gemzar) is the most common drug used to treat pancreatic cancer. It has many side effects but can be efficacious in some patients. Some physicians use a combination of two therapies at a time, such as combining gemcitabine with radiation treatment.

If surgery is performed, and all or most of the pancreas is removed, patients will develop diabetes and chronic digestive disorders, such as diarrhea and cramping.

Pancreatic cancer is usually diagnosed at a late stage, when it is impossible to overcome with mainstream treatments. For this reason, many patients are encouraged to join a clinical trial when they are diagnosed, in which they may have an opportunity to try medications and treatments that are not available to most patients.

pancreatitis Inflammation of the pancreas, which may be acute or chronic. If acute, the condition may be life threatening, and the individual should be hospitalized so that he or she can receive immediate and careful treatment. Experts report that about 10 percent of cases of patients with acute pancreatitis become life threatening, with a high death rate. If pancreatitis is a chronic problem rather than an acute one, the patient may be treated outside the hospital.

The most common causes of pancreatitis are gallstones or chronic alcohol abuse (together they represent the etiology of about 80 percent of all the cases of pancreatitis). However, some metabolic medical problems can also lead to pancreatitis; for example, HYPERTRIGLYCERIDEMIA, which refers to elevated blood triglycerides levels (usually greater than 1,000 mg/dl may induce pancreatitis). In some cases, congenital defects of the pancreas or biliary duct system may cause pancreatitis. Very infrequently, HYPERPARATHYROIDISM with its associated HYPERCALCEMIA may cause pancreatitis. In addition, some medications may cause the condition.

Risk Factors

Obesity is a major risk factor for developing pancreatitis, mainly due to its association with gallstones and hypertriglyceridemia. The other major risk factor is alcohol abuse.

Some infections are also associated with the development of pancreatitis, particularly hepatitis A and B. Patients with acquired immune deficiency syndrome (AIDS) have a greater risk than others of developing the condition. This occurs partly because AIDS patients are more likely to develop infections that can affect the pancreas (such as cytomegalovirus, cryptococcus, and other infections) and partly because AIDS patients are more likely to take medications, such as pentamidine and sulfa drugs, that can cause pancreatitis directly.

Pancreatitis can also be genetic. Hereditary pancreatitis is a rare condition that has been linked to chromosome 7. Symptoms and signs of hereditary pancreatitis usually occur before the child is 10 years old but are often mild at first, with increasingly difficult bouts that may occur on a weekly or more frequent basis.

Signs and Symptoms of Pancreatitis

Severe nausea with or without vomiting and abdominal pain, often around the umbilicus and radiating toward the back, are the most common indicators of pancreatitis. Patients with pancreatitis are often so ill that they present at hospital emergency rooms.

Diagnosis and Treatment

If the patient's signs and symptoms indicate the possible presence of pancreatitis, the diagnosis can be confirmed with blood tests, specifically, tests for the pancreatic enzymes lipase and amylase. Imaging tests, such as COMPUTERIZED TOMOGRAPHY (CT) scans or ULTRASOUND tests, may help corroborate the diagnosis by revealing gallstones or changes within the pancreas.

In severe cases of pancreatitis, plain X-rays will show indications of pancreatitis, such as pancreatic calcifications. Blood tests are also ordered to determine if triglyceride levels are elevated. A special type of endoscopy (ERCP) may be ordered to evaluate the condition of the pancreas, which may also include removal of stones or insertion of prostheses to widen closed ducts. This is a very specialized procedure that should be performed only by an experienced gastroenterologist.

The treatment of pancreatitis depends on the identified cause as well as the treatment for pain. In most cases, patients are given bowel rest, which means they are not allowed to eat, as this would stimulate the secretion of digestive enzymes from the pancreas and worsen the situation. Patients are also given intravenous fluids during this period

If an infection is identified, antibiotics or other drugs specific for the particular infection are indicated. If gallstones have caused pancreatitis, gallbladder surgery may be indicated. If the pancreatitis stems from chronic alcoholism, patients are urged to stop drinking altogether and are warned that continued consumption of alcohol could lead to their death. In some cases, medications can cause pancreatitis. If so, they are discontinued or the dosages are decreased. When high triglyceride levels are the cause of the pancreatitis, the patient is given dietary recommendations and appropriate medications to lower triglyceride levels.

Acutely severe pancreatitis can lead to endocrine dysfunction, leading to the need for insulin therapy to normalize glucose levels. The chronic use of insulin and pancreatic enzyme supplements are needed when 80 percent of the pancreas is damaged.

See also AIDS; DIABETES MELLITUS; OBESITY; PANCREAS.

Blomgren, Kerstein B., et al. "Obesity and Treatment of Diabetes with Glyburide May Both Be Risk Factors for Acute Pancreatitis." *Diabetes Care* 25, no. 2 (February 2002): 298–302.

Minocha, Anil, M.D., and Christine Adamec. *The Encyclopedia of Digestive Diseases and Disorders.* New York: Facts On File, Inc., 2004.

Steinberg, William, and Scott Tenner. "Acute Pancreatitis." *New England Journal of Medicine* 330, no. 17 (April 28, 1994): 1,198–1,210.

parathyroid cancer A rare form of cancer that stems from the parathyroid glands and that also may cause HYPERCALCEMIA (excessive levels of calcium in the blood). Only a few hundred cases per year of parathyroid cancer are reported in the United States, at most. The five-year survival rates among parathyroid cancer patients are variable, ranging from 40–86 percent.

Parathyroid cancer cases represent less than 1 percent of all cases of patients who are diagnosed with primary HYPERPARATHYROIDISM. The risk for developing parathyroid cancer appears to be slightly increased among patients who are undergoing treatment for end-stage renal disease (kidney failure). Parathyroid cancer is also associated with MULTIPLE ENDOCRINE NEOPLASIA, type 1 (MEN 1).

Diagnosis and Treatment

Patients with parathyroid cancer usually have higher calcium levels on average than patients with benign causes of hyperparathyroidism. These patients are much more likely than patients with benign hyperparathyroidism to have a neck mass, bone disease, and kidney problems. As the calcium levels are much higher than normal, they can also present as parathyroid crisis. This occurs when the patients have severe hypercalcemia, with mental status changes as well as dysfunction of other organ systems. The pathologist often has difficulty distinguishing between a benign parathyroid adenoma and parathyroid cancer.

When identified, the treatment for parathyroid carcinoma is the surgical removal of the cancerous parathyroid gland and a thorough evaluation of the other three parathyroids for any indication of cancer. If cancer is found in the other glands, they should also be surgically excised. In addition, parts of the thyroid gland or the entire thyroid may also need to be excised. Depending upon the location of the tumor, wide surgical excision may necessitate removal of lymph nodes, the thymus gland, and muscle tissue in the neck.

Postoperatively, the patient must be watched very carefully, because he or she may experience severe HYPOCALCEMIA (unusually low levels of calcium in the blood) and may need large doses of intravenous calcium until the body stabilizes to normal. This occurs because these patients may develop hungry bone syndrome, a situation that develops when there has been a long period of excessive parathyroid hormone exposure of the bone with attendant micro- and macrostructural changes.

After recovery occurs, most patients can be maintained on daily oral doses of calcium and prescribed CALCITRIOL (vitamin D). After all surgical options have been exhausted, medical treatment of parathyroid cancer revolves around the control of hypercalcemia, with adequate hydration and the use of BISPHOSPHONATES and gallium nitrate. Drugs that mimic the effects of calcium have been used experimentally. Radiation therapy has also been used, although the results have been variable. The National Cancer database reported a 10-year survival rate of 49 percent in a cohort of 286 patients.

See also CALCIUM BALANCE; PARATHYROID GLANDS.

Hundahl, S. A., et al. "Two Hundred Eight-Six Cases of Parathyroid Carcinoma Treated in the U.S. Between 1985–1995: A National Cancer Data Base Report. The American College of Surgeons Commission on Cancer and the American Cancer Society." *Cancer* 86, no. 3 (August 1, 1999): 538–544.

Shane, Elizabeth. "Parathyroid Carcinoma." *Journal of Clinical Endocrinology & Metabolism* 86, no. 2 (2001): 485–493.

parathyroid glands Refers to the four endocrine glands located in the neck around the thyroid gland and that control the exchange of calcium into the bloodstream and the bones. On occasion, a person may have three or even five or six parathyroid glands. At times, parathyroid glands develop within the thyroid gland or even migrate down into the chest.

Sometimes a parathyroid gland or glands may become cystic and these cysts may be functional (still able to secrete some parathyroid hormone). These cystic glands can also form in the lateral neck as an embryological remnant. They can also form from the degeneration of very large parathyroid adenomas.

They are usually discovered as small, soft neck masses. Aspiration of these cysts may resolve them. Parathyroid hormone can be measured in the cyst fluid from those cysts that are functional.

See also CALCIUM ABSORPTION; HYPERCALCEMIA; HYPERPARATHYROIDISM; HYPOCALCEMIA; HYPOPARATHYROIDISM.

parathyroid hormone (parathormone or PTH) The protein hormone, secreted by the parathyroid glands in the neck, that helps to regulate calcium and phosphorus balance in the bloodstream. When the blood calcium level in the body dips even slightly, this dip is sensed by the parathyroid glands, which then increase their secretion of parathyroid hormone. At that point, PTH travels via the bloodstream to the gut, bone, and the kidney to exert its effects. Parathyroid hormone also affects the bone. At the site of the bone, PTH activates OSTEOCLASTS and also helps to remove a small amount of calcium from the bone to return the blood level to normal.

Parathyroid hormone also helps to stimulate the conversion of vitamin D to a more active form, which works at the gut to help increase calcium absorption. In the kidneys, PTH stimulates the reabsorption of the calcium that is filtered, thus increasing the amount of calcium in the bloodstream.

As the calcium level in the blood returns to its previous level, this change is sensed by the parathyroid glands, which will then decrease their secretion of PTH. If the level of calcium in the blood becomes too low or too high, the parathyroid glands will react and change their secretion of PTH hormone to normalize the blood calcium levels.

An excessive continued secretion of PTH is called HYPERPARATHYROIDISM, a disease that is subdivided into primary, secondary, and tertiary hyperparathyroidism.

PTH can be measured in the blood. When measured, intact PTH is most frequently measured, as is the level of calcium. The endocrinologist needs to compare the relative values of both PTH and calcium in order to interpret the patient's clinical situation appropriately.

Conversely, an inadequate secretion of parathyroid hormone leads to a condition called HYPOPARATHYROIDISM. This condition may be caused by neck surgery, particularly of the thyroid gland. It results from damage to the parathyroid glands and/or to their blood supply. In addition, severe deficiencies of magnesium, which are seen in malnourished patients and especially alcoholics, can lead to a state of hypoparathyroidism and HYPOCALCEMIA (abnormally low blood levels of calcium).

Recombinant PTH is now available as an injectable drug called TERIPERATIDE (Forteo) and is used for the treatment of severe OSTEOPOROSIS.

Parathormone-related peptide, or PTH-rp is a protein or peptide that is secreted by some malignant tumors. It can lead to the development of HYPERCALCEMIA. PTH-rp is similar in structure to PTH, but it can be specifically measured to help physicians determine if a patient's elevated blood calcium levels are due to excessive PTH (high calcium, high PTH, and low or normal PTH-rp) or to PTH-rp (high calcium, low PTH and high PTH-rp).

See also PARATHYROID GLANDS.

pheochromocytoma A tumor, usually of the medulla of the adrenal gland. Most (90 percent) of pheochromocytomas occur in the adrenal gland. However, they can also be found anywhere along the midline of the body along the sympathetic nervous system chain, from near the bladder up to the carotid arteries.

Most pheochromocytomas are benign (about 90 percent), but some are cancerous. The pheochromocytoma leads to secretion of excessive amounts of catecholamines (adrenaline, noradrenalin), leading to severe paroxysms of hypertension (only 5 percent of patients with pheochromocytomas have normal blood pressure), ORTHOSTATIC HYPOTENSION, headaches, and episodes of flushing. Other symptoms include palpitations, rapid heart rate, anxiety, chest pain, and sweating.

On rare occasions, pheochromocytomas also secrete other hormones, including CALCITONIN, neuropeptide y, PTH-rp, and adrenocorticotropic hormone (ACTH).

If undiagnosed, pheochromocytomas will lead to death even in very healthy young individuals, especially if they undergo surgery with general anesthesia and the condition is not recognized and treated ahead of time.

Pheochromocytomas may occur spontaneously or may be associated with other endocrine and genetic disorders, such as MULTIPLE ENDOCRINE NEOPLASIA, type 2 syndrome, familial pheochromocytoma, von Hippel-Lindau disease, NEUROFIBROMATOSIS, and von Recklinghausen disease.

The majority of these tumors are unilateral (on one side), but 5–10 percent may be bilateral. About 10 percent of the cases occur in children.

When they occur, pheochromocytomas most commonly appear among patients in their 40s and 50s. They are a secondary cause of hypertension (representing 1 percent or less of the cases of hypertension).

Diagnosis and Treatment

The standard approach when a patient has signs and symptoms suggestive of a pheochromocytoma is to measure catecholamines and their metabolites in a 24-hour urine collection. The measurement of plasma metanephrines may become a standard test in the future. When the diagnosis is in doubt, the clonidine suppression test may be ordered. This test measures levels of epinephrine, norepinephrine, and dopamine. If the hormone levels are abnormally high, this indicates the presence of a pheochromocytoma.

Once a diagnosis is made, the tumor is localized with COMPUTERIZED TOMOGRAPHY (CT) scanning of the abdomen, and elsewhere if necessary. If the tumor cannot be found with standard imaging modalities, a special nuclear medicine imaging test called a METAIODOBENZYLGUANIDINE SCAN (MIBG scan) may be obtained.

The ultimate treatment is excision of the tumor. However, prior to anesthesia and surgery, the excess catecholamines are controlled, usually with a combination of alpha-blockers (phenoxybenzamine, prazosin (Minipress), doxazosin (Cardura), terazosin (Hytrin), and phentolamine) and beta-blockers (labetalol, propranolol (Indera, Inderal-LA), atenolol (Tenormin) and metoprolol (Lopressor, Toprol-XL). When needed, calcium channel blockers and volume repletion can also be used prior to surgery.

See also ADRENAL GLANDS; CANCER; CLONIDINE SUPPRESSION TEST.

Klinger, H. Cristoph, et al. "Pheochromocytoma." *Urology* 57, no. 6 (2001): 1,025–1,032.

Young, W. F. "Pheochromocytoma and Primary Aldosteronism: Diagnostic Approaches." *Endocrinology and Metabolism Clinics of North America* 26, no. 4 (1997): 801–827.

physical examination   The physician's review of the patient's medical history, including a history of the chief complaint and present illness, a review of systems, a social history, a past medical history, and a family history, as well as an examination of any parts of the body that appear to have signs of disease or about which the patient complains.

Most physical examinations include annual routine tests after a given age, such as a rectal examination, a breast check for lumps, and so forth. Endocrine diseases and disorders (as well as other medical problems) are often identified during an annual health check. For example, the physician may notice that a patient has an enlarged neck or staring, protruding eyes, which may indicate HYPERTHYROIDISM and ophthalmopathy caused by GRAVES' DISEASE.

See also COMPUTERIZED TOMOGRAPHY; MAGNETIC RESONANCE IMAGING; ULTRASOUND.

pineal gland   An endocrine gland whose function is largely unknown. However, it is known that the pineal gland secretes natural melatonin, which is involved in the sleep-wake cycles of humans. The secretion of melatonin is mainly controlled by cycles of light and dark (day and night). Melatonin can be taken as a supplement to prevent jet lag.

Some studies indicate that melatonin secreted by the pineal gland may have a protective effect against the development of some forms of cancer. A malfunction of the pineal gland may cause sleep disorders because of the insufficient release of melatonin. Studies of elderly individuals with decreased melatonin levels have shown that the patients improved with supplemental melatonin.

On rare occasions, benign and malignant tumors as well as cysts of the pineal gland may form.

See also ELDERLY; MELATONIN.

pituitary adenomas   Benign tumors of the pituitary gland. The most common pituitary adenomas secrete prolactin (PROLACTINOMA) or are nonsecreting. They are usually detected by MAGNETIC RESONANCE IMAGING (MRI) of the pituitary gland. Tumors that measure between one and nine millimeters are called microadenomas, and those that are 10 millimeters or greater are called macroadenomas. They may be detected because they make one of several hormones and cause some sort of clinical syndrome that brings the patient to medical attention. Instead of secreting complete functional hormones, some adenomas secrete only the alpha or beta subunits of pituitary hormones and they have no endocrine activity.

Sometimes pituitary adenomas are found when an MRI or COMPUTERIZED TOMOGRAPHY (CT) scan of the brain is performed for another reason. These tumors are often referred to as incidentalomas, and often they cause no symptoms.

In some autopsy series, as many as 25 percent of the deceased patients had a small pituitary adenoma, usually one that was not detected prior to death.

Treatment of these tumors is directed at the underlying disorder and can include medications, surgery, and radiation therapy. Much modern pituitary surgery is performed via the transsphenoidal approach. This surgery requires the cooperation of a neurosurgeon as well as an otorhinolaryngologist (a specialized ear, nose, and throat doctor).

With this procedure, the pituitary is approached from below, through the sinuses that are centered above the upper teeth. Mortality rates range from 0.25–3 percent, depending upon the type and size of the tumor as well as other illnesses that the patient has. Complications can include bleeding, infection (meningitis), cerebrospinal fluid leak, visual disturbance, and taste and smell changes.

See also HYPOPITUITARISM; PITUITARY FAILURE; PITUITARY GLAND.

pituitary failure   A total breakdown of the pituitary gland. Pituitary failure is also known as hypopituitarism. The failure can be partial or total. This clinical syndrome is rare. The most common causes of pituitary failure are PITUITARY ADENOMAS (either due to the size of the tumor itself or secondary to therapy, including surgery, medications, or radiotherapy). It may also be caused by trauma, inflammation, or vascular problems including POSTPARTUM PITUITARY NECROSIS (Sheehan's syndrome).

There can be deficiencies of any of the six anterior pituitary hormones, including PROLACTIN, LUTEINIZING HORMONE (LH), FOLLICLE-STIMULATING HORMONE (FSH), GROWTH HORMONE, adrenocorticotropic hormone (ACTH), and THYROID-STIMULATING HORMONE (TSH). These pituitary hormones fail in a typical pattern. First, the gonadotropins (LH, FSH) will fail, then growth hormone and TSH, and finally ACTH. Prolactin deficiency is rare unless there is a vascular etiology.

More commonly, partial failure of the pituitary gland occurs. Treatment of the cause (tumor, trauma to the pituitary, and so forth) may enable the patient to recover. Because pituitary failure will result in the inability of the body to produce needed hormones, patients will need to take supplements of LEVOTHYROXINE (to replace thyroid not produced by the thyroid), hydrocortisone (to replace cortisol not produced by the adrenal glands), and other medications.

See also HYPOPITUITARISM.

pituitary gland   An endocrine gland that is composed of two lobes: the anterior pituitary (the adenohypophysis) and the posterior pituitary (the neurohypophysis). Many experts call the anterior pituitary the *master gland* because it produces hormones used by another endocrine gland. For example, it releases adrenocorticotropic hormone (ACTH), which is used by the adrenal glands, and thyroid-stimulating hormone (TSH), which is used by the thyroid gland. The pituitary gland also releases luteinizing hormone (LH), follicle-stimulating hormone (FSH), prolactin (PRL), growth hormone (GH), and pro-opiomenalnocortin (POMC). These seven hormones are essential to normal functioning.

If the pituitary malfunctions, it can cause a secondary endocrine disorder in another endocrine gland, because it causes that gland to malfunction also. (A primary endocrine disorder occurs when the disease originates in the endocrine gland itself.)

See also ACROMEGALY; ACTH; FOLLICLE-STIMULAT-
ING HORMONE; GROWTH HORMONE; HYPOPITUITARISM;
PROLACTIN; THYROID-STIMULATING HORMONE.

pituitary insufficiency   See HYPOPITUITARISM; PITU-
ITARY FAILURE.

polycystic ovary syndrome (PCOS)   A metabolic
syndrome that affects about 8 percent of women of
reproductive age. Its clinical manifestations range
from minimal to severe. It is characterized by menstrual irregularities, hyperandrogenism (excess
male hormones, leading to acne, alopecia, and/or
hirsutism), anovulation with infertility, and miscarriages. Polycystic ovary syndrome appears to be
caused by or tightly associated with insulin resistance syndrome. Thus those affected with PCOS are
predisposed to IMPAIRED GLUCOSE TOLERANCE, DIA-
BETES MELLITUS, OBESITY, and HYPERLIPIDEMIA, with
all the attendant risks of these health problems.

Women with PCOS also have a much higher-
than-average risk of developing cardiovascular
problems; the risk of a heart attack is seven times
greater among patients with PCOS compared with
women who do not have this syndrome. In addition, patients with PCOS have an increased risk for
developing endometrial cancer and breast cancer.

Polycystic ovary syndrome was originally
known as Stein-Leventhal syndrome and was first
discussed in 1935. At that time, the diagnosis
required hirsutism (unusual hairiness), obesity,
and amenorrhea (failure to menstruate). Later, a
National Institute of Health consensus revised the
diagnostic criteria to include hyperandrogenism
with ovulatory dysfunction as well as the exclusion
of CUSHING'S SYNDROME, nonclassical CONGENITAL
ADRENAL HYPERPLASIA, hyperprolactinemia, and
androgen-secreting tumors. In 2004, the presence
of polycystic ovaries were considered consistent
with the diagnosis of PCOS but were not necessary
to make the diagnosis.

The condition may present as early as puberty.
Some studies indicate that women with PCOS have
a low-grade chronic inflammation of the lining of
their blood vessels as measured by the increased
levels of high-sensitivity C-reactive protein (CRP)

concentrations in their blood. This is seen in
patients with insulin resistance syndrome.

Risk Factors

Women with Type 2 diabetes are at greater risk for
developing PCOS than those without glucose intolerance. PCOS is also found more commonly among
women who are overweight or obese. Other diseases that may present along with PCOS are ACAN-
THOSIS NIGRICANS and hypertension.

Many women with PCOS also have abnormal
cholesterol and triglyceride levels, typically mildly
increased low-density lipoprotein (LDL) levels, low
high-density lipoprotein (HDL) levels, and elevated
triglyceride levels (hyperlipidemia). These risk
associations may signify that the underlying cause
is insulin resistance, as these risk factors are all
associated with or caused by insulin resistance.

Signs and Symptoms

PCOS usually comes to the attention of physicians
when their female patients present to them with
menstrual irregularities, hirsutism, and/or infertility. As mentioned, these women are often overweight, and may have acanthosis nigricans. The
two main conditions necessary to diagnose PCOS
are hyperandrogenism and anovulation. In severe
cases of PCOS, the physician may find large ovarian cysts during a pelvic examination, although
cysts are not necessary to make the diagnosis.

Hyperandrogenism

The excessive levels of male hormones found
among women with PCOS are mainly synthesized
by the ovaries, although the adrenal glands may
also contribute. Most women with PCOS have elevated blood levels of testosterone, with the manifestations of acne and/or hirsutism. However, some
racial groups, such as Asians, may not present with
acne or hirsutism. Physicians will typically measure
the patient's levels of total and free testosterone as
well as dehydroepiandroesterone sulfate (DHEAS)
that is made by the adrenal glands.

Anovulation

Many patients with PCOS do not menstruate at all.
However, some women continue to menstruate yet
do not ovulate, while others have irregular men-

struation without ovulation. Anovulation can be ascertained by the measurement of hormone levels, such as LUTEINIZING HORMONE (LH), FOLLICLE-STIMU-LATING HORMONE (FSH), and ESTRADIOL. It can also be determined by measuring basal body temperature.

Polycystic Ovaries

The third historic sign of PCOS is the polycystic ovary, which is diagnosed with ultrasound. The ovary is usually enlarged as well as cystic. This sign is not necessary to make the diagnosis.

Diagnosis and Treatment of PCOS

Blood tests can determine if androgen levels are unusually high, and doctors also note the presence of hirsutism. An ultrasound will reveal the presence of polycystic ovaries. Anovulation is more difficult to pinpoint.

Treatment is aimed at lowering insulin resistance (the body's inability to use the body's natural insulin). Medication, nutritional therapy, and exercise are tried first. After that, medications are used, such as metformin, rosglitazone, or pioglitazone, although none of these drugs are approved by the Food and Drug Administration (FDA) for this indication. An overweight woman who has not menstruated or who has menstruated only erratically and is then placed on one of these drugs is advised to use birth control unless pregnancy is her intention because sometimes the drugs may alleviate years of infertility. Some women have been known to ovulate and become fertile within one month of initiating metformin therapy.

Some patients are treated with low doses of ORAL CONTRACEPTIVES to stabilize their menstrual cycle and lower their androgen levels. The excess androgen effects can also be treated with spironolactone (Aldactone), which blocks the androgen receptor, or with dexamethasone (Decadron), which decreases the synthesis of adrenal androgens. Neither of these drugs is FDA approved for these particular indications, although both have been used clinically in this manner for years.

Obese women are advised to lose weight, which may help to normalize hormonal function. In some cases, weight reduction may resolve anovulation.

See also AMENORRHEA; HIRSUTISM IN WOMEN; INFERTILITY.

For further information, contact the following organization:

Polycystic Ovarian Syndrome Association
P.O. Box 3403
Englewood, CO 80111
(877) 775-PCOS
http://www.pcosupport.org

Diamanti-Kandarakis, Evanthia, et al. "Increased Endothelin-1 Levels in Women with Polycystic Ovary Syndrome and the Beneficial Effect of Metformin Therapy." *Journal of Clinical Endocrinology & Metabolism* 86, no. 10 (2001): 4,666–4,673.

Franks, Stephen, M.D. "Polycystic Ovary Syndrome." *New England Journal of Medicine* 333, no. 13 (September 28, 1995): 853–861.

Kelly, Chris C. J., et al. "Low Grade Chronic Inflammation in Women with Polycystic Ovarian Syndrome." *Journal of Clinical Endocrinology & Metabolism* 86, no. 6 (2001): 2,453–2,455.

Lobo, Rogerio A., M.D., and Enrico Carmina, M.D. "The Importance of Diagnosing the Polycystic Ovary Syndrome." *Annals of Internal Medicine* 132, no. 12 (2000): 989–993.

Tsilchorozidou, T., C. Overton, and G. S. Conway. "The Pathophysiology of Polycystic Ovary Syndrome." *Clinical Endocrinology* 60, no. 1 (2004): 1–17.

postpartum pituitary necrosis Pituitary failure caused by severe hypotension during or after giving birth, usually due to severe blood loss. This condition is also known as Sheehan's syndrome or postpartum hypopituitarism. Because an end artery nourishes the pituitary gland, when blood pressure drops significantly, only a minimal amount of blood may reach the pituitary, causing the gland to die. This rare condition may occur in an estimated one in 10,000 deliveries.

When a woman is pregnant, her pituitary gland nearly doubles in size and thus is at risk for postpartum complications. If tissue within the anterior pituitary is destroyed because of severe postpartum bleeding from a vaginal delivery or caesarean section, the woman's hormones are thrown into disarray, including her thyroid hormone, adrenal hormone, growth hormone, prolactin, and all the other hormones that the pituitary normally oversees. The posterior pituitary usually survives, and in most cases, the patient does not need replacement of the antidiuretic hormone desmopressin acetate (DDAVP).

According to author Mark E. Molitch, M.D., although the frequency of postpartum pituitary problems is not known for certain, an estimated 25 percent of women who die in the first 30 days after delivery have indications of pituitary infarction.

Diagnosis and Treatment

An acute case of this syndrome should be suspected in a woman who has had severe blood loss and/or hypotension in the peripartum period. She may have persistent low blood pressure, headache, nausea, and vomiting and may develop fluid and electrolyte abnormalities. Within several weeks, the patient may be unable to lactate (fail to produce breast milk) and experience malaise, fatigue, nausea, and a loss of both underarm (axillary) hair and pubic hair. If women are successful at lactating after delivery, then postpartum pituitary necrosis can usually be ruled out.

The diagnosis of postpartum pituitary necrosis can be confirmed by a computerized tomography (CT) scan and/or magnetic resonance imaging (MRI) of the pituitary as well as by measurement of appropriate hormone levels (CORTISOL, THYROXINE, THYROID-STIMULATING HORMONE (TSH), ESTRADIOL, FOLLICLE-STIMULATING HORMONE (FSH), insulin-like growth factor 1 (IGF-1), and PROLACTIN). Because there is total infarction of the anterior pituitary gland, this syndrome is also a cause of EMPTY SELLA SYNDROME.

In acute cases of postpartum pituitary necrosis, patients are treated with intravenous doses of hydrocortisone as well as normal saline with dextrose solution. When the patient's condition has stabilized, treatment for the chronic illness can be started. Hydrocortisone, cortisone acetate, or prednisone is given to replace glucocorticoids. Thyroxine is given to replace natural thyroid hormone. Estrogen and progesterone that were formerly produced by the body may be replaced with oral contraceptives or medications that are given to women during menopause. Growth hormone may also be replaced if it is found to be deficient, although its use is considered controversial in adults.

In many cases, however, the condition is not initially severe and dramatic. Some patients develop a chronic form of hypopituitarism that occurs weeks or even years after giving birth. In such cases, assessment of the pituitary's ability to secrete its hormones in appropriate amounts, which is performed immediately in the case of acute postpartum necrosis, is done at a later date. Typically, a cortrosyn stimulation test is also administered and levels of free T4, TSH, estradiol, FSH, LUTEINIZING HORMONE, and IGF-1 are measured.

See also HYPOPITUITARISM; PITUITARY FAILURE; PITUITARY GLAND.

Molitch, Mark E., M.D. "Sheehan Syndrome," in *NORD Guide to Rare Diseases*. Philadelphia, Pa.: Lippincott Williams & Wilkins, 2003.

Sheehan, H. L. "The Recognition of Chronic Hypopituitarism Resulting from Postpartum Pituitary Necrosis." *American Journal of Obstetrics and Gynecology* 111, no. 6 (November 1971): 852–854.

postpartum thyroid disease   Thyroid disease that is diagnosed after giving birth. An estimated 5–10 percent of new mothers develop some form of postpartum thyroid disease, including THYROIDITIS, GRAVES' DISEASE, and thyroid adenomas.

Because so many women also develop postpartum depression, researchers have studied whether there was a link between the development of thyroid disease and depression in the postpartum period. They reported on their findings in a 2001 issue of *Clinical Endocrinology.*

The researchers studied 641 women who did not have either thyroid disease or diabetes initially and followed up with them before and after delivery until one year after their babies were born. The researchers found that 11 percent of the women developed postpartum thyroid disease. Interestingly, the researchers found that women with postpartum thyroid disease did not experience an increased risk for developing depression compared with women without thyroid disease.

See also HYPERTHYROIDISM; HYPOTHYROIDISM; PREGNANCY; THRYOID NODULES; THYROTOXICOSIS.

Lucas, A., et al. "Postpartum Thyroid Disease Is Not Associated with Postpartum Depression." *Clinical Endocrinology* 55, no. 6 (2001): 809–814.

Prader-Willi syndrome (PWS)   An inherited medical condition characterized by mental developmental delay, behavioral problems (irritability and tantrums), OBESITY, short stature, decreased muscle mass, and genital abnormalities (hypogonadatropic hypogonadism). Prader-Willi syndrome was named after the Swiss pediatricians Andrea Prader and H. Willi, who first described this condition in 1956.

Prader-Willi syndrome occurs in one in 10,000–16,000 births. Most adult patients with PWS cannot live independently. Consequently, they live with their families or in group homes.

In many patients with PWS (as many as 75 percent), the syndrome is caused by a genetic defect: the deletion of a segment on chromosome 15q11-q13, which was inherited from the father. In some cases, the genetic problem is inherited from the mother.

Signs and Symptoms of Prader-Willi Syndrome

Infants with Prader-Willi syndrome have symptoms as newborn babies. They have poor sucking reflexes and difficulties with swallowing, and they may require tube feeding. Babies with PWS also have poor muscle tone and below-normal weight, partially due to their feeding problems.

Most children and adults with Prader-Willi syndrome have small hands and feet. They often exhibit constant scratching because of a severe itching problem and may be physically scarred because of their chronic scratching behavior. Individuals with this syndrome may also have an unusually high tolerance to pain.

Most patients with Prader-Willi are also developmentally delayed, with intelligence quotients in about the 70s. (An IQ of 100 is considered normal in the general population.)

Prader-Willi syndrome is also characterized by an extreme and ravenous appetite, which leads to obesity. This excessive appetite usually starts in early childhood, around the age of three years old, and is generally attributed to a disorder in the central nervous system. The compulsive overeating (hyperphagia) is so extreme and intense that individuals with PWS will seek out food that has been left in the garbage or will eat the food of their household pets. In many households, the refrigerator and the kitchen cabinets must actually be locked up because of this complete lack of appetite control.

Short stature is another common feature of PWS. Most patients (90 percent) are below normal in height. They also generally experience a DELAYED PUBERTY due to hypogonadatropic hypogonadism. When they do experience puberty, their voices will usually not change.

Many patients with Prader-Willi also have abnormal glucose tolerance or diabetes mellitus, at least in part because of their extreme obesity. About a third of patients with this syndrome are about twice the expected normal weight for their height.

Other common characteristics of Prader-Willi syndrome include the following signs and symptoms:

- Sleep disorders, especially sleep apnea
- Poor muscle tone
- Almond-shaped eyes
- Small mouth

Some patients also have kyphosis or scoliosis (skeletal deformities), OSTEOPOROSIS, and body temperature control problems. It has also been reported that some patients are unusually adept at putting together jigsaw puzzles.

Treatment of Prader-Willi Syndrome

Until recent years, the symptoms of patients with this syndrome could not be treated but only managed, which was extremely difficult for both the individual and the families, particularly in the case of hyperphagia behavior. Some studies indicate that treatment with growth hormone may help some patients with PWS. For example, the findings of a two-year study of 54 children with the syndrome, ages four to 16 years old when they joined the study, was reported in a 2002 issue of *Pediatrics*. Some of the children (35 children) were given growth hormone, while the rest were used as a control group.

In all but one child who received growth hormone, the children showed considerable improvement. The treated children became more energetic and active, and their moods improved markedly. The memory of most of the treated children (85 percent) improved. In addition, 89 percent of the children became much more sociable. Growth hormone did not make the children become "normal," but it did dramatically improve the lives of both the children and their families. Some families said that their other children, who did not have PWS, reported that they were no longer embarrassed to be seen by others in the company of their sibling who had Prader-Willi syndrome.

Growth hormone therapy was also found to accelerate growth and decrease the percentage of body fat in the PWS patients. Unfortunately, no increase occurred in the resting energy expenditure. Patients who were given growth hormone therapy had increased respiratory muscle strength as well as an increase in their overall physical strength and agility.

Growth hormone treatment is not without risk. A study reported in a 2004 issue of the *Journal of Pediatrics* discussed the case of a four-year old boy with Prader-Willi syndrome who was being treated with growth hormone and who suddenly died from bronchopneumonia while asleep. Before his death, the boy's snoring had become worse. Several other cases have indicated that growth hormone may increase the risk of respiratory infection, obstructive apnea, and sudden death. More research needs to be done on the use of growth hormone with Prader-Willi patients.

Preliminary research indicates that some patients with PWS have abnormal levels of GHRELIN, a weight- and appetite-regulating hormone. Manipulation of the ghrelin levels may help to improve the uncontrollable eating, although more research needs to be performed on this aspect of the illness. The lives of many families that include a child with PWS would be much happier if the excessive eating could be brought under greater control.

Because patients with Prader-Willi have hypogonadism, experts suggest that sex hormone replacement, including testosterone for males and estrogen for females, should be administered. These drugs could protect against bone mineral diseases such as osteoporosis. In one study of patients with PWS, 41 percent of males and 18 percent of females received hormone replacement. Families of the patients who did not receive hormone replacement may not have wished to encourage sexuality among their developmentally delayed relatives with Prader-Willi syndrome. Physicians may also be reluctant to provide hormone replacement drugs because of the health controversies that surround these drugs.

See also GROWTH HORMONE; TYPE 2 DIABETES.

For further information on Prader-Willi syndrome, contact the following organizations:

The Foundation for Prader-Willi Research
6407 Bardstown Road
Suite 252
Louisville, KY 40291
(502) 254-9375
http://www.pwsresearch.org

Burman, Pia, E. Martin Ritzen, and Ann Christin Lindgren. "Endocrine Dysfunction in Prader-Willi Syndrome: A Review with Special Reference to GH." *Endocrine Reviews* 22, no. 6 (2001): 787–799.

Carrel, A. L., et al. "Growth Hormone Improves Body Composition, Fat Utilization, Physical Strength and Agility in Prader-Willi Syndrome." *Journal of Pediatrics* 134, no. 2 (1999): 215–221.

Vliet, G. V, et al. "Sudden Death in Growth Hormone-Treated Children with Prader-Willi Syndrome." *Journal of Pediatrics* 144, no. 1 (2004): 129–131.

Whitman, Barbara Y. "The Behavioral Impact of Growth Hormone Treatment for Children and Adolescents with Prader-Willi Syndrome: A 2-Year, Controlled Study." *Pediatrics* 109, no. 2 (February 2002). Available online. URL: http://pediatrics.aappublications.org/cgi/content/full/109/2/e35?maxtoshow=&HITS=10&HITS=10&RESULTFORMAT=&fulltext=PraderWilli&searchid=1093574871920_18858&storedsearch=&FIRSTINDEX=0&sortspec=relevance&journalcode=pediatrics. Downloaded November 15, 2003.

precocious puberty   See EARLY PUBERTY.

prediabetes   A new term created by the AMERICAN DIABETES ASSOCIATION and the NATIONAL INSTITUTES OF HEALTH to distinguish abnormalities of blood glucose from normal levels and from overt DIABETES MELLITUS. The previously used and technically correct terms of *impaired fasting glucose* and *impaired glucose tolerance* were not well understood by the public. As a result, the American Diabetes Association and the National Institutes of Health sought to impress upon the general public the fact that these metabolic abnormalities were quite serious and should not be ignored. The newly created term *prediabetes* was believed to convey this concept.

Not all patients with prediabetes syndrome will actually develop diabetes. However, even those who do not develop overt diabetes have an extremely high risk of suffering from heart attack, stroke, other atherosclerotic abnormalities, and premature death. Patients with prediabetes who have a family history of diabetes are more likely to develop the disease. However, many patients who are diagnosed with prediabetes may either prevent or delay the development of diabetes by losing weight (if they are overweight), exercising, and adopting a healthy and nutritious diet.

In the Diabetes Prevention program, a study in the United States that ended in 2001, patients with impaired glucose tolerance were treated with diet and exercise or with the medication metformin to determine the effects on their progression to diabetes. The diet and exercise group lost an average of 7 percent of their baseline weight and walked an average of 150 minutes per week, and they decreased their risk of progressing from prediabetes to overt diabetes by 58 percent.

The group treated with about 1,700 mg of metformin decreased their risk of progression to diabetes by 31 percent. The results achieved with this study regarding diet and exercise have been duplicated in similar trials in China and Finland. Data also suggests that the use of other drugs, such as thiazolidinediones, angiotensin-converting enzyme inhibitors, alpha glucosidase inhibitors, and statins may also lower the rate of progression from prediabetes to diabetes mellitus.

pregnancy Gestation of an infant. Some pregnant women have endocrine diseases or disorders before they become pregnant (such as diabetes, thyroid disease, and many other medical problems). Some women develop endocrine diseases or disorders during pregnancy or the postpartum period directly after the delivery of the baby. These endocrine illnesses need to be identified and treated for the health of both the mother and the child. For example, women with GESTATIONAL DIABETES (a form of diabetes mellitus that occurs only during pregnancy) are at risk for having many medical problems, as are their children. Such women need to be under the close supervision of an obstetrician as well as an ENDOCRINOLOGIST during their pregnancies.

Screening During Pregnancy

Virtually all obstetricians screen women for diabetes mellitus between the 24th and 28th weeks of pregnancy. Screening pregnant women for thyroid disease would also be advisable (which is not routinely done). Significant numbers of pregnant women are hypothyroid or hyperthyroid, both conditions that could be harmful to mother and child if not treated.

Endocrine Diseases May Prevent Pregnancy

Women with some endocrine diseases may have difficulty achieving a pregnancy, such as women with HYPOTHYROIDISM, POLYCYSTIC OVARY SYNDROME, and hyperprolactinemia. The elevated prolactin levels can be treated with bromocriptine during pregnancy to decrease the levels of prolactin as well as the size of the pituitary microadenoma.

See also BREAST-FEEDING; FERTILITY; HYPERTHYROIDISM; INFERTILITY; POSTPARTUM PITUITARY NECROSIS; PROLACTIN.

Kovacs, Christopher S., and Henry M. Kronenbergy. "Maternal-Fetal Calcium and Bone Metabolism During Pregnancy, Puerperium, and Lactation." *Endocrine Reviews* 18, no. 6 (1997): 832–872.

prolactin A hormone produced by the anterior pituitary gland that is directly involved in stimulating breast milk for breast-feeding infants. Men and nonlactating women produce very low levels of prolactin, but these levels become elevated in breast-feeding and pregnant women. Pregnant women do not lactate, despite their high levels of prolactin, because their levels of estrogen and progesterone are high enough to block milk production. After the baby is born, the estrogen and progesterone levels in the mother drop dramatically, enabling her milk production to commence, which usually occurs within three days from the child's birth. Lactation is further stimulated by the infant's suckling on the breasts.

Prolactin is unusual in that its production is inhibited by the hypothalamic secretion of dopamine. This is in contrast to all the other anterior pituitary cells, where the hypothalamus secretes hormones that stimulate the secretion of pituitary hormones rather than inhibit them.

Prolactin levels may become elevated in non-nursing individuals who are hypothyroid or who have a benign tumor of the pituitary (prolactinoma). Patients with kidney failure or liver failure may experience elevated levels of prolactin.

Medications may also increase the blood levels of prolactin. These medications include psychiatric medications (haloperidol, risperidone, and medications in the tricyclic antidepressant and monoamine oxidase (MAO) inhibitor categories of medications) and antinausea drugs such as metoclopramide (Reglan). Verapamil, a blood pressure and heart medication, may also increase prolactin levels. Typically, these medications increase the levels of prolactin from the normal range to the range of 30–100 mcg/l.

High levels of prolactin may cause decreased libido and infertility in men as well as headaches and cranial nerve abnormalities. It may cause some secretion of milk in nonnursing women (galactor-rhea). Unusually low levels of prolactin do not appear to cause any disease or disorder other than a woman's inability to breast-feed a child.

See also BREAST-FEEDING; HORMONES; PREGNANCY; PROLACTINOMA.

prolactinoma   A benign tumor of the pituitary gland and the most common form of tumor in the pituitary. The prolactinoma accounts for 40 percent of all pituitary tumors. It is so-named because the pituitary gland produces a hormone called PRO-LACTIN, which is at low levels in most individuals except nursing mothers, in whom prolactin promotes the production of breast milk. Prolactinomas are estimated to be a significant problem in only about 14 of 100,000 people, according to the NATIONAL INSTITUTES of HEALTH. Both men and women may develop prolactinomas.

Signs and Symptoms

Women with prolactinomas may develop problems such as irregular menstruation, AMENORRHEA (failure to menstruate), or infertility. Some women who are not pregnant or nursing an infant may develop breast milk production (galactorrhea), which is seen in four out of five women with prolactinomas.

Other indicators of excessive levels of prolactin are a decreased interest in sex and an increase in vaginal dryness. Since all of these signs and symptoms are common to other medical problems, with the exception of the production of breast milk, diagnosis can be difficult for most physicians. A prolactinoma may be diagnosed after oral contraceptives are discontinued, but there is no evidence that the use of birth control pills leads to the development of these tumors.

Among males with prolactinomas, symptoms include eye problems or headaches because the pituitary gland, which is located in the head, begins to press on the optic nerves. Men may also have a decreased sex drive (libido). Often these tumors are diagnosed much later in men than in women; even small increases in prolactin will lead to changes in menstruation, which women generally notice. No corresponding sign occurs in men.

Diagnosis and Treatment

Patients are treated based on their signs, symptoms, and laboratory results, specifically, their blood levels of prolactin. Initially, prolactin can be measured at any time. If the level is only mildly increased, the laboratory test should be repeated in the morning prior to the patient eating any meals since proteins (amino acids), exercise, and breast stimulation can all increase prolactin levels.

Some drugs may increase the production of prolactin in the absence of tumors, such as the antipsychotic drugs Stelazine (trifluoperazine) and Haldol (haloperidol) as well as the antinausea drug Reglan (metoclopramide). The doctor will also test for thyroid function levels because sometimes people with HYPOTHYROIDISM have elevated prolactin levels. Magnetic resonance imaging (MRI) of the pituitary gland will identify the tumor in the pituitary as well as any other lesion that may be compressing the pituitary stalk.

The lactotroph cells that secrete prolactin are different from the other pituitary cells in that they are inhibited by dopamine that comes from the hypothalamus. In contrast, hormones from the hypothalamus stimulate all the other pituitary hormones. Thus, any lesion that interrupts the flow of dopamine from the hypothalamus can lead to an increased level of prolactin. As a result, other disorders, such as ACROMEGALY, granulomatous disorders, and craniopharyngiomas may lead to hyperprolactinemia. In many cases, however, no specific cause can be determined. In such patients, one of every three will become normal without any therapy.

When a prolactinoma is diagnosed, endocrinologists use medications to decrease the amount of prolactin secreted. Typically, BROMOCRIPTINE or CABERGOLINE is used. These medications are not antitumor agents, although they seem to help stabilize the size of the tumor and, in some cases, to shrink it.

If the medication does not work to reduce prolactin levels and the tumor, other means will be used, such as surgery or radiation therapy. Transsphenoidal surgery should not be the therapy of choice, because it does not reliably lead to a cure. Surgery is often used for macroadenomas (tumors greater than 10 millimeters in size), especially if the tumors are pushing on the optic nerve or are extending into the cavernous sinuses and other cranial nerves. Patients who need surgery or radiation therapy for a prolactinoma will usually need to receive this treatment from a neurosurgeon who operates on many pituitary tumor patients. In most cases, such neurosurgeons practice at major medical centers rather than at local hospitals.

Doctors should also monitor the estrogen levels of women who have had prolactinomas because hyperprolactinemia (excess levels of prolactin in the bloodstream) can lead to reduced estrogen levels and then to OSTEOPOROSIS.

For further information, contact the following organization:

Pituitary Network Association
P.O. Box 1958
Thousand Oaks, CA 91360
(805) 499-9973
http://www.pituitary.com

Schlette, J. A. "Prolactinoma." *New England Journal of Medicine* 349, no. 21 (2003): 2,035–2,041.

prolactin-secreting tumors   See PROLACTINOMA.

pseudohypoparathyroidism   A condition that resembles HYPOPARATHYROIDISM, which is caused by abnormally low levels of parathyroid hormone. However, with pseudohypoparathyroidism, the body is actually producing sufficient amounts of parathyroid hormone but is unable or resistant to use all that is produced. Patients may present with low serum calcium levels (HYPOCALCEMIA) and high phosphate levels (HYPERPHOSPHATEMIA).

Pseudohypoparathyroidism is primarily caused by one of two abnormal genes and occurs in two forms: type Ia and type Ib. Individuals with type Ia pseudohypoparathyroidism present with round faces, short hand and foot bones (and they often appear to be missing a knuckle), and short stature. This condition is also known as Albright's hereditary osteodystrophy.

Individuals with type Ib pseudohypoparathyroidism have normal physical appearances and experience a resistance of their kidneys to parathyroid hormone. If a father with an abnormal gene transmits the gene to a child who also gets a normal gene from the mother, the child can have what is known as pseudopseudohypoparathyroidism, with the Albright's hereditary osteodystrophy and no hypocalcemia.

There is also a type II form of pseudohypoparathyroidism, which is very rare. It causes hypocalcemia, hyperphosphatemia, and increased levels of serum parathyroid hormone levels. The mechanism of action of parathyroid hormone in the kidney is different from what is seen with patients with type Ib.

Diagnosis and Treatment

If the physician suspects the patient has pseudohypoparathyroidism, he or she will order laboratory tests. Indications of pseudohypoparathyroidism include low serum calcium, elevated serum phosphorus, elevated intact parathyroid hormone, and an abnormal urinary cAMP (cyclic adenosine monophosphate) response to a parathyroid challenge test. In addition, a COMPUTERIZED TOMOGRAPHY

(CT) scan or a MAGNETIC RESONANCE IMAGING (MRI) scan will show calcification of the basal ganglia.

Patients with pseudohypoparathyroidism are treated with supplements of calcium and vitamin D. Doctors should also check for other endocrine disorders, such as HYPOGONADISM or HYPOTHYROIDISM, because the defective response to hormones can also include THYROID-STIMULATING HORMONE (TSH), FOLLICLE-STIMULATING HORMONE (FSH), and LUTEINIZING HORMONE (LH).

Vlaeminck-Guillen, Virginie, et al. "Pseudohypoparathyrodism Ia and Hypercalcitoneinemia." *Journal of Clinical Endocrinology & Metabolism* 86, no. 7 (2001): 3,091–3,096.

radioactive iodine   A substance used for both diagnostic purposes and therapeutic reasons in suspected or known cases of thyroid disease. The iodine isotopes I-123, I-125, and I-131 can all be used for radioactive iodine uptake studies and scans of the thyroid gland. Typically I-123 is chosen, although technetium pertechnetate is also often used as it is less expensive and more readily available. For uptake purposes, only an iodine isotope can be used.

The Procedure

Radioactive iodine is given orally. It is absorbed from the gut and then trapped by the thyroid gland. The more active the thyroid is, the more iodine trapped in the gland. Thus, a radioisotope uptake scan will provide an excellent measure of the physiological activity of the thyroid.

The patient is brought into the nuclear medicine department, and the amount of radioactive activity taken up by the thyroid is counted and reported as a percentage. The typical normal range in the United States is from 15–30 percent. With GRAVES' DISEASE, the percentages usually range from 40–100 percent. In THYROIDITIS, however, the percentage is usually very low, in the 0–5 percent range.

The amount of iodine that is trapped by the thyroid depends on the diet and the amount of iodine available in the food supply, and it also varies greatly around the world; however, it is fairly consistent throughout the United States.

Technetium is more often used to scan the thyroid gland or, in essence, to obtain a picture of the thyroid. It can also help to determine if a palpable abnormality is a nodule; whether the activity in the thyroid gland is homogenous or heterogeneous; if there is other active thyroid tissue around the thyroid gland or elsewhere; and whether functional and/or nonfunctional hot nodules are present. Nodules that take up iodine or technetium are known as hot nodules and are rarely malignant. Nonfunctional or cold nodules may have a 5–15 percent risk of malignancy.

Radioactive Iodine as a Therapy

Radioactive iodine is also used as a therapy. For this application, I-131 is used, as it emits enough energy to damage and kill thyroid cells. It is the most commonly used form of therapy for Graves' disease in the United States, although it is less favored in Europe and other parts of the world. I-131 can also be used to ablate toxic hyperfunctioning thyroid nodules as well as attempt to decrease the size of large, multinodular GOITERS.

It is a safe and effective therapy but can cause some acute tenderness in the thyroid, which can often be treated with simple analgesics or anti-inflammatory medications, up to and including GLUCOCORTICOIDS. If a patient with hyperthyroidism is treated with radioactive iodine, damage to the gland can cause the release of already-synthesized thyroid hormones and thus can temporarily exacerbate the hyperthyroidism.

Effects of Radioactive Iodine

The major, long-term effect of radioactive therapy is HYPOTHYROIDISM that necessitates the use of lifelong thyroid hormone therapy. Concern has been raised that the use of radioactive iodine therapy may lead to an exacerbation of Graves' ophthalmopathy (bulging eyes), although most endocrinologists do not feel this is a significant problem. When there is concern about the possible worsening of these EYE PROBLEMS, patients are often pretreated with a glucocorticoid medication, such as prednisone, to help minimize the impact.

Very large doses of radioactive iodine can be used to ablate thyroid tissue left behind in a THY-ROIDECTOMY performed for THYROID CANCER. It can also be used to treat metastases (cancer spread) from papillary and follicular thyroid cancers.

recombinant thyroid-stimulating hormone (thyrogen)   A hormone available for the evaluation of patients with THYROID CANCER. In the past, after a near-total or total THYROIDECTOMY, patients had to be taken off thyroid hormone replacement medication to allow their thyroid-stimulating hormone (TSH) to increase, typically to greater than 30 microunits/ml. These patients developed symptoms of HYPOTHYROIDISM and felt poorly. Now when a RADIOACTIVE IODINE thyroid scan is planned as a follow-up for thyroid cancer patients, in order to look for thyroid cells in the neck or elsewhere, thyroid hormone can be introduced. The patient can be given recombinant TSH by injection.

This synthetic TSH increases TSH levels in the blood and helps to improve the uptake of iodine into the thyroid cells, if any are present. Thus, the scan can be performed without the necessity of causing hypothyroid symptoms. In addition to the iodine scan, endocrinologists will often measure the patient's thyroglobulin levels to help determine if any thyroid cells remain behind. Typically, Thyrogen is given in two or three intramuscular doses over the course of three to five days.

reproductive endocrinology   The science of studying endocrine conditions that may impede fertility. For example, women with hypothyroidism may have difficulty becoming pregnant, as may women with disorders of the ovaries such as POLY-CYSTIC OVARY SYNDROME. Men with TESTOSTERONE deficiencies are often unable to create a pregnancy with their wives. It is also true that for most men and women, fertility declines with age. For women, fertility ends with the onset of MENOPAUSE. Men may continue to have the ability to father a child for the rest of their lives, although with a less robust facility than was present in their earlier years.

Many individuals in the United States and other developed countries choose to delay childbearing

while they concentrate on their careers. When they decide they wish to start a family in their 30s or 40s, they may be shocked to learn that it is difficult and sometimes impossible to achieve a pregnancy. For this reason, they consult with reproductive specialists to see if the cause of the infertility can be determined and corrected.

Most of these physicians are obstetricians with extra training in endocrinology, and they often work together with internal medicine endocrinologists. Evaluation of an infertile couple includes a medical history and a physical examination. The physician may order imaging tests, initially made to look for structural abnormalities, if indicated by the physical examination. He or she will also conduct laboratory tests to determine whether the individuals' hormone levels are normal. Hormones tested may include estradiol, progesterone, testosterone, prolactin, thyroxine, and others. Women are tested for evidence of ovulation, while men receive evaluations to test for the normal function of sperm and for the numbers of spermatozoa.

Physicians who are expert at resolving infertility problems will perform in-depth analyses to try to pinpoint where the problem lies. Sometimes a simple surgical procedure can resolve the infertility. Other times, women or men who are infertile must undergo complex surgery. In some cases, physicians are unable to determine the cause of the infertility. In other cases, doctors know what the problem is but are unable to correct it.

See also FERTILITY; INFERTILITY; PREGNANCY; TURNER SYNDROME.

reverse T3 (rT3)   An inactive thyroid hormone derived from thyroxine (T4). T4 is usually converted to the physiologically active form of thyroid hormone T3 by the removal of specific iodine from one of the tyrosine rings. If the iodine is removed instead, then reverse T3 is created. Some reverse T3 is always present. When more than normal levels are present, however, it may indicate a nonthyroid illness, such as pneumonia or heart attack. Typically, T4 (thyroid hormone) is converted to T3 by the body at rates that allow adequate T3 to be present, such that individuals have just enough thyroid hormone present to function normally.

When people become ill, however, their bodies convert more T4 to reverse T3 instead of to T3. Many experts believe this happens because the body is trying to slow itself down and preserve itself in times of increased stress.

In addition to nonthyroid illnesses, the medication amiodarone, which is used to treat irregular heart rhythms, can also increase the levels of reverse T3. With EUTHYROID SICK SYNDROME, levels of rT3 can also be elevated.

Reverse T3 levels typically mirror the T3 levels. For instance, in a nonthyroid illness, T3 levels will usually begin to fall, while rT3 levels will rise. Reverse T3 levels are rarely needed to diagnose and treat patients and are typically measured in complex ill patients who are hospitalized for other reasons.

If measurement of rT3 is taken, it can help physicians determine the exact thyroid state of the patient and whether further treatment is needed. With significant medical illness, both T3 and T4 levels decline and rT3 levels increase.

Camacho, Pauline M., M.D., and Arcot A. Dwarkanathan, M.D. "Sick Euthyroid Syndrome." *Postgraduate Medicine* 105, no. 4 (April 1999): 215–228.

rickets A bone abnormality of childhood. The term refers to a group of disorders in which there is a defect in the mineralization of bone matrix or osteoid. In adults, the disorder is referred to as OSTEOMALACIA, as the defect occurs only in the matrix and the growth plates have already sealed. In children, the disorder is referred to as *rickets* because the mineralization abnormality is located at the growth plate. Rickets is often classified as calcium- or phosphate-deficient rickets.

The major skeletal problems are seen at sites in the body where there is rapid bone growth, such as in the forearm, knee, and the costochondral junctions. Thus, the child with rickets may have bone abnormalities, such as a bowing of the legs and the wrists. Abnormalities may also be seen at the ends of ribs, such as a beading known as *rachitic rosary*. Rickets can cause growth abnormalities as well as be associated with abnormalities of nerve and muscle function, depending on the cause. Children with severe metabolic abnormalities have bone pain, sweat excessively, and are more prone to developing infections.

Vitamin D-Dependent Rickets

Type 1 and type 2 rickets are caused by rare congenital errors of vitamin D metabolism. With type 1 rickets, there is a defect in the enzyme in the kidney that coverts vitamin D stores to its most active form. Children with type 1 rickets typically have symptoms in their first two years of life. Calcium and 1,25-dihydroxyvitamin D levels are low, while parathyroid hormone levels are elevated. Large doses of vitamin D preparations are used to treat this condition.

In children with type 2 rickets, the children are resistant to the effects of vitamin D. Their vitamin D blood levels are normal or elevated. This disorder is usually diagnosed in children before they reach age two. Rarely, this condition has been diagnosed in adults. Very large doses of vitamin D are needed by patients to correct their low calcium levels and to lead to normal bone mineralization.

Hypophosphatemic Rickets

Another form of rickets is hypophosphatemic rickets. This disorder causes an abnormal reabsorption of phosphorus from the kidneys. Typically, male children are affected. They present with growth problems, low blood phosphorus levels, and lower-leg abnormalities. The abnormal gene that causes this disorder has been named *PHEX*. There have been rare reports of females with a mild form of this disorder. Growth hormone has been effectively used with patients to improve growth, although these children are not growth hormone deficient.

See also BONE AGE; BONE DISEASES; BONE MASS MEASUREMENT; OSTEOPENIA; OSTEOPOROSIS; VITAMIN D; VITAMIN D RESISTANCE.

Carpenter, T. O., et al. "24-25-Dihydroxyvitamin D Supplementation Corrects Hyperparathyroidism and Improves Skeletal Abnormalities in X-Linked Hypophosphatemic Rickets: A Clinical Research Center Study." *Journal of Clinical Endocrinology & Metabolism* 81, no. 6 (1996): 2,381–2,388.

Seikaly, M. G., et al. "The Effect of Recombinant Human Growth Hormone in Children with X-Linked Hypophosphatemia." *Pediatrics* 100, no. 5 (1997): 879–884.

risk factors   Genetic or environmental conditions that predispose an individual to illness. Race, for example, plays a role in risks for many diseases. For instance, African Americans have a higher risk for developing TYPE 2 DIABETES than Caucasians. Obesity is a condition also linked to the development of diabetes (and some experts believe that it has a genetic basis as well). Thus, if a person is African American and also obese, he or she has a higher risk for developing diabetes than Caucasians or than nonobese African Americans.

Age is another factor in the likelihood of developing a range of illnesses. The probability of developing many different endocrine diseases and disorders, such as osteoporosis, Type 2 diabetes, and other medical problems, usually increases with age.

Sometimes gender alone is a risk factor. Women or men are more likely to develop a particular endocrine disease and disorder. For example, women are more likely to develop hypothyroidism.

Family medical history is another key factor in the development of many endocrine problems. People whose parents or siblings have had thyroid disease or cancer usually face an increased risk for these diseases themselves. This is why doctors usually ask patients about other family members and their problems so they can be alert to possible signs and symptoms of this disease in the patient.

See also GENETIC RISKS.

secondary hypothyroidism Hypothyroidism (low thyroid levels) caused by a defect or problem at the level of the PITUITARY GLAND. If there is a problem at the level of the HYPOTHALAMUS that causes hypothyroidism, that condition is referred to as tertiary hypothyroidism.

Secondary hypothyroidism causes the same symptoms as primary hypothyroidism, although here, symptoms may be more subtle. Patients with secondary hypothyroidism must be treated as if they had primary hypothyroidism with loss or destruction of the thyroid gland. The usual treatment is the replacement of thyroid hormone with LEVOTHYROXINE (T4).

Patients with secondary hypothyroidism may have a low or a normal level of THYROID-STIMULATING HORMONE (TSH) when their blood is tested. As a result, the diagnosis must be suspected based on the totality of the patient's clinical symptoms, the physician's clinical observations, and some laboratory testing. Free thyroxine levels may be low normal or just below normal.

Once diagnosed with secondary hypothyroidism, patients are given levothyroxine supplements, starting at a low level, with the dosage titrated based on the patient's clinical symptoms as well as the free thyroxine level. Patients are evaluated clinically before any increases in the medication are prescribed. Once clinically stable levels are reached, the patient should be rechecked once every six to 12 months. The physician must also be alert to other symptoms that might indicate other pituitary deficiencies, because typically patients have more than one problem.

See also HYPOTHYROIDISM.

Sheehan's syndrome See POSTPARTUM PITUITARY NECROSIS.

skin The largest organ of the body. Many endocrine diseases and disorders have a direct and noticeable effect on the patient's skin. For example, a key feature of ADDISON'S DISEASE is to cause hyperpigmentation, typically causing the skin to change to a darker color. This color change is due to the excess of pro-opiomelanocortin (POMC) secreted from the brain, stemming from the glucocorticoid deficiency that the disease causes. Undiagnosed and poorly controlled DIABETES MELLITUS may cause the skin to itch. It may also cause a thickening of the skin (waxy contractures or scleroderma) due to excess deposits of carbohydrate/protein complexes.

People with HYPOTHYROIDISM may have very dry, coarse, and thickened skin that can be cold to the touch. The skin may also appear yellow due to excess carotene. These patients may also have decreased perspiration. Patients with HYPERTHYROIDISM may have warm, moist skin and excessive sweating.

The skin of the patient with CUSHING'S DISEASE is thin and subject to easy bruising. This is due to the effects of the excess glucocorticoids on the protein synthesis of collagen that is needed to strengthen and stabilize the subcutaneous layers of capillaries and tissues. Patients with Cushing's disease may also have severe acne, alopecia (balding), fungal infections of the skin, and HIRSUTISM (excessive hairiness). The patient with ACROMEGALY has sweaty and oily skin and may also have excessive skin tags (loose pieces of skin). Women with POLYCYSTIC OVARY SYNDROME (PCOS) often have acne.

Another condition, ACANTHOSIS NIGRICANS, causes a fine, velvety hyperpigmentation of the skin, often seen at the back of the neck, under the arms, and in the breast and groin creases. Acanthosis nigricans is often seen in patients with INSULIN RESISTANCE SYNDROME.

Sometimes the appearance of the skin is the first clue to the patient or the physician that an illness is present, because there are few or no other symptoms or signs of disease. Upon further exploration with a physical examination and the careful taking of the patient's medical history, as well as the ordering of laboratory or imaging tests, as needed, the physician may be able to identify an illness that would otherwise have gone undetected had the skin changes not been observed.

Levin, Nikka A., and Kenneth E. Greer. "Cutaneous Manifestations of Endocrine Disorders." *Dermatology Nursing* 13, no. 3 (June 1, 2001): 189–196.

somatostatin A pancreatic protein hormone synthesized and secreted from endocrine-like D cells. When first discovered, somatostatin was found to inhibit growth hormone release, thus its name *somato,* referring to growth, and *statin* referring to stopping or inhibiting. It is now known to affect a variety of gastrointestinal secretions and to affect the secretion of a number of hormones in addition to growth hormone. Somatostatin is produced in paracrine cells throughout the gastrointestinal tract as well as in nervous tissue, including the hypothalamus. In the gut, somatostatin generally decreases secretions. Most of its effects are paracrine in nature—secreted in a tissue—and they have local effects.

When synthetic somatostatin is injected intravenously, 50 percent is gone within two to three minutes. Somatostatin inhibits the secretion of DDAVP (desmopressin acetate), growth hormone, thyroid-stimulating hormone (TSH), insulin, glucagons, gastrin, and many other hormones.

Somatostatin has also been artificially synthesized as octreotide acetate (Sandostatin and Sandostatin LAR) and is used as a growth hormone suppressant in treating ACROMEGALY. It is often used to treat carcinoid syndrome and chronic secretory diarrhea syndromes when other therapies have failed. In addition, it has been used to treat TSH and adrenocorticotropic hormone (ACTH)-secreting tumors, Zollinger-Ellison syndrome, vasoactive intestinal peptide (VIP)-producing tumors or VIPomas, insulinomas, and glucagonomas. It has also been used to treat diabetic diarrhea.

Some endocrine tumors have somatostatin receptors on their surface. Radioactive somatostatin can be used to attempt to image these tumors (an octreotide scan).

subclinical hypothyroidism/hyperthyroidism Recently discovered entities in which thyroid function tests are abnormal but the patient is clinically well and without obvious signs and symptoms of thyroid disease. This condition has become more common as the measurement of THYROID-STIMULATING HORMONE (TSH), the gold standard thyroid test, has become more sensitive, with third-generation assays now able to measure TSH levels as low as 0.01 microunit/ml of blood.

In the case of subclinical hypothyroidism, these patients have elevated TSH levels and free T4 and total T3 levels that are normal or only minimally abnormal. In the hyperthyroid state, patients have a lower-than-normal or even a completely suppressed (immeasurable) TSH level and normal or slightly elevated free T4 and T3 levels.

A review of this topic in 2004 in the *Journal of the American Medical Association* noted that TSH levels that were minimally elevated to greater than 10 microunits/ml were associated with elevated cholesterol levels but that the benefits of treating with thyroid hormone were unproven.

In the situation in which the TSH was lower than 0.01 microunits/ml (indicating hyperthyroidism), there was good evidence suggesting that there was a high prevalence of atrial fibrillation (rapid irregular heart rate) as well as a greater rate of progression to overt hyperthyroidism. Unfortunately, again the study could find no evidence that early therapy impacted outcomes.

Because little data supports routine treatment in the general population when a patient is diagnosed with subclinical hyperthyroidism or hypothyroidism, the authors advised against routine screening with THYROID BLOOD TESTS in the general population. However, they said, "Aggressive case finding is appropriate in pregnant women, women older than 60 years, and others at high risk for thyroid dysfunction."

See also GRAVES' DISEASE; HYPERTHYROIDISM; HYPOTHYROIDISM.

Surks, M. I., et al. "Subclinical Thyroid Disease: Scientific Review and Guidelines for Diagnosis and Management." *Journal of the American Medical Association* 291 no. 2 (January 13, 2004): 228–238.

surgery   Procedure involving an incision and some action taken on the body, usually when material is excised. Some endocrine diseases may require surgery, particularly OVARIAN CANCER, TESTICULAR CANCER, and other forms of cancer. Patients with ADDISON'S DISEASE may need to have their adrenal glands surgically excised. Some patients with thyroid disease have near-total thyroidectomies, although this surgery is rarely done except in cases of THYROID CANCER.

See also THYROIDECTOMY.

Tanner stages   Five stages of adolescent sexual development, originally derived by J. M. Tanner in 1962. For example, with Stage 1, the preadolescent, there is no pubic hair present in either males or females. In Stage 2, males have some slightly pigmented hair around the base of the penis, while females have some sparse, slightly pigmented hair around the labia. In addition, at Stage 2, the male's testes and scrotum begin to enlarge, as does the penis. In the female, breast buds start to form. In stage 3, the male penis has an increased growth in length, as do the scrotum and testes. The pubic hair of the male becomes coarser and curlier. In females at stage 3, the breast mound becomes enlarged further, and the pubic hair is darker and coarser than at stage 2. At stage 4, the male penis has grown further from stage 3, and the testes and scrotum have also enlarged. The male pubic hair is at the adult level. Among females at stage 4, the areola and papilla together form a mound above the breast and the pubic hair is at the adult level. Stage 5 is the most mature stage of development. In this stage, the genitalia have a fully adult appearance. Tanner stages are also known as Tanner scales.

Some individuals experience a puberty that is precocious (EARLY PUBERTY), while others have a DELAYED PUBERTY. The Tanner stages chart enables physicians to determine the stage of development of a particular patient, despite his or her chronological age.

See also ADOLESCENTS.

Marshall, W. A., and J. M. Tanner. "Variations in the Pattern of Pubertal Changes in Boys." *Archive of Disease in Childhood* 45, no. 239 (1970): 13–23.

———."Variations in Pattern of Pubertal Changes in Girls." *Archives of Disease in Childhood* 44, no. 235 (1969): 291–303.

Tanner, J. M., M.D. *Growth at Adolescence with a General Consideration of the Effects of Hereditary and Environmental Factors Upon Growth and Maturation from Birth to Maturity,* 2d ed. Springfield, Ill.: Charles C. Thomas, 1962.

teriparatide (Forteo)   A recombinant human parathyroid hormone, approved by the Food and Drug Administration (FDA) in November 2002, for the treatment of postmenopausal women who are at high risk of developing fractures as a result of osteoporosis. Teriparatide is also used to treat men who are experiencing primary hypogonadism and who are at high risk for developing fractures.

Teriparatide is given as a daily subcutaneous injection via a penlike device. The standard dose of teriparatide as of this writing is 20 mcg, and patients also must take adequate oral dosages of calcium and vitamin D.

The drug has been successful in decreasing fractures in osteoporotic women by 65 percent and increasing their bone mineral density by nearly 10 percent in the spine.

In general, the side effects of teriparatide are mild and do not cause most patients to discontinue the drug.

See also FRACTURES; HYPOGONADISM; PARATHYROID GLANDS.

testes/testicles   Refers to the reproductive organs in men that are located in the scrotum, the sac beneath the penis, and that make the sperm needed to create a pregnancy when combined with a woman's egg from her ovary. (One testicle is a *testis,* while two are referred to as *testes.* Most males have two testes.) The testes also create most of the TESTOSTERONE, a hormone needed by the male body. (The ADRENAL GLANDS generate about 5 percent of a man's testosterone.)

In the male, testosterone is responsible for sex drive, muscle mass, the male pattern of hair distribution (such as facial hair and chest hair), and other key aspects of masculinity. In addition to testosterone, the testes produce other hormones, such as dehydroepiandrosterone (DHEA) and androstenedione. The testes are made up in part of Leydig's cells, which provide enzymes that enable androgens to be synthesized by the body. The testes also secrete limited amounts of estrogen hormones.

Very rarely, the testes are unseen and are located in the intra-abdominal area, resulting in an infant of indeterminate sex and who may have a MICROPENIS. Sometimes the child may have the sexual characteristics of both sexes, which is called HERMAPHRODITISM.

During puberty, the male undergoes a variety of body changes, including enlargements of the testes (the first sign of puberty in boys) and the penis, as well as other changes. Some males may experience a DELAYED PUBERTY, undergoing puberty several years later than their peers, while others may have an EARLY PUBERTY, also known as precocious puberty.

Examination of the Testes

Upon physical examination, the testes should be of a certain size, shape, and consistency. Typically, they are 15–25 cubic centimeters each. Endocrinologists use a device known as an orchidometer to compare the sizes of the testes. It is a chain of sphere-shaped beads that range from one to 30 cubic centimeters in size.

Most testes are firm and smooth to the touch, and they are not tender.

Infertility and the Testes

Some adult males experience problems with INFERTILITY related to insufficient sperm production or the absence of sperm altogether. In some cases, such problems can be resolved through treatment. Males may also develop cancer in the testicle area. TESTICULAR CANCER is highly treatable, in most cases, when it is identified. Some men also have problems with partial or total ANDROGEN RESISTANCE, which means that their bodies are unable to use all of the androgens (male hormones) they produce.

See also HYPOGONADISM; HYPOGONADOTROPISM; KLINEFELTER SYNDROME; MALE REPRODUCTION.

testicular cancer Malignant tumor of the testicle. According to the American Cancer Society, an estimated 8,980 men were diagnosed with testicular cancer in 2004 in the United States. The death rate is relatively low, and only about 360 men were predicted to die of testicular cancer in 2004. The five-year survival rate for men diagnosed with testicular cancer is 99 percent for men with localized cancer and 76 percent for testicular cancer that has spread, both very favorable rates. Testicular cancer represents less than 1 percent of all cancers diagnosed in the United States.

In Canada, according to the National Cancer Institute of Canada, 800 men were diagnosed with testicular cancer in 2003. In addition, about 35 men died of testicular cancer in 2003 in Canada.

Risk Factors

Caucasian males have a greater risk for developing testicular cancer than men of other races, although why this is true is unknown (see table). Testicular cancer is most common among men between the ages of 20 and 35 and is very rare among men over age 40.

Studies have also revealed that men who have had testicular cancer also face an increased risk for the next 20 years of developing another form of cancer, such as prostate cancer, colon cancer, bladder cancer, pancreatic cancer, thyroid cancer, kidney cancer, and other cancers. In a study reported in a 1997 issue of the *Journal of the National Cancer Institute*, researchers analyzed 29,000 testicular cancer survivors and found that 1,406 men had developed second cancers.

Signs and Symptoms

Men with early testicular cancer may have no symptoms or may experience swelling in the scrotum. They may also have pain and a feeling of heaviness and hardness in the area.

CANCER OF THE TESTES: INVASIVE CANCER INCIDENCE COUNTS BY
U.S. CENSUS REGION AND DIVISION, STATE AND METROPOLITAN AREA AND RACE, 2000

	All Races	Caucasian	African American		All Races	Caucasian	African American
Northeast				Atlanta	80	72	*
New England				Maryland	125	112	*
Connecticut	105	96	*	North Carolina	189	173	*
Massachusetts	198	189	*	South Carolina	81	73	*
New Hampshire	61	60	*	West Virginia	46	44	*
Rhode Island	31	21	*				
Vermont	21	21	*	East South Central			
				Alabama	82	72	*
Middle Atlantic				Kentucky	103	101	*
New Jersey	230	215	*				
New York	440	387	25	West South Central			
Pennsylvania	350	337	*	Louisiana	90	79	*
Midwest				**West**			
East North Central				Mountain			
Illinois	292	272	*	Arizona	139	133	*
Indiana	165	157	*	Colorado	160	158	*
Michigan	252	235	*	Idaho	44	44	*
Detroit	96	88	*	Montana	35	33	*
Ohio	299	280	*	Nevada	53	51	*
Wisconsin	160	152	*	New Mexico	44	41	*
				Utah	71	70	*
West North Central				Wyoming	19	19	*
Iowa	96	93	*				
Kansas	70	67	*	Pacific			
Minnesota	220	207	*	California	928	854	23
Missouri	113	109	*	San Francisco–Oakland	126	103	*
Nebraska	37	37	*	San Jose–Monterey	54	44	*
North Dakota	20	20	*	Los Angeles	243	227	*
				Hawaii	24	*	*
South				Oregon	119	113	*
South Atlantic				Washington	211	193	*
Florida	356	330	18	Seattle–Puget Sound	146	136	*
Georgia	168	154	*				

* Fewer than 16 cases in this category
Note: Data is not available for all states in the U.S.
Source: U.S. Cancer Statistics Working Group. *United States Cancer Statistics: 2000 Incidence.* Department of Health and Human Services, Centers for Disease Control and Prevention and National Cancer Institute, 2003.

Patients with advanced testicular cancer may experience the following signs and symptoms:

- Abdominal pain
- Unintended weight loss
- GYNECOMASTIA (growth of excess breast tissue in men and seen in 5 percent of men with germ cell tumors and 25 percent of males who have Leydig's cell tumors)
- Urinary obstruction
- Headaches
- Seizures

Gynecomastia is the most common endocrine abnormality seen in men with testicular cancer. With the Leydig's cell form, when seen in boys ages five to 12 years old, gynecomastia is usually associated with EARLY PUBERTY. It is also seen in men ages 25–35 who have erectile dysfunction in addition to the testicular mass. The gynecomastia is often associated with increased levels of human chorionic gonadatropin (HCG). In addition, the hormone levels of prolactin, estrogens, and androgens, may be altered. Interestingly, men with very high levels of HCG may develop HYPERTHYROIDISM due to the ability of the HCG to interact with the thyroid-stimulating hormone (TSH) receptor on the surface of the thyroid gland, which then subsequently leads to an overproduction of thyroid hormone.

Diagnosis and Treatment

If the physician suspects that a man has testicular cancer, he or she will usually order an imaging test—either a COMPUTER TOMOGRAPHY (CT) scan or a MAGNETIC RESONANCE IMAGING (MRI) scan. The doctor will also order laboratory tests, such as blood tests for serum alpha-feto protein (AFP) and serum beta-HCG, both of which are markers for testicular cancer. A biopsy is usually not performed.

The treatment for testicular cancer is an inguinal orchiectomy, which is the removal of the testis and spermatic cord. If only one testis is removed, the man may continue to be fertile. It may be advisable, however, to store his sperm before the surgery so that it can be used later to create a pregnancy, if desired. In most cases, surgery is sufficient to treat

and cure the cancer. If the cancer has advanced, which is unusual, chemotherapy may be necessary to extend life.

See also CANCER; TESTES/TESTICLES.

Bishop, Philippe C., and Barnett S. Kramer. "Testicular Carcinoma," in *Bethesda Handbook of Clinical Oncology.* Philadelphia, Pa.: Lippincott Williams & Wilkins, 2001.

Travis, Lois B., et al. "Risk of Second Malignant Neoplasms Among Long-term Survivors of Testicular Cancer." *Journal of the National Cancer Institute* 89, no. 19 (October 1, 1997): 1,429–1,439.

Tseng, A. Jr., et al. "Gynecomastia in Testicular Cancer Patients: Prognostic and Therapeutic Implications." *Cancer* 56, no. 10 (1985): 2,534–2,538.

testosterone　The male sex hormone and the most important androgen. It is synthesized by the testes and is converted in target tissues by 5-alpha reductase to dihydrotestosterone, a more potent form of testosterone. Testosterone production increases at the beginning of puberty and contributes to the changes in androgen-dependent tissues such as beard growth, pubic hair growth, increased muscle mass, deepening of the voice, and decrease in body fat content. Testosterone is believed to be the primary determinant of libido. Testosterone affects many aspects of a man's life, including sex drive, energy levels, and physical attributes such as muscle mass and strength.

Low levels of testosterone partially define HYPO-GONADISM. The other part of the definition is the inability to produce adequate levels of spermatozoa.

Women also have low levels of testosterone.

Testosterone Declines with Aging

In general, testosterone production declines with aging. The Baltimore Longitudinal Study of Aging revealed that hypogonadal levels of testosterone are present in 20 percent of men over 60 years of age, 30 percent of men over 70 years of age, and 60 percent of men over 80 years of age. The numbers are higher if the measurement is of free testosterone as opposed to total bound testosterone. Whether physiological declines in testosterone levels should be treated remains an area of controversy.

Treatment of Low Testosterone Levels

If treatment for low testosterone levels is given, testosterone may be replaced by the intramuscular (injection) or topical (applied to the skin) route. The intramuscular form is given every 10–28 days in the form of testosterone enanthate or cypionate. With this method, the levels of testosterone are often high for the first week and then below normal after two or three weeks. As a result, dosing every 10–14 days is best. The topical forms of testosterone, either by patch or gel, provide much more stable and normal levels.

Raising hypogonadal levels through testosterone replacement therapy will increase energy, a sense of well-being, muscle strength, libido, and general sexual function. Side effects of this therapy include irritation, impatience, acne, oily skin, increased prostate size, and a greater risk for prostate cancer and polycythemia (increased red blood cell mass).

See also ANABOLIC STEROIDS; HORMONES.

Harman, S. Mitchell, et al. "Longitudinal Effects of Aging on Serum Total and Free Testosterone Levels in Healthy Men." *Journal of Clinical Endocrinology & Metabolism* 86, no. 2 (2001): 724–731.

tetany   A form of uncontrollable muscle spasms that can be focal or diffuse. It is a form of severe neuromuscular irritability caused by repetitive, high-frequency discharges from the nerve endings, muscles, and spinal cord. Tetany may be caused by extremely low levels of calcium, magnesium, or potassium in the bloodstream. Thus, hypocalcemia tetany can be seen in HYPOPARATHYROIDISM (a condition of low levels of parathyroid hormone in the blood) or a hypocalcemic form of RICKETS.

Tetany often leads to what is known as carpal-pedal spasm, which is severe muscle contractions in both the hands and feet. The condition can be quite painful. TROUSSEAU'S SIGN is a form of limited tetany, in which hand and forearm tetany is induced by raising the blood pressure of a patient and changing the local acid-base balance (pH) so that the calcium level is low.

Tetany may occur shortly after a THYROIDECTOMY or other neck surgery. If the condition causing tetany is not treated immediately, the symptoms of tetany will worsen and the individual will die, although this cause of death occurs very rarely. Hypocalcemic tetany is usually reversed by administering intravenous calcium. After the patient is stabilized, the parathyroid glands may resume partial function. If the hypoparathyroidism does not improve, patients may need to take lifelong doses of both calcium and vitamin D.

See also CHVOSTEK'S SIGN; HYPOCALCEMIA.

Tohme, J. F., and J. P. Bilezikian. "Hypocalcemic Emergencies." *Endocrinology and Metabolism Clinics of North America* 22, no. 2 (1993): 363–375.

thirst   The need for fluid. Constant thirst may be a sign of dehydration or of a disease such as uncontrolled TYPE 1 DIABETES or TYPE 2 DIABETES, caused by high levels of glucose in the bloodstream. Excessive thirst may also be seen in DIABETES INSIPIDUS, in which there is a lack of the hormone DDAVP (desmopressin acetate) or a lack of effectiveness of the kidney, which leads to constant urination (polyuria). Thirst can also be a consequence of pituitary or hypothalamic lesions caused by tumors or after neurosurgery or radiation therapy to the brain.

See also DIABETES MELLITUS.

thymus gland   A small, anterior mediastinal gland (a gland in the upper anterior chest cavity) that weighs about 15 grams at birth and increases to 40 grams by puberty. It then decreases in size over time to an atrophic state. The thymus (from the Greek for "life force") assists the immune system by helping the development of T lymphocytes, which are used in cell-mediated immunity to fend off infection. The thymus gland contains thymic epithelial cells and lymphocytes. The epithelial cells may sometimes become cancerous. The thymus also contains neuroendocrine cells that may release hormones. Sometimes these cells may also become cancerous.

Until the 1960s, researchers had no idea what function, if any, was performed by the thymus. It is now known that the thymus is important in the immune system of the fetus and the young infant. However, some researchers believe the thymus may continue to be more important than is currently known or generally accepted. Chemotherapy for cancer can impede the actions of the thymus in producing T lymphocytes.

Some infants have DiGeorge syndrome, a disorder that affects the thymus, the parathyroid glands, and the heart. In the worst case of DiGeorge syndrome, the infants have significantly impaired immune systems because of their reduced T cell function related to the thymus malfunction. This is a very rare disease. However, in one case, researchers transplanted postnatal thymus tissue into five infants with complete DiGeorge syndrome. Two of the patients survived and their immune system was restored. The researchers concluded, in their 1999 article in the *New England Journal of Medicine*, "In some infants with profound immunodeficiency and complete DiGeorge syndrome, the transplantation of thymus tissue can restore normal immune function."

The Thymus and Longevity

Some researchers believe that the thymus and the pineal gland together have significant effects in extending longevity and that they are geroprotective.

Researchers in Russia and the Ukraine, who reported on their findings in a 2003 issue of *Neuroendocrinology Letters,* treated subjects with thymalin, a peptide regulator from the thymus, and also with epithalamin, another peptide regulator that stems from the pineal gland. They administered these drugs to 266 elderly individuals who were older than age 60 over the course of six to eight years. The researchers found a significant decrease in respiratory disease, heart disease, hypertension, osteoarthritis, and osteoporosis compared with subjects in the control group. They also found a decreased mortality rate among the treated subjects. Further research is needed to confirm or refute these findings.

Cancer of the Thymus

The thymus can become cancerous, which is known as thymoma and thymic carcinoma. Thymoma is usually a slow-growing tumor that remains inside the thymus gland. Most people with thymoma have another immune system disease, such as myasthenia gravis, a disease that causes weak muscles. Thymic carcinoma, in contrast, often spreads to other parts of the body. Thymic tumors do not usually cause any symptoms until they begin to compress the trachea and cause shortness of breath. Sometimes facial swelling is also noted. According to the American Cancer Society, patients may also experience flushing, asthma, and diarrhea.

Most patients are treated with surgery. Radiation therapy may also be used. The oncologist (cancer doctor) may employ chemotherapy and/or hormone therapy to treat thymic tumors.

Carcinoid tumors may also develop in the thymus.

Khavison, Vladimir Kh., and Vyacheslav Morozov. "Peptides of Pineal Gland and Thymus Prolong Human Life." *Neuro Endocrinology Letters* 24, no. 3/4 (June/August 2003): 233–240.

Markert, M. Louise, M.D., et al. "Transplantation of Thymus Tissue in Complete DiGeorge Syndrome." *New England Journal of Medicine* 341, no. 16 (October 14, 1999): 1,180–1,189.

thyroid blood tests   Generally refers to blood tests obtained to determine the level of thyroid hormone in the patient's bloodstream. These tests help the physician to know whether disease is present and if the thyroid is functioning at an appropriate level. They may be used to diagnose illness or to follow-up with patients already known to have thyroid disease to determine whether the medical treatment is appropriate and effective. Patients may receive blood tests to check their THY-ROID-STIMULATING HORMONE (TSH) levels, T3 or T4 levels, as well as their "free" thyroid levels of T3 and T4.

The TSH test, described in more detail in this entry, is the primary test employed when a physician is screening for a thyroid disorder. It is also the test of choice when determining whether a patient is taking an appropriate amount of thyroid hormone replacement for the treatment of any one of the many causes of HYPOTHYROIDISM. For other conditions, the TSH level must be measured and other tests performed to make a determination of the patient's status.

Helpful though they are, thyroid blood tests should not be the only tool doctors rely upon to diagnose thyroid disorders. Prior to making a diagnosis, an experienced ENDOCRINOLOGIST will always take into account the patient's history, the findings from the physical examination, as well as any thyroid function tests, ultrasounds, nuclear scans, or biopsy data.

Nonetheless, researchers using thyroid blood tests have clearly demonstrated that thyroid disease is very common. For example, in 2000, the researchers in the Colorado Thyroid Disease Prevention Study reported findings of elevated TSH levels in 9.5 percent of nearly 26,000 patients who had not previously been diagnosed with thyroid disease. Thus, they found a significant number of people who were biochemically hypothyroid and untreated.

This study is even more compelling when considering that the researchers used an upper limit of 5.1 microunits/ml as the top normal TSH value. As of 2003, based on recent data, the American Association of Clinical Endocrinologists narrowed the normal range for TSH levels to between about 0.3 and 3.04 microunits/ml. Thus, if the Colorado Thyroid Disease Prevention team had repeated their study using current guidelines for the diagnosis of hypothyroidism, utilizing a tighter TSH range, they would have found an even greater percentage of undiagnosed people with hypothyroidism.

Additionally, the researchers in this study found below-normal TSH levels (indicating hyperthyroidism) among about 2 percent of the individuals tested, using lower limits of 0.3 microunits/ml. This value is about what most laboratories continue to use today for a lower normal limit of TSH.

A variety of laboratory tests other than the TSH test are used to help physicians determine if a patient has thyroid disease and to assess the severity of any existing illness. These tests include the T3 test, the T4 test, the TSI test, and the anti-TPO test.

The TSH Test

The most commonly used thyroid test is the TSH blood test. This is a measurement of a hormone produced by the pituitary gland. As the name implies, this hormone stimulates the thyroid gland. TSH is necessary in small amounts for the thyroid to function well at baseline. TSH is under the control of thyrotropin-releasing hormone (TRH), pro-

duced in the hypothalamus. The usual feedback loop is that T4 and T3 thyroid hormones travel via the blood to the pituitary and the hypothalamus. In both places, if the thyroid hormone levels are inadequate, the synthesis of TRH and, in turn, TSH are increased. This increased TSH travels via the blood to the thyroid to stimulate more thyroid hormone production.

When thyroid hormone levels are adequate, the hypothalamus and the pituitary detect them, and the TRH and the TSH levels both return to baseline. The body modulates the amount of thyroid hormones from minute to minute as well as over the course of an individual's life.

Note that some individuals who are ill may have TSH levels within the normal range. For example, patients with EUTHYROID SICK SYNDROME often have a normal TSH. Many ELDERLY individuals with hypothyroidism may have a normal TSH level. Thus, as previously discussed, the doctor must consider the patient's medical history, physical examination results, as well as the laboratory findings in order to make an appropriate diagnosis.

Because increased TSH levels indicate underactive thyroid function (hypothyroidism) while low TSH levels are usually seen with HYPERTHYROIDISM, a discussion with patients about TSH levels often causes confusion. This apparent contradiction is due to the FEEDBACK LOOP that is in play involving the thyroid gland, the pituitary, and the hypothalamus.

If either low or high levels of TSH are found in a blood test for the first time, the test should be performed again to make sure that the findings were not in error. Administering thyroid hormone to a person based on one TSH test alone would be a bad idea. Some medications can affect the TSH blood test result, such as dopamine, glucocorticoid drugs, and octreotide.

The T3 Test

The T3 test measures the concentration of total T3, which is all T3 that is bound to proteins in the blood and consists mainly of albumin and thyroid-bonding globulin. Typically, T3 is measured with a process known as radioimmunoassay. An estimated 20 percent of T3 is synthesized in the thyroid gland, and the balance is created in nonthyroid tissues. Total T3 is not commonly measured but is useful in the assessment of hyperthyroidism. It is not helpful at all in the diagnosis of hypothyroidism.

In the most common form of hyperthyroidism, GRAVES' DISEASE, T3 can be preferentially produced in the thyroid gland. Production of T3 can also be seen in toxic multinodular goiters as well as with single toxic nodules or adenomas (also called autonomously functioning thyroid nodules). Very low levels of T3 can be seen in severe hypothyroidism, chronic illness, or starvation.

Physicians may also request a test of free T3 level. This refers to the concentration of unbound T3 able to get into cells and move to the nucleus to interact with that cell's DNA and to cause its myriad effects. Free T3 is rarely measured as it is more difficult to assay and because free T3 tests are more expensive than other thyroid tests. It is occasionally ordered by endocrinologists when there is a complex issue involving binding proteins and an attempt to determine the level of hyperthyroidism.

The T4 Test

The physician may order a test for total T4, or thyroxine. Nearly 100 percent (99.7 percent) of T4 is found in the bound form. Thyroxine is produced solely by the thyroid gland. In patients who are hypothyroid, synthetic thyroxine, known as levothyroxine (T4), enables them to achieve a normal level of thyroid functioning.

Some patients take preparations of DESSICATED THYROID, which is a prescribed drug that includes both T3 and T4. The TSH test can be used regardless of the type of thyroid supplement (if any) that is taken by patients, although the interpretation of thyroid function is more complicated when patients are taking a combination of T4 and T3 medications than when they are taking just T4 alone. Note that three prospective studies have failed to show any advantage to the use of the combination of T4 and T3 medications versus the use of T3 alone.

Researchers have made assessments based on objective and subjective parameters, such as patient strength, energy levels, sense of well-being, weight, blood pressure, and cognitive function. Patients on T4 alone did as well as those on combination therapy.

Normal values for total T4 vary slightly from laboratory to laboratory, but the typical normal range is approximately 4.5–11 micrograms per deciliter (mcg/dl). Greater-than-normal levels of T4 may indicate the patient has a form of hyperthyroidism, such as Graves' disease. It may also indicate elevated levels of binding proteins, as is seen in women taking oral contraceptives or patients who have liver disease. Thus, these patients have high concentrations of total T4, but they are clinically euthyroid (normal). They have normal TSH levels and no signs or symptoms of hyperthyroidism.

Other drugs in addition to oral contraceptives may cause elevated total T4 levels, including estrogens, methadone, amiodarone, and clofibrate. Some medications decrease T4 absorption, such as aluminium hydroxide, ferrous sulfate, sucralfate, cholestyramine, and colestipol. Other drugs affect the metabolism of both T3 and T4, including phenobarbital, rifampin, phenytoin, and carbamazepine, and cytokines such as interferon or interleukin-2. The effects will show up on thyroid tests, but only the physician can determine potential causes for the laboratory results. This is why it is very important for the doctor to obtain a complete medical history, including all medications that the patient takes for any reason.

Lower-than-normal levels of total T4 may indicate the patient has a form of hypothyroidism, such as a later stage of HASHIMOTO'S THYROIDITIS. It may also indicate malnutrition or a serious systemic illness that has caused a decrease in proteins that bind to T4. In addition, some medications cause below-normal T4 levels, such as lithium, iodine, methimazole, interferon alpha, interleukin-2, amiodarone, dexamethasone, propranolol, and propylthiouracil.

Many radioimmunoassay kits now allow laboratories to measure the amount of free thyroxine (free T4) in the blood. They are relatively easy to use but have some variability from laboratory to laboratory and are not as precise, as of this writing, as the TSH test.

These radioimmunoassay kits are helpful in sorting out issues related to illness, especially when that illness affects the levels of thyroid binding. These assays have made it less common for laboratories to have to measure the total T4 as well as some measure of binding proteins and then to calculate a free T4 level. In various laboratories, these free T4 tests have been given different names, such as the free thyroxine index, calculated free thyroxine, effective thyroxine, or estimated free thyroxine. Individuals with a lower-than-normal level of free T4 may have hypothyroidism, while above-normal levels often indicate hyperthyroidism.

The TSI Test

The thyroid-stimulating immunoglobulin (TSI) test, also known as the TSH receptor antibody test, may also be ordered for patients who are suspected of or known to have Graves' disease. It provides a rough estimate of how much of this antibody is present as well as how active it is.

The TSI test is most commonly used for women in their third trimester of pregnancy to help predict neonatal Graves' disease in the fetus. In cases in which it is unclear whether the patient has Graves' disease, a positive TSI assay may indicate the diagnosis of this autoimmune illness. The test is also given to infants, children, and adolescents to predict thyroid disease.

The Anti-TPO Test

The most commonly assayed thyroid antibody test is the anti-thyroid peroxidase antibody, or anti-TPO test. Peroxidase is a protein, specifically an enzyme, that is present in thyroid cells. As a protein, it can function as an antigen, which means the immune system can respond to it. In patients with Hashimoto's thyroiditis, the body mistakenly makes an antibody (also known as an immunoglobulin) to combat the peroxidase protein. This antibody binds to the thyroid. If enough of these antibodies bind, they can damage the thyroid gland. This can cause transient hyperthyroidism and then eventually cause hypothyroidism.

The anti-TPO test is now the gold standard for determining whether a patient has Hashimoto's thyroiditis. However, test results may also show mild elevation for other forms of thyroiditis as well as for Graves' disease. After many years of damage to the thyroid gland, the levels of anti-TPO antibodies can be quite low. Thus its absence does not completely rule out autoimmune thyroid disease. This test has replaced the older and less specific antimicrosomal antibody test and the antithyroglobulin test. The antiglobulin test still has some value when monitoring patients with THYROID CANCER.

See also HASHIMOTO'S THYROIDITIS; THYROIDITIS.

Canaris, Gay J., M.D., et al. "The Colorado Thyroid Disease Prevalence Study." *Archives of Internal Medicine* 160, no. 4 (2000): 526–534.

Demers, Lawrence M., and Carole A. Spencer. *Laboratory Medicine Practice Guidelines: Laboratory Support for the Diagnosis and Monitoring of Thyroid Disease.* National Academy of Clinical Biochemistry, 2002. Available online. URL: http://www.nacb.org/lmpg/thyroid lmpg pub.stm. Downloaded January 15, 2004.

Surks, Martin I., M.D., and Rubens Sievert, M.D. "Drugs and Thyroid Function." *New England Journal of Medicine* 333, no. 25 (1995): 1,688–1,694.

thyroid cancer Malignant tumor of the thyroid gland. Thyroid cancer is not a rare form of cancer, and most patients with the disease have a very good prognosis. According to the American Cancer Society, an estimated 22,000 new cases of thyroid cancer were diagnosed in the United States in 2003, 16,300 females and 5,700 males. Clearly, thyroid cancer is a greater risk for women, and it represents 3 percent of all cancers in women. An estimated 1,400 people died of thyroid cancer in 2003, including 800 women and 600 men. In considering middle-aged adults with thyroid cancer, from 80–95 percent of them will survive 10 years or more.

There are four major types of thyroid cancer, including papillary thyroid cancer, follicular thyroid cancer, medullary thyroid cancer, and anaplastic thyroid cancer. Of these, papillary thyroid cancer is the most common, representing from 70–80 percent of all thyroid cancers. The least common is anaplastic thyroid cancer, which represents less than 3 percent of all thyroid cancers. There are also rare lymphomas of the thyroid gland as well as metastases (spread) to the thyroid from other primary tumors.

In the Surveillance, Epidemiology and End Results (SEER) government database of nearly 16,000 patients, the 10-year survival rate for the epithelial thyroid cancers were as follows: 98 percent for papillary type, 92 percent for the follicular type, and 13 percent for the anaplastic type.

In a study of 336 patients whose thyroid cancer was known to have spread, reported in a 2003 issue of the *Journal of the American College of Surgery,* researchers found that those with the best survival outcomes were patients who were under age 45 years old.

According to the National Cancer Institute of Canada, thyroid cancer has the most rapidly increasing rate of incidence among both men and women in Canada, although the reasons for this is unknown.

Risk Factors

Thyroid cancer occurs among all age groups, although it is more commonly found among individuals over age 30. Women have about a two to three times greater risk of developing thyroid cancer than men. Distinctive racial differences occur in the incidence of thyroid cancer.

In the United States, high rates have been identified among Asian women, with Filipino women (14.6 per 100,000 women) experiencing the highest rates, followed by Vietnamese women (10.5 per 100,000) and Hawaiian women (9.1 per 100,000). Caucasians are more likely than African Americans to develop thyroid cancer. The lowest rates of thyroid cancer occur among African-American women (3.3 per 100,000).

People who were exposed to excessive radiation have an increased risk for developing thyroid cancer. From the 1920s to the 1950s, many doctors routinely used X-rays to diagnose and treat children with tonsillitis, acne, an enlarged thymus, and other medical problems of the head and neck. According to the National Cancer Institute, scientists later discovered that this increased radiation exposure made patients more vulnerable to thyroid cancer. (Experts report that radiation from dental X-rays is not risky for children and adults, although shields should be used to protect the body below the head, whenever possible.) Experts are currently studying patients who were exposed to radioactive fallout in Hanford, Washington, and Chernobyl in the Ukraine in the former Soviet Union.

People who have goiters have an increased risk for developing thyroid cancer. The incidence among such patients is 10–15 percent.

A lack of iodine in the diet may lead to thyroid cancer. Because iodine is added to salt in the United States, thyroid cancer is rarely caused by iodine deficiencies in this country.

Thyroid cancer may also have a genetic basis. Some researchers have found that an alteration in the *RET* gene may be transmitted from a parent to a child, causing medullary thyroid cancer. If several people in a family are diagnosed with thyroid cancer, other members may wish to be tested for a mutation of the *RET* gene. This syndrome, when present, is also called *familial medullary thyroid cancer* or multiple endocrine neoplasia, type 2 (MEN 2). Individuals who have MEN 2 syndrome are also at risk for developing other types of cancer.

Symptoms of Thyroid Cancer

As with many other forms of cancer, most people in the early stages of thyroid cancer have no symptoms or signs of disease. When symptoms or signs occur, they may include the following:

• Hoarseness

• A lump near the Adam's apple of the neck

• Swollen lymph nodes in the neck or nearby

• Dysphagia (difficulty swallowing)

• Pain in the neck or throat

Medullary carcinoma of the thyroid secretes CALCITONIN and thus can cause symptoms due to the presence of this hormone, such as flushing, nausea, and diarrhea. In addition, medullary carcinoma of the thyroid is often inherited. Family members can be screened by measuring their calcitonin levels or by looking for abnormal chromosomes, such as *RET*.

Anaplastic carcinoma typically presents in older men as a very hard mass in the neck. It is often incurable at the time of diagnosis, as it does not concentrate iodine, and thus radioactive iodine (RAI) therapy cannot be used. It is poorly responsive, if at all, to chemotherapy and external radiation therapy.

Diagnosis and Treatment

If symptoms are present (though in the early stages of thyroid cancer, they usually are not), the doctor will perform a physical examination of the neck to check for nodules or swelling. (Most patients with thyroid nodules do *not* have thyroid cancer, but it needs to be ruled out.)

When a thyroid nodule is discovered, the first step should be a fine needle aspiration biopsy of the thyroid gland. In this procedure, a very small needle, usually 21–27 gauge, is inserted into the thyroid in order to obtain small numbers of thyroid cells that can be viewed under a microscope. This procedure can be done in the doctor's office. Ultrasound guidance may be used if the nodule is difficult to palpate or if multiple nodules are present.

The ultrasound can also be used to follow up and check on the size of a nodule accurately. If a specific kind of calcification is seen on the ultrasound, it can be a marker for a malignancy, although the presence of this calcification is not sensitive or specific enough to be used as a screening technique.

If the biopsy results are unclear, the endocrinologist may order a technetium or iodine scan of the thyroid to determine if the nodule is functional (warm), nonfunctional (cold), or hyperfunctional (hot). Cold nodules have the highest risk of malignancy, although the majority of them (70–85 percent) are still benign. Hot nodules are very rarely malignant.

Blood tests may also indicate the presence of thyroid cancer. For example, calcitonin is considered a tumor marker for medullary carcinoma of the thyroid. It is always elevated when the patient has thyroid cancer.

With papillary and follicular thyroid cancers, measurement of serum thyroglobulin is used to help physicians track the disease. Thyroglobulin is a protein that is composed of only thyroid cells. If a person has had his or her entire thyroid removed as well as follow-up RAI therapy, then usually no detectable thyroglobulin is in the blood. If thyroglobulin is detected, this is an indication of cancer spread that should be treated with further radiation therapy.

To stage the cancer (determine how advanced it is and whether it has spread to other organs), whole-body radioactive iodine scans are used to look for thyroid tissue in the thyroid bed and elsewhere. Other imaging techniques such as ULTRASOUND, COMPUTERIZED TOMOGRAPHY (CT) scans, MAGNETIC RESONANCE IMAGING (MRI) scans, or positron emission tomography (PET) scans are required for some thyroid cancers and may be used to help determine the extent of the spread of the tumor.

The treatment of the cancer depends on the severity of the disease. Severity is a function of the type of cancer (papillary being the least aggressive and anaplastic being the most aggressive), the size of the tumor, and whether or not there is metastases. For small, nonaggressive cancers, a hemithyroidectomy, which is a near-total thyroidectomy, may suffice. If there is concern that small amounts of cancer may have been left behind in the thyroid bed or if there are metastases, then radioactive iodine is used to kill the remaining cells. A thyroidectomy *must* be done prior to the use of RAI therapy. Giving a dose that is large enough to wipe out the entire thyroid is not practical or safe. Thus the majority of the thyroid cells (most of which are benign) must be removed surgically prior to the use of RAI.

The isotope iodine-131 is used. It is very safe in small-to-moderate doses with little risk to the recipient. However, when large doses are used, such as greater than 200 millicuries, bone marrow is affected. Its ability to function must be monitored by physicians. In addition, if there is a large amount of metastases in the lung, large doses of RAI can cause scarring (fibrosis) of the lung, damaging its ability to function.

In the past, in order to use RAI therapy effectively, thyroid hormone therapy was withdrawn to allow the body's endogenous level to rise. This would then maximize the efficacy of the RAI therapy, and an elevated thyroid-stimulating hormone (TSH) level would help drive the RAI into the remaining thyroid cells. However, the patients necessarily became very hypothyroid during this time and felt miserable. Recombinant TSH (thyrogen) is now used.

In most cases, two or three doses of Thyrogen are given to the patient intramuscularly several days prior to the RAI uptake scan and therapy. The Thyrogen increases the overall level of TSH in the system while the patient is still taking thyroid hormone replacement. Both the scan and the treatment can be done effectively without causing the patient to become hypothyroid.

For tumors that do not concentrate iodine, other forms of chemotherapy may be used, although most are fairly ineffective. Another option for patients with advanced thyroid cancer is to join a clinical study, in which they may have the opportunity to try a new drug or treatment that is under study and that otherwise would not be available to them.

See also CANCER; MULTIPLE ENDOCRINE NEOPLASIA.

For further information on thyroid cancer, contact the following organizations:

American Cancer Society
1599 Clifton Road NE
Atlanta, GA 30329
(404) 320-3333 or (800) 227-2345 (toll-free)
http://www.cancer.org

Light of Life Foundation
P.O. Box 163
Manalpan, NJ 07726
(877) 565-6325 (toll-free)
http://www.lightoflifefoundation.org

National Cancer Institute
Building 31, Room 11A16
9000 Rockville Pike
Rockville, MD 20892
(800)-4-CANCER (toll-free)
http://www.cancer.gov

ThyCa: Thyroid Cancer Survivors Association, Inc.
P.O. Box 1545
New York, NY 10159
(877) 588-7904 (toll-free)
http://www.thyca.org

Abraham, Jame, and Tito Fojo. "Endocrine Tumors." in *Bethesda Handbook of Clinical Oncology.* Philadelphia, Pa.: Lippincott Williams & Wilkins, 2001.

Gilliland, F. D., et al. "Prognostic Factors for Thyroid Carcinomas: A Population Based Study of 15,698 Cases from the Surveillance, Epidemiology and End Results (SEER) Program 1973–1991." *Cancer* 79, no. 3 (1997): 564–573.

Shoup, M., et al. "Prognostic Indicators of Outcomes in Patients with Distant Metastases from Differentiated Thyroid Carcinoma." *Journal of the American College of Surgery* 197, no. 2 (August 2003): 191–197.

thyroidectomy   Partial or total surgical removal of the diseased thyroid gland, often due to nodular thyroid disease, GRAVES' DISEASE, or THYROID CANCER.

The thyroidectomy is described as partial (any part), hemi (half), isthmusectomy (excision of the isthmus), and total or near-total thyroidectomy. Thyroid surgery is best done by a surgeon with extensive experience in performing this procedure. Typically, a necklace-type incision is used. As with all surgeries, complications are possible as well as possible complications due to anesthesia, blood loss, and infection, although complications from blood loss and infection are rare.

The thyroid must be carefully excised by the surgeon because the parathyroids can be temporarily or permanently damaged or disrupted by the surgery. (If the parathyroids are damaged or destroyed, the resulting HYPOPARATHYROIDISM will necessitate the use of vitamin D and calcium, and possibly of magnesium supplement, for the remainder of the patient's life.) In addition, the recurrent laryngeal nerves are located very close to the thyroid gland and can become damaged during surgery, which would lead to partial or complete vocal cord paralysis.

If a total or near-total thyroidectomy is performed, the patient will need to take replacement thyroid medication for the rest of his or her life.

See also THYROID GLAND.

thyroid gland   A very important, butterfly-shaped organ, located in the neck, that controls the body's overall METABOLISM and energy levels through its production of thyroid hormone.

The thyroid has two lobes and a connecting section called the isthmus. Embryologically, the thyroid descended from an area near the tongue. Sometimes, remnants of thyroid tissue can be left behind and can form what is known as a thyroglossal duct cyst in the middle of the neck. In addition, this migration of the thyroid as the fetus develops also causes the recurrent laryngeal nerves to be pulled along. A surgeon performing thyroid surgery must be very careful to avoid damaging these vital structures that control the vocal cords and the ability to speak and sing properly.

The thyroid gland can be inspected from the front of the neck. The endocrinologist will check it by palpating the thyroid from the front and often from the rear. The thyroid is fairly superficial, but it is partially covered by a thick layer of the anterior neck strap muscles.

During an examination, the physician will often want the patient to swallow to see that the thyroid moves properly up and down. Sometimes it is situated a bit lower than usual and is behind the mannerism (the top part of the sternum, or the breastbone), and thus it can be felt only when the person swallows. At times, the thyroid gland is completely behind the breastbone and can be seen only with imaging techniques.

A substantial goiter is not uncommon in the thyroid gland. The four parathyroid glands are located close to the right and left thyroid lobes and at times actually lie within the thyroid gland itself.

The thyroid gland has active transporters to take up iodine from the circulation and combine it with tyrosine, an amino acid, in order to make various thyroid hormones. The thyroid gland synthesizes T4 (LEVOTHYROXINE), T3 (tri-iodothyronine), thyroglobulin, and various other forms of thyroid hormone that are relatively unimportant. The thyroid's ability to take up iodine from the circulation actively is utilized in thyroid scanning with radioactive iodine and technetium to create images of the gland and to measure its biological activity. In addition, the ENDOCRINOLOGIST can use this ability of the gland to import iodine actively to treat patients with GRAVE'S DISEASE and THYROID CANCER with the appropriate therapeutic dosages of radioactive iodine.

When the thyroid gland functions normally, the energy levels of a person are consistent with the needs of the individual and the overall metabolism is within normal ranges. When it malfunctions, individuals may have HYPOTHYROIDISM, with low levels of thyroid hormone, or they may have HYPERTHYROIDISM, with excessively high levels of thyroid hormone. Thyroid hormone should be thought of as a permissive hormone, or one that is required in appropriate amounts to allow each cell and organ system to function properly. It is not that these systems will not function at all without thyroid hormone but, rather, that they will not function as well as they should function.

The most common forms of thyroid disease are two autoimmune disorders: Graves' disease, which causes hyperthyroidism, and HASHIMOTO'S THYROIDITIS, which causes hypothyroidism. Some individuals develop THYROID NODULES, which might need to be evaluated for the presence of thyroid cancer.

See also GOITER; THYROID BLOOD TESTS; THYROIDECTOMY; THYROIDITIS; THYROID-STIMULATING HORMONE; THYROXINE.

thyroiditis   A general term indicating an inflammation of the thyroid gland. Thyroiditis may cause excessively low (hypothyroid) or high (hyperthyroid) levels of thyroid hormone. HASHIMOTO'S THYROIDITIS, the most common cause of hypothyroidism, is also the most common cause of chronic thyroiditis. Other forms of thyroiditis, which may be acute or subacute, include painless lymphocytic thyroiditis (which is the cause of the thyroiditis and is also known as painless sporadic thyroiditis and postpartum thyroiditis), subacute thyroiditis (which is painful), suppurative thyroiditis, and drug-induced thyroiditis. The treatment of the thyroiditis depends on the particular cause.

Hashimoto's Thyroiditis

An autoimmune disorder that can occur at any age, Hashimoto's thyroiditis is most common among patients between the ages of 30 and 50 years. It is more frequently found among smokers. Hashimoto's thyroiditis may also cause a GOITER (enlargement of the thyroid gland).

In the early phases of the illness, the patient maintains normal thyroid function. As the gland enlarges, portions of it become damaged and do not function as well. Thus, early on, the thyroid gland may be slightly enlarged and firmer than usual. The patient may have increased levels of antithyroid peroxidase antibodies but yet have completely normal levels of thyroid hormone.

Many endocrinologists choose to treat patients early in the course of this disease with prescribed thyroid hormone. They hope that the thyroid hormone, which decreases the amount of thyroid-stimulating hormone (TSH), will prevent the thyroid gland from enlarging. They prefer to avoid waiting for the overt symptoms of hypothyroidism to occur.

Later in the course of the disease, due to ongoing damage to the thyroid gland, it may shrink and become fibrotic (scarred).

Hashimoto's thyroiditis is chronic and slow developing. Consequently, it is painless, causing no tenderness nor redness. Patients with Hashimoto's thyroiditis are at an increased risk for developing a lymphoma of the thyroid, although such a development is very rare.

Painless Lymphocytic Thyroiditis (Postpartum Thyroiditis and Painless Sporadic Thyroiditis)

Postpartum thyroiditis, also an autoimmune disorder, is fairly common and occurs in as many as 10 percent of women within several months of childbirth. It is more common among women with TYPE 1 DIABETES, other autoimmune disorders, or a family history of autoimmune disorders, especially autoimmune thyroid disorders. THYROTOXICOSIS may occur within one to six months after the delivery and may last for one to four months, although most patients who experience thyrotoxicosis have it for one to two months. The patient then enters a euthyroid (normal thyroid phase) for one to two months.

After this phase, the patient may then become hypothyroid (underactive thyroid) for four to six months. About 80 percent of women with painless postpartum thyroiditis eventually regain normal thyroid function.

With all the many changes that women face after delivering a child (fatigue, disrupted sleep, hair loss, and other symptoms), this thyroid condition can be misdiagnosed or missed completely. If diagnosed, the physician needs to be fully aware of the course of postpartum thyroiditis since sequential thyroid tests can give confusing results and may be elevated, then normal, and finally, low.

Physicians may elect to use a 24-hour iodine uptake test to differentiate painless lymphocytic thyroiditis from GRAVES' DISEASE. With painless lymphocytic thyroiditis, the iodine uptake is very low. In contrast, with most patients with Graves' disease, it is high.

Painless sporadic thyroiditis is essentially the same disease as painless postpartum thyroiditis, without a pregnancy having occurred. The therapy is the same as well.

Many patients do not require any medication for painless lymphocytic thyroiditis. Symptoms of hyperthyroidism, such as rapid heartbeat (tachycardia), nervousness, palpitations, tremors, and anxiety can be diminished with the use of beta-blockers such as propranolol (Inderal), atenolol (Tenormin), and metoprolol (Lopressor and Toprol-XL).

Painful Subacute Thyroiditis

This disease is also an autoimmune disorder. Painful subacute thyroiditis is rare and represents only about 5 percent of all diagnosed thyroid diseases. It is most commonly seen in the summertime after the patient has had an upper-respiratory viral infection. Patients present with a sore throat and neck, general body aches and pains, fatigue, and low fevers.

Many patients are misdiagnosed because the condition is not considered or the gland is not palpated, nor is it noted to be tender. As many as half of these patients may also have thyrotoxicosis for several weeks, after which their thyroid function will be normal for several months, possibly followed by the patient becoming hypothyroid for about four to six months. About 95 percent of patients with painful subacute thyroiditis ultimately regain normal thyroid function.

Patients with painful subacute thyroiditis have an elevated level on the erythrocyte sedimentation rate (ESR) blood test, antithyroid antibodies, and also have high rates of C-reactive protein blood concentration.

Treatment is aimed at helping the patient cope with pain. Most patients are treated with aspirin or nonsteroidal anti-inflammatory medications (NSAIDs) to provide pain relief. If the pain is extreme, patients may be treated with corticosteroids such as prednisone, which are generally tapered down over four to six weeks.

Suppurative Thyroiditis

This form of thyroid inflammation is usually caused by a bacterial infection, but it may also be caused by fungal, mycobacterial, or parasitic infections. Infections of the thyroid gland are rare. They may be found in patients with preexisting thyroid disease as well as among those who are immunocompromised, such as elderly individuals, patients with acquired immune deficiency syndrome (AIDS), and recipients of organ transplants.

Patients with suppurative thyroiditis have trouble swallowing (dysphagia), fever, and neck pain. Their sedimentation rates and white blood cell counts are elevated. The illness is usually diagnosed with a fine-needle aspiration and a culture of the tissue. Antibiotics are used, and the thyroid is drained of any abscess that may be present.

Medication-Induced Thyroiditis

The primary types of medications that may cause thyroiditis are amiodarone (a heart medication), lithium (a psychiatric medication), and interferon alpha or interleukin-2 (medications given to boost the immune system).

Amiodarone-Induced Thyroiditis

Thyroid disease caused by taking amiodarone is often very difficult to treat. Amiodarone may cause hypothyroidism (may be treated with thyroid hormone) and hyperthyroidism. However, when hyperthyroidism is induced by amiodarone, life becomes very difficult for patients, their cardiologist, and their endocrinologist. This is because amiodarone is used to treat significant heart arrythmias (such as atrial fibrillation, ventricular tachycardia, and other life-threatening heart rhythm disturbances), and must be maintained for life.

Because amiodarone is 37 percent iodine by weight, antithyroid drugs and radioactive iodine will not work. Antithyroid drugs work by blocking the uptake of iodine and decreasing thyroid hormone synthesis. Radioactive iodine kills thyroid cells. Neither works because the amiodarone has filled the thyroid full of iodine.

Two types of amiodarone-induced thyrotoxicosis occur. Type I is more commonly seen among patients with preexisting thyroid disease. Treatment with antithyroid medications, such as methimazone or propylthiouracil, can be attempted but often fails. Type II thyroiditis may be treated with high doses of corticosteroids, which may help. In addition, perchlorate may be used to try to discharge the excess iodine from the thyroid gland. However, this is not a Food and Drug Administration-approved use of perchlorate. In resistant cases, the symptoms can be diminished with beta-blockers and the patient can undergo a thyroidectomy.

Lithium-Induced Thyroiditis

Thyroiditis caused by a patient taking lithium usually causes hypothyroidism. In a few cases, the lithium may induce Graves' disease, the dominant form of hyperthyroidism. When hypothyroidism occurs, treatment with thyroid hormone is usually used. When hyperthyroidism occurs, and if it cannot be successfully treated, patients must confer with their psychiatrist, neurologist, or primary care physician to consider therapies other than lithium to treat their underlying disorders.

Immune Medication-Caused Thyroiditis

Interferon alpha, when used as therapy to treat hepatitis B and hepatitis C, can cause thyroid dysfunction within three months of beginning therapy. This form of thyroiditis is most likely to occur among patients with a preexisting thyroid abnormality, such as those who have a predisposition to developing an autoimmune thyroid disease and who have only positive thyroid peroxidase antibodies. Interferon alpha can induce both hypothyroidism and hyperthyroidism.

Interleukin-2, which is used in the treatment of leukemia and other malignancies, can cause thyroid dysfunction in about 1–3 percent of those treated.

Patients with thyroiditis who continue on the interferon alpha or interleukin-2 may also receive beta-blocker medications or corticosteroids. If they are hypothyroid, they will also be treated with levothyroxine.

Other Forms of Thyroiditis

Radiation-induced thyroiditis can occur after the use of radioactive iodine for the treatment of hyperthyroidism, at which point there is elevated thyroid iodine uptake. The destructive effects of radioactive iodine can lead to a brief exacerbation of hyperthyroidism that can usually be treated symptomatically with beta-blockers. Pain that has been caused by damage to the thyroid gland can be treated with simple analgesics (painkillers), nonsteroidal anti-inflammatory medications (NSAIDs), and sometimes corticosteroids.

Palpation-induced thyroiditis is caused by an overly vigorous palpation of the thyroid gland. It is rare and usually mild and can be treated with over-the-counter analgesics, ice, and NSAIDs.

Fibrous thyroiditis is a very rare condition that is part of a primary fibrosing (scarring) syndrome. It is treated with corticosteroids and surgery to avoid compressive symptoms that prevent swallowing or breathing properly.

Pearce, Elizabeth N., M.D., Alan P. Farwell, M.D., and Lewis E. Braverman, M.D. "Thyroiditis." *New England Journal of Medicine* 348, no. 26 (June 26, 2003): 2,646–2,655.

thyroid nodules   Any focal enlargement of a portion of the thyroid gland as detected by palpation upon physical examination, ULTRASOUND, or another imaging modality such as nuclear thyroid scanning, COMPUTED TOMOGRAPHY (CT) scan, or MAGNETIC RESONANCE IMAGING (MRI).

Thyroid nodules are very common. In a study from Framingham, Massachusetts, the prevalence of clinically detected nodules was 6.4 percent in women and 1.5 percent in men.

Concern About Cancer

The biggest fear when patients have thyroid nodules is whether they represent cancer. Up to about 90 percent of thyroid cancers in the United States are papillary, follicular, or mixed thyroid cancers, (usually papillary-follicular) all of which have very good long-term survival rates.

The incidence of cancer in nonselected nodules (nodules that are randomly detected) is in the 3–6 percent range in the United States. The presence of microcarcinomas of the thyroid (less than 10 millimeters in diameter) is very common and may be as high as 15 percent.

Endocrinologists will assess the individual's cancer risk based on the patient's medical history and risk factors. Cancer is more likely to be found in nodules in patients who are younger than age 30 as well as in male patients and in those who have experienced radiation exposure.

Single or Multiple Nodules

There may be a solitary nodule or multiple nodules. A solitary nodule, if greater than one centimeter in diameter, is considered to be a clinically significant nodule. (This definition continues to evolve as imaging modalities become better and are able to detect smaller and smaller nodules.) In cases of multiple nodules, if one nodule is clearly larger than the others, it is considered a dominant nodule. Dominant nodules have a higher risk of cancer. On occasion, when multiple nodules are present and two are much larger than all the rest, these two nodules are considered to be codominant. Thus, if nodules were present that were five millimeters, three millimeters, six millimeters, seven millimeters, three millimeters, 15 millimeters, and 19 millimeters in diameter, the 15-millimeter and 19-millimeter nodules would be considered codominant.

Nodules may be simple or complex and solid or cystic. They may also be consistent throughout (homogeneous) or partially cystic, containing some fluid and partly solid (heterogeneous).

Growth of Nodules Does Not Ensure Cancer Presence

Most thyroid nodules grow, whether they are benign or malignant. So increased growth is not necessarily an indication of thyroid cancer.

In a study reported in a 2003 issue of the *Annals of Internal Medicine*, researchers analyzed the outcomes for all patients referred to the Brigham and Women's Hospital Thyroid Nodule Clinic in Boston, Massachusetts, between 1995 and 2000 who requested a follow-up ultrasound examination within one month to five years after their initial examination. There were a total of 268 patients with 338 nodules. The majority were female patients.

The researchers found that the majority of patients (89 percent) had thyroid nodules that grew by at least 15 percent. They also found that solid nodules were more likely to grow than cystic ones. Of the nodules that the researchers reaspirated with fine-needle aspiration, only one in 74 was malignant.

Diagnosis and Treatment

The patient and/or the physician may notice the presence of a single nodule, multiple nodules, or goiter (a general term, meaning enlargement of the thyroid gland). Many nodules are found accidentally by the physician. For example, a patient may be sent for an ultrasound of the carotid arteries and a nodule is detected, or a patient may have a CT scan of the neck or chest and a nodule is seen. Endocrinologists often refer to nodules detected in this manner as incidentalomas. However, because thyroid cancer is relatively common, these nodules must be evaluated.

The first step in the evaluation of a single nodule, many nodules, or a dominant or codominant nodule should be to biopsy the patient with a fine-needle aspiration. In the past, when a multinodular goiter was detected, many endocrinologists did not pursue a biopsy. However, it is now known that the presence of a multinodular goiter does not protect a patient from thyroid cancer.

In this procedure, which is typically performed at the endocrinologist's office without any anesthesia, a very small needle is inserted through the skin into the thyroid gland. The needle is usually a 23–27 gauge needle, much smaller than the needles used to draw blood. Anywhere from one to six passes are made into the nodule. The needle and the syringe are also rinsed in a solution to enable the retrieval of as many cells as possible.

Sometimes a small amount of local numbing medicine may be injected under the skin prior to the fine-needle biopsy. However, most patients feel that the prick and burning from this anesthetic (typically a form of novocaine) is worse than the biopsy itself.

If a nodule is not easily palpable (the physician cannot feel it with the fingers), it could be biopsied with ultrasound guidance. Often with a multinodular goiter, the biopsy must be done in this way to be sure that the appropriate nodule is biopsied.

A fairly small number of cells are shaved off by the beveled end of the needle and squirted onto a slide. The solution is spun down to make a small pellet of cells. The slide is examined by cytopathologists much as Pap smears in women are studied. The pathologist must be experienced in this specific form of pathology, because the analysis can be very tricky. If the local pathologist is not trained or experienced in this field, the slides are usually forwarded to another pathologist who has the requisite skills.

In general, one of four conclusions can be reached about the biopsy sample:

1. The specimen is inadequate for analysis and the biopsy must be repeated
2. The specimen is suspicious for cancer or is consistent with a cancer diagnosis, and the patient is referred for surgery
3. The specimen appears clearly benign, and the patient can be followed conservatively
4. The specimen is indeterminate, and other tests must be factored in to allow the physician to reach a treatment decision

Laboratory tests should *not* be used first to evaluate a nodule. Laboratory tests should be obtained specifically when called for, especially if the patient has any signs and/or symptoms of thyroid overactivity (hyperthyroidism) or underactivity (hypothyroidism). Typically, the risk of cancer is lower in a hyperthyroid patient than in a patient who is hypothyroid or euthyroid (having normal thyroid levels), but it is still not zero. If the patient has hyperthyroid signs and symptoms or he or she is found to be hyperthyroid by laboratory tests and also has a thyroid nodule, this does not yet rule out the diagnosis of cancer.

If a fine-needle aspiration biopsy of a thyroid nodule gives indeterminate results, the options for follow-up include watchful waiting (observing and monitoring the patient but taking no action), surgical excision of the thyroid gland, a repeat biopsy, or a thyroid scan. The thyroid scan will determine whether the nodules are functional (warm or hot) or nonfunctional (cold). Cold nodules have a higher risk of cancer. Warm nodules have a lower risk, and hot nodules have a very low risk of cancer. Although nodules that grow do not necessarily indicate cancer, patients should be carefully followed by their physicians in the event that the nodule does become cancerous.

See also GOITER; HYPERTHYROIDISM; HYPOTHYROIDISM; THYROID CANCER.

Alexander, Erik K., M.D., et al. "Natural History of Benign Solid and Cystic Thyroid Nodules." *Annals of Internal Medicine* 138, no. 4 (February 2003): 315–318.

Mortensen, J. D., L. B. Woolner, and W. A. Bennett. "Gross and Microscopic Findings in Clinically Normal Thyroid Glands." *Journal of Clinical Endocrinology & Metabolism* 15, no. 10 (1955): 1,270–1,280.

Tan, G. H., and H. Gharib. "Thyroid Incidentalomas: Management Approaches to Nonpalpable Nodules Discovered Incidentally on Thyroid Imaging." *Annals of Internal Medicine* 126, no. 3 (1997): 226–231.

Vander, J. B., E. A. Gaston, and T. R. Dawber. "The Significance of Non-Toxic Thyroid Nodules. Final Report of a 15-Year Study of the Incidence of Thyroid Malignancy." *Annals in Internal Medicine* 69 (1968).

thyroid-stimulating hormone (TSH) A hormone produced by the anterior pituitary to stimulate the thyroid gland. It is under the control of the hypothalamus, which stimulates the pituitary with thyrotropin-releasing hormone (TRH). Both the hypothalamus and the pituitary are part of a feedback loop with the thyroid gland. The hypothalamus and the pituitary gland can both detect low levels of thyroid hormone and then increase their secretion of TRH and TSH to normalize those levels.

TSH also refers to an assay for thyroid-stimulating hormone. This blood test is the gold standard as a single test to measure thyroid function and indicates whether a patient has low, normal, or high TSH levels. The measurement of thyroid-stimulating hormone concentration is the most sensitive barometer of thyroid function in the body. The usual range for TSH is 0.3–3.4 microunits/ml, according to the AMERICAN ASSOCIATION OF CLINICAL ENDOCRINOLOGISTS (AACE). This is a change from the past recommended range of 0.5–5 microunits/ml.

With the TSH test, a below-normal level generally indicates that the patient may have HYPERTHYROIDISM (high levels of thyroid hormones and excess thyroid function), while an above-normal level indicates HYPOTHYROIDISM (low levels of thyroid hormones and inadequate thyroid function). Although the TSH assay tends to be very accurate, the test will be repeated if the results are abnormal in case a laboratory error has occurred.

The TSH is the best test to use in patients with primary hypothyroidism. With chronically hypothyroid patients, the American Academy of Clinical Endocrinologists now recommends titrating the amount of thyroid hormone given to maintain a TSH level between 0.5 and 2.0 microunits/ml.

See also GRAVES' DISEASE; HASHIMOTO'S THYROIDITIS; POSTPARTUM THYROID DISEASE; THYROID BLOOD TESTS.

thyroid storm A life-threatening condition in which the patient has extremely high levels of thyroid hormone and multiple clinical abnormalities, including fever and dysfunction of an organ system other than the thyroid gland. Thyroid storm is the most extreme case of THYROTOXICOSIS. Because GRAVES' DISEASE is the most common cause of hyperthyroidism and thyrotoxicosis, it is also the most common cause of thyroid storm.

Thyroid storm tends to occur in patients who have underlying hyperthyroidism, that is, either untreated or partially treated hyperthyroidism. There is often a precipitating event. Some precipitating events include infection, heart attack, surgery, and the use of intravenous contrast material that contains large amounts of iodine.

Thyroid storm is the extreme opposite of the MYXEDEMA COMA, in which patients have so little thyroid hormone that they lapse into unconsciousness. Both conditions are very severe. Patients are usually cared for in an intensive care unit with input from the intensive care staff, cardiologists, pulmonologists, and endocrinologists.

The symptoms and signs of thyroid storm are fever, very rapid heartbeat (tachycardia), and other organ system dysfunctions. These often include but are not limited to congestive heart failure, delirium/psychosis, or respiratory failure.

The treatment for thyroid storm is first aimed at decreasing the patient's rapid heart rate and controlling the fever. Thus, acetaminophen (Tylenol), cooling blankets, and intravenous beta-blocker medications are usually employed. Many patients may require invasive monitoring of their cardiopulmonary status and may also need mechanical ventilation (artificial breathing devices).

The underlying cause of the thyroid storm must be sought and appropriate therapy begun. If the cause is nondestructive, such as Graves' disease, then toxic nodule or goiter antithyroid drugs are begun in very high doses. Occasionally, iodine is used in the form of a supersaturated solution of potassium iodine (Lugol's solution) or iopanoic acid. If the cause of the thyroid storm is a destructive lesion of the thyroid gland, such as a form of thyroiditis, then therapy is aimed at decreasing the effects of the excess thyroid hormone.

See also HYPERTHYROIDISM.

Thyrolar (liotrix tablets) A thyroid hormone replacement medication that contains synthetic T4 and T3. The 60 mg or 1-grain tablet contains about 50 mg of T4 and 12.5 mg of T3, or about the equivalent of 100 mcg of LEVOTHYROXINE.

thyrotoxicosis The clinical syndrome resulting from an excess of thyroid hormones in the bloodstream. In extreme cases, known as THYROID STORM, the patient is in a life-threatening situation and requires immediate medical treatment. Thyroid storm is defined as thyrotoxicosis and fever plus dysfunction of one other organ system. Thyrotoxicosis is similar to HYPERTHYROIDISM but implies a more severe clinical situation with more signs and symptoms of excess thyroid hormones.

In most cases (about 80 percent) the cause of thyrotoxicosis is GRAVES' DISEASE. However, some patients with HASHIMOTO'S THYROIDITIS, a form of HYPOTHYROIDISM, can develop thyrotoxicosis. An estimated 5–10 percent of women develop thyrotoxicosis after childbirth (postpartum thyrotoxicosis), typically due to postpartum thyroiditis, also known as painless lymphocytic thyroiditis (see POSTPARTUM THYROID DISEASE). Other causes include a toxic multinodular goiter or a toxic single nodule. In rare cases, lithium therapy can cause thyrotoxicosis.

Signs and Symptoms

Patients with thyrotoxicosis typically have accentuated symptoms of hyperthyroidism, including rapid heartbeat (tachycardia), heat intolerance, nervousness, disrupted sleep, tremulousness, weight loss, and a variety of other symptoms. The patient may or may not have an enlarged thyroid GOITER. Menstruating women may have a diminished menstrual flow or may have no menstrual flow (AMENORRHEA). Elderly patients with thyrotoxicosis may present with apathy rather than with hyperactivity and may appear to have an underactive gland.

Diagnosis and Treatment

Thyrotoxicosis is usually suspected based on clinical symptoms. It is diagnosed by blood samples that test for thyroid-stimulating hormone (TSH), free thyroxine, and in some cases, triiodothyronine levels (T3).

Treatment of thyrotoxicosis is directed at the underlying cause. It generally involves watchful waiting and the use of beta-blocker medications (for thyroiditis), antithyroid drugs (for Graves' disease, toxic nodule, or goiter), or surgery in any case in which the other therapies cannot be utilized safely or effectively.

Fisher, Joseph N., M.D. "Management of Thyrotoxicosis." *Southern Medical Journal* 95, no. 5 (2002): 493–505.

thyroxine (T4) Natural thyroid hormone produced by the thyroid gland. It is also known as T4 due to the four iodine molecules attached to the amino acid tyrosine that make up this hormone. Thyroxine acts as a prehormone. The body uses an enzyme to cleave one iodine and to create the more active hormone, which is T3, also known as triiodothyronine. Most of T4 that circulates in the blood is bound to proteins, mostly albumin and thyroid-binding globulin (TBG). Thyroxine can be measured as the bound hormone or total T4. A bound hormone is attached to a binding protein in the blood to be transported around the body, as well as used for storage purposes. It can also be measured as the unbound or free form, free T4, which typically provides a more accurate assessment.

Most patients with HYPOTHYROIDISM must rely upon supplemental LEVOTHYROXINE, a synthesized form of thyroid hormone, to bring their thyroid blood levels up to normal.

See also DESSICATED THYROID; THYROID BLOOD TESTS; THYROLAR.

triiodothyronine (T3)   The active form of thyroid hormone in the body. The thyroid actually makes more THRYOXINE, (T4), another thyroid hormone, than T3. The body uses enzymes to take one iodine off the T4 and covert it to T3 as it is needed. This is why deficient thyroid hormone is usually replaced with T4; thryoxine can be dosed once a day as opposed to 2–4 times per day with triiodothryonine. Thyroxine also provides prove stable levels and less side effects than when T3 is used to replace deficient thyroid hormone. In some disease states, such as GRAVES' DISEASE and toxic thyroid nodules, the thyroid may produce more T3 than T4 and lead to symptoms of HYPERTHYROIDISM/THYROTOXICOSIS.

Trousseau's sign   An indicator of low levels of circulating calcium (HYPOCALCEMIA) that was originally discovered and described by 19th-century French physician Armand Trousseau. It is generally considered to be a more reliable indicator of possible hypocalcemia than CHVOSTEK'S SIGN. Even if Trousseau's sign is positive, however, the physician should order laboratory blood levels of calcium before diagnosing hypocalcemia, because there are false positives with this sign. In addition, Trousseau's sign does not screen all individuals with hypocalcemia. Patients can test negative for Trousseau's sign and yet still have hypocalcemia.

To check for Trousseau's sign and possible hypocalcemia, the physician inflates a blood pressure cuff above the patient's systolic blood pressure level. Patients who are positive for Trousseau's sign will experience an involuntary wrist flexion toward the body and flexion of the fingers, with the thumb moving toward the palm. The patient will also experience paresthesias (numbness and tingling or pins and needles) in the fingers and may experience an involuntary twitching of the fingers.

According to author Frank Urbano in his 2000 article for *Hospital Practice*, the Trousseau-von Bonsdorff test is another test that can be used in concert with Trousseau's sign. If Trousseau's sign is positive, the Trousseau-von Bonsdorff test is performed directly after the sphygmomanometer (blood pressure device) is deflated. The patient will breathe deeply, at about 40 breaths per minute, and then the physician will check for the same spasm that is seen in Trousseau's sign.

See also HYPOPARATHYROIDISM; TETANY.

Urbano, Frank L., M.D. "Signs of Hypocalcemia: Chvostek's and Trousseau's Signs." *Hospital Physician* 36, no. 3 (March 2000): 43–45.

Turner syndrome   A genetic disorder with endocrine features that is found in about one in 2,500 girls born in the United States. About 60,000 girls and women in the United States have Turner syndrome. The syndrome was named after Dr. Henry Turner, an American physician who reported its traits in 1938 in the journal *Endocrinology*. Dr. C. Ford identified the major chromosomal abnormality that causes Turner syndrome in 1959.

The most common feature of Turner syndrome, affecting an estimated 95 percent of all patients, is short stature. The average adult height of a patient with Turner syndrome is four feet and eight inches. Other common features are the lack of the development of secondary sexual characteristics (such as pubic hair and breasts) and the presence of INFERTILITY. Most females with Turner syndrome are born without ovaries. Most patients have normal intelligence and can expect to live average life spans.

Turner syndrome is usually accompanied by a variety of medical problems, most prominently heart defects (aortic valve problems and coarctation), INSULIN RESISTANCE (an increased relative risk for both TYPE 1 DIABETES and TYPE 2 DIABETES), kidney defects contributing to hypertension, celiac sprue, and a greater risk than normal for autoimmune HYPOTHYROIDISM. (An estimated 10–30 percent of patients with Turner syndrome have hypothyroidism.) Many patients with Turner syndrome also have hearing difficulties, such as hearing loss, chronic middle ear infections, and inner ear hearing loss. Speech problems are also common.

Signs and Symptoms

Physical traits of females with Turner syndrome include a shield-shaped chest, webbed neck, low-set ears, a lower-than-normal hairline, eye abnormalities (amblyopia, strabismus, ptosis, and red-green color blindness, among others), and puffy feet and hands. About 10 percent of patients with Turner syndrome develop scoliosis. Patients with Turner syndrome are prone to developing keloid scars (very puffy and raised scars) if they are injured or have surgery. Thus elective surgery should be used on a limited basis only. Even simple ear piercing can create scars in a patient with Turner syndrome.

Diagnosis and Treatment

Turner syndrome is diagnosed based on the characteristic signs and symptoms of this medical problem and may also be confirmed by genetic testing. Patients typically lack part or all of one of the two X chromosomes, although there are cases of mosaicism in which there are a mix of some normal and abnormal chromosomes, thus the syndrome may not be as severe or obvious. There is no specific genetic treatment for Turner syndrome as a whole, but many of the medical problems that are caused by or are related to it can be treated. For example, the patient with Turner syndrome who has hypertension can be treated for this ailment. Hypothyroidism can be treated with thyroid supplements. Girls and women with Turner syndrome who have speech and hearing difficulties should receive a referral to an ear, nose, and throat clinic and a speech therapist.

Because many girls with Turner syndrome have dental abnormalities, they should see a dentist and, if appropriate, an orthodontist as well.

Girls with unusually short stature may be treated with growth hormone, although there are many pros and cons to administering growth hormone therapy. Only a pediatric endocrinologist should initiate and monitor this form of therapy.

The efficacy combining a growth hormone and a low dose of estrogen was tested in a study reported in a 2002 issue of the *Journal of Clinical Endocrinology & Metabolism*. In this study, 232 patients with Turner syndrome who were at least five years old and had a bone age of less than 12 years old were placed into two groups. The subjects came from sites throughout the United States.

In one group, the patients received growth hormone and a low dose of estrogen. The other group received a placebo. The researchers found a significant increase of growth among the study subjects who were given growth hormone, and 29 percent of them achieved a height greater than five feet (60 inches), compared with the placebo group, in which only 5 percent achieved this height. The researchers also found that subjects with younger age and lower bone age were more likely to have increased growth. They also found that estrogen administration did not improve the growth rate.

Physicians have also noted an increasing incidence of osteoporosis and fractures in women with Turner syndrome as they age. Many of these women often had not previously received estrogen therapy.

See also GROWTH HORMONE.

For more information, contact:

The Endocrine Society
8401 Connecticut Avenue
Suite 900
Chevy Chase, MD 20815
(301) 941-0200
http://www.endo-society.org

Turner Syndrome Society
14450 T. C. Jester
Suite 260
Houston, TX 77014
(800) 365-9944 (toll-free)
http://www.turner-syndrome-us.org

Quigley, Charmian A., et al. "Growth Hormone and Low Dose Estrogen in Turner Syndrome: Results of a United States Multi-Center Trial to Near-Final Height." *Journal of Clinical Endocrinology & Metabolism* 87, no. 5 (2002): 2,033–2,041.

Saenger, P., et al. "Recommendations for the Diagnosis and Management of Turner Syndrome." *Journal of Clinical Endocrinology & Metabolism* 86, no. 7 (2001): 3,061–3,069.

Saenger, Paul, M.D. "Turner Syndrome." *New England Journal of Medicine* 335, no. 23 (December 5, 1996): 1,749–1,754.

Turner, H. D. "A Syndrome of Infantilism, Congenital Webbed Neck, and Cubitus Valgus." *Endocrinology* 28, no. 23 (1938): 566–574.

Type 1 diabetes   One of the two prevailing forms of diabetes (the other being Type 2 diabetes). Type 1 diabetes was formerly known as *insulin-dependent diabetes mellitus* or *juvenile-onset diabetes*. Patients with Type 1 diabetes represent about 5–10 percent of all cases of diabetes found in North America. In the United States, about 900,000 children and adults have Type 1 diabetes, and about 13,000 new cases are diagnosed every year. The disease is more common among Caucasians than among other racial groups.

Type 1 diabetes is an autoimmune disease in which the afflicted individual's own immune system destroys the beta cells in the pancreas that make insulin. Consequently, patients with Type 1 diabetes need to administer insulin in order to live, either through injecting it with needle, a pen-like device, or with an insulin pump. Patients must carefully monitor their blood glucose levels at least several times daily, depending on the advice provided by their physicians. They also need to act on the information the blood tests provide, in some cases changing their diet, getting more rest, or taking other actions.

A landmark study published in 1993 demonstrated that tightly controlled blood glucose levels with maintenance of hemoglobin A1c levels to 7.0 percent decreased the risk of complications such as DIABETIC NEPHROPATHY, DIABETIC NEUROPATHY, and DIABETIC RETINOPATHY by 30–70 percent.

Typical signs of Type 1 diabetes, due to hyperglycemia, are as follows:

- Extreme thirst
- Frequent urination
- Unexplained weight loss
- Extreme hunger
- Wounds that heal slowly

These signs can appear suddenly, and patients who have them should see their physicians as soon as possible for diagnosis and treatment.

See also DIABETES MELLITUS; GESTATIONAL DIABETES; TYPE 2 DIABETES.

Petit, William A. Jr., and Christine Adamec. *The Encyclopedia of Diabetes*. New York: Facts On File, Inc., 2002.

Type 2 diabetes   The most prevalent form of diabetes, representing about 90–95 percent of all cases. (The other most common form is Type 1 diabetes.) Type 2 diabetes was formerly called *non-insulin-dependent diabetes* (NIDDM) or *adult-onset diabetes*. Individuals with Type 2 diabetes produce insulin, but their bodies are unable to use insulin effectively due to insulin resistance.

Type 2 diabetes is caused by two problems. First, there is a genetic predisposition for insulin resistance. Second, there is beta cell dysfunction in the pancreas, which means that the patient cannot make enough insulin to overcome this resistance and thus, the blood glucose level increases.

Risk Factors

Based on 2004 estimates, approximately 17 million patients in the United States have Type 2 diabetes. Type 2 diabetes is more common among certain racial groups, such as African Americans or Native Americans, particularly the Pima Indians of Arizona. The risk for developing Type 2 diabetes also rises with advancing age. OBESITY and lack of exercise are also linked to Type 2 diabetes.

There is also a hereditary aspect to Type 2 diabetes. If a parent or sibling has the disease, the risk is increased for other family members.

Signs and Symptoms

The most common signs and symptoms of Type 2 diabetes are constant thirst (polydipsia), frequent urination (polyuria), blurred vision, slowly healing wounds, and, on occasion, unexplained/unintentional weight loss. The lessons of the United Kingdom Prospective Diabetes Study (UKPDS), a very large clinical study of diabetes patients in the United Kingdom, showed that the metabolic dysfunction leading up to Type 2 diabetes generally goes on for 10–12 years prior to the patient being diagnosed. This is why some patients can have complications of diabetes, such as DIABETIC NEUROPATHY and DIABETIC RETINOPATHY at the same time they are diagnosed. Thus, these patients should begin to have their eyes checked on a yearly basis, starting at the time of diagnosis. They should also check their feet on a daily basis, because a small wound can become a severe medical problem if untreated.

Diagnosis and Treatment

If physicians suspect the presence of Type 2 diabetes based on signs and symptoms, the disease may be diagnosed with a fasting blood glucose level (greater than or equal to 126 mg/dl on two separate occasions) or an oral glucose tolerance test, with a two-hour glucose level that is equal to or greater than 200 mg/dl.

The cornerstone of therapy is nutritional guidance along with exercise, with the aim of weight loss. Even small amounts of weight loss, such as 5–10 percent of body weight, will lead to significant improvements in glucose levels. If possible, all patients should be referred to a registered dietitian for education. In addition, all patients with diabetes require education about the disease, typically held in a class and lead by certified diabetes educators. Most insurance companies will reimburse for at least some diabetes education, and Medicare will cover all of it.

If Type 2 diabetes is diagnosed, patients must be instructed on how to test their blood, which should be done at least several times each day. They must also be trained about what to do based on the blood test results. For example, if the blood sugar level is low (hypoglycemia), they should raise their glucose levels by eating a food high in sugar or using a product specifically designed for patients with diabetes. If patients find that their blood levels are high in blood sugar, they must avoid products with high glucose contents so that the blood levels stabilize downward.

There is some controversy over which medications to administer first. As most patients with Type 2 diabetes are overweight, the biguanide metformin drug (Glucophage, Glucophage-XR) is often used first. It is chosen because it does not lead to any weight gain and sometimes leads to some weight loss. It decreases the liver's production of glucose and indirectly leads to a decrease in resistance to insulin. Metformin cannot be used in patients with kidney or liver dysfunction. It will not lead to hypoglycemia when used by itself (monotherapy) as it does not increase insulin secretion.

If the patient is of normal weight or is thin, often a sulfonylurea drug is utilized, as these patients often have decreased insulin secretion. These drugs include glipizide (Glucotrol, Glucotrol XL), glimepiride (Amaryl), and glyburide (Micronase, Diabeta, and Glynase). They directly stimulate the beta cell in the pancreas to secrete more insulin. This can lead to hypoglycemia if not dosed appropriately. Sulfonylurea medications must be used with caution in the elderly and in patients with liver and kidney dysfunction.

Two more rapid-acting agents also increase insulin secretion, and they are repaglinide (Prandin) and nateglinide (Starlix). These drugs are taken prior to each meal and act over only a short time. Thus, they are useful in patients with variable eating habits, a susceptibility to hypoglycemia, or mild kidney problems. These drugs can also cause hypoglycemia.

The newest class of medications as of this writing are the glitazones or thiazolidinediones, which include rosiglitazone (Avandia) and pioglitazone (Actos). This type of medication can also be used as initial therapy. Often one of these drugs is chosen to treat patients with significant insulin resistance or in those with kidney problems. These drugs work by directly decreasing resistance to insulin, affecting mainly muscle and fat. They are the slowest-working medications for Type 2 diabetes and may take 12–16 weeks to get to maximal effect. They cannot be used in patients with significant liver disease, those with congestive heart failure, or those with any form of significant edema.

Common adverse effects with rosiglitazone and pioglitazone are edema and some weight gain (typically three to eight pounds in the first year), although not all patients will gain weight.

Research indicates that these drugs also have direct effects on the lining of blood vessels, (the endothelium) and may help to prevent atherosclerosis. They appear to have a wide range of effects other than those on glucose, such as increasing high-density lipoprotein (HDL) or "good" cholesterol, decreasing protein loss in the urine, decreasing triglyceride levels, and decreasing levels of mediators of clotting and inflammation, such as plasminogen activator inhibitor-1 (PAI01) and interleukins.

As of this writing, there are also two glucosidase inhibitors. These drugs slow the absorption of carbohydrates into the bloodstream and are used by some patients with Type 2 diabetes. Two examples are acarbose (Precose) and miglitol (Glyset). They are typically titrated slowly, as a rapid dose escalation will lead to significant flatulence and diarrhea. These drugs will not cause hypoglycemia when used alone.

Most patients with Type 2 diabetes, however, require more than one medication. There are now several combination medications on the market, such as Glucovance (metformin and glyburide), Metaglip (metformin and glipizide), and Avandamet (rosiglitazone and metformin).

Most patients with Type 2 diabetes can control their illness by taking oral medications along with maintaining careful control over their diets. However, approximately 7 percent of these patients will require insulin each year, either because their bodies stop making any insulin or because they are no longer able to maintain adequate control using diet, exercise, and oral medications. Patients will learn how to perform these injections from their physician or nurse.

Preventing or Delaying Type 2 Diabetes

Large clinical studies such as the Diabetes Prevention Program have clearly demonstrated that lifestyle changes, such as a modest weight loss (5–7 percent) and exercise (equivalent to 150 minutes of brisk walking per week) will decrease the risk of progression from prediabetes to overt diabetes by 58 percent. The use of metformin alone will decrease the risk by 31 percent. A study of women who had gestational diabetes and who were given thiazolidinedione medications after the pregnancy showed that the women decreased their risk of developing diabetes. Another study showed about a 30 percent decrease in progression to diabetes when patients were treated with acarbose. The HOPE (Heart Outcomes Prevention Evaluation) trial, in patients at high risk for cardiac problems, demonstrated a decrease in the risk of diabetes using the blood pressure drug armorial (Altace).

See also DIABETES MELLITUS; TYPE 1 DIABETES.

American Diabetes Association and National Institute of Diabetes and Digestive and Kidney Diseases. "The Prevention or Delay of Type 2 Diabetes." *Diabetes Care* 25, no. 4 (April 2002): 742–749.

Petit, William A. Jr., and Christine Adamec. *The Encyclopedia of Diabetes.* New York: Facts On File, Inc., 2002.

ultrasound   A noninvasive imaging test that uses painless sound waves to form a shadowy picture of internal organs. It is used to diagnose many different medical conditions and problems, and it sometimes accompanies medical procedures that doctors perform. Ultrasound was first used to detect the medical status of the fetus to provide information to pregnant women. It was later adapted to collect information about virtually every internal organ.

Most ultrasound tests are external, but probes allow studies to be done within the vagina of a woman or the rectum of man to assess for disease. There are also very small probes that allow for ultrasound within blood vessels.

Ultrasound is commonly used in the evaluation of thyroid disorders to determine if one or many nodules are present and whether there is a dominant nodule (one that is significantly larger than the others). Ultrasound can also be used to follow a thyroid nodule or cyst over time to see if further growth or other changes occur. It can also be used to guide a fine-needle aspiration biopsy of the thyroid when the nodule is difficult to feel by hand or if the nodule is located under the collarbone or even slightly substernal (under the breastbone).

Ultrasound is helpful in evaluating the testes and ovaries for structural abnormalities. It is used on occasion to evaluate the pancreas but has generally been replaced in this function by computerized tomography (CT) scanning.

See also COMPUTERIZED TOMOGRAPHY; MAGNETIC RESONANCE IMAGING.

vasoactive intestinal peptide producing tumor (vipoma)   An islet cell tumor of the pancreas that leads to severe watery diarrhea (80 percent of patients exceed three liters of diarrhea per day) and decreased potassium and chloride in the bloodstream. Also known as pancreatic cholera syndrome, Verner-Morrison syndrome, WDHA (watery diarrhea, hypokalemia, achlorhydria), or WDDH (watery diarrhea, hypokalema) syndrome. A large number (40 percent) of vipomas are malignant.

Diagnosis and Treatment

Patients present with generalized weakness and diarrhea. They have low levels of potassium, chloride, and magnesium and elevated glucose levels (likely due to the severe losses of potassium that, in turn, lead to the inability to secrete adequate insulin) and calcium. On rare occasions, vipoma is associated with MULTIPLE ENDOCRINE NEOPLASIA (MEN) syndrome. Vipoma is difficult to detect in the plasma.

Therapy is surgery to remove the tumor. If the patient has hyperplasia and not a tumor, a total pancreatectomy is considered. A drug called octreotide is quite useful in treating this syndrome.

vitamin D   The vitamin that helps the body to maintain normal levels of calcium and phosphorus in the blood and bones, mainly by its effects in increasing calcium absorption from the gastrointestinal tract.

The body uses sunshine (specific ultraviolet rays) to make vitamin D (cholecalciferol or vitamin D3). It is estimated that casual sun exposure leads to the synthesis of the equivalent of ingesting about 200 IU of vitamin D. There can be wide variations in vitamin D levels of individuals, depending on the season. In some very northern countries with long winters and little sunshine, supplements of exposure to appropriate artificial ultraviolet light is critical.

Vitamin D can also be obtained from foods. Many foods are also fortified with vitamin D (vitamin D2 or ergocalciferol), such as milk and breakfast cereals. Few foods are naturally high in vitamin D. Those that are include cod liver oil, cooked salmon, cooked mackerel, sardines, and eels.

CALCITRIOL is a human-made form of vitamin D that is taken by people who are deficient in vitamin D and/or calcium, such as patients with HYPOPARATHRYROIDISM (a rare condition in which the parathyroid glands have been damaged by an autoimmune reaction or have been surgically damaged). Supplemental vitamin D boosts the levels of calcium in the blood and bones by increasing the absorption from the gastrointestinal tract. High doses are available by prescription only.

Deficiencies of Vitamin D (Hypovitaminosis)

Deficiencies of vitamin D may be more common than is generally realized. In one study, physicians studied 290 hospitalized patients of all ages to determine if they were deficient in vitamin D. These findings were reported in a 1998 issue of the *New England Journal of Medicine*. The researchers obtained information on diet and medical histories and also obtained measures of the serum parathyroid hormone levels of the patients. They found that 57 percent of the patients had hypovitaminosis D, or very low levels of vitamin D. The conditions most often associated with hypovitaminosis were kidney disorders, glucocorticoid (steroid) therapy, cirrhosis, anticonvulsant therapy, and gastric or bowel resections. The study also pointed out that vitamin D deficiencies are more common among acutely ill individuals than had been realized in the past.

The researchers concluded, "Because of the potential adverse effects of vitamin D deficiency on the skeleton and other organ systems, widespread screening for vitamin D deficiency or routine vitamin D supplementation should be considered."

People can also become deficient in vitamin D if they have little or no sunlight exposure, although some people need vitamin D supplements even if they obtain normal levels of sunlight. This is particularly true for individuals older than age 65 and/or for hospitalized patients. It is also true that some people's bodies cannot absorb vitamin D from the gastrointestinal tract. In addition, sometimes the kidney is unable to make adequate vitamin D (1,25-dihydroxy-vitamin D).

The most commonly known deficiencies of vitamin D are RICKETS and OSTEOMALACIA. Rickets is a childhood disease that causes weak bones and skeletal abnormalities. Osteomalacia involves muscle weakness as well as weak bones. This condition is often suspected in a high-risk group if the calcium level is low. The diagnosis can be made if a 25-hydroxy vitamin D level is measured. Typically, healthy people have vitamin D levels greater than 30 ng/dl, even though the normal range is often stated to be about 9–52 ng/dl. To determine if the level is physiologically effective, the endocrinologist will often measure a 24-hour urine test for creatinine (to check that the collection has been correct and to calculate the kidney function as well). The calcium levels should be between two and four mg of calcium/kg body weight.

People older than age 50 have a greater risk of being deficient in vitamin D than younger individuals and may need to take supplemental vitamin D. Some categories of people who may become deficient in vitamin D include the following groups:

- People with Crohn's disease
- Individuals with kidney disease
- People with celiac sprue (gluten enteropathy)
- Individuals with chronic liver diseases (cirrhosis)
- People with pancreatic enzyme deficiencies (due to pancreatitis)
- Elderly individuals

- Infants without adequate Sun exposure or supplementation
- Strict vegetarians, especially in the winter

Hypervitaminosis with Vitamin D

Having too much vitamin D in the bloodstream is also possible. Having toxic levels of vitamin D from diet alone is almost impossible. Instead, most people with excessively high levels of vitamin D are taking supplements, either prescribed or over-the-counter drugs. Too much vitamin D in the body can cause the following signs and symptoms:

- Nausea and vomiting
- Constipation
- Increased thirst and urination
- Itching
- Weakness
- Poor appetite
- Weight loss
- Mental confusion

Hypervitaminosis of vitamin D is treated by discontinuing, or at least decreasing, the supplements of vitamin D. A low-calcium diet is another treatment. Sometimes corticosteroid medications (such as prednisone) are given.

See also ALTERNATIVE MEDICINE.

Haddad, J. G. "Vitamin D—Solar Rays, the Milky Way, or Both?" *New England Journal of Medicine* 326, no. 18 (1992): 1,213–1,215.

Heaney, Robert P., M.D., and Connie M. Weaver. "Calcium and Vitamin D." *Endocrinology and Metabolism Clinics of North America* 32, no. 1 (2003): 181–194.

Lamberg-Allardt, C., et al. "Low Serum 25-Hydroxyvitamin D Levels and Secondary Hyperparathyroidism in Middle-Aged White Strict Vegetarians." *American Journal of Clinical Nutrition* 58, no. 5 (1998): 684–689.

Lips, Paul. "Vitamin D Deficiency and Secondary Hyperparathyroidism in the Elderly: Consequences for Bone Loss and Fractures and Therapeutic Implications." *Endocrine Reviews* 22, no. 4 (2001): 477–501.

Reichler, H., H. P. Koeffler, and A. W. Norman. "The Role of the Vitamin D Endocrine System in Health and Disease." *New England Journal of Medicine* 320, no. 15 (1989): 980–991.

Thomas, Melissa K., M.D. "Hypovitaminosis D in Medical Inpatients." *New England Journal of Medicine* 338, no. 12 (March 19, 1998): 777–783.

vitamin D resistance   A medical condition in which a person has a normal level of vitamin D in the blood but the body is unable to use this vitamin D appropriately and thus develops signs and symptoms of Vitamin D deficiency. The cause may be a genetic defect that prevents CALCITRIOL (a form of Vitamin D) from binding to the vitamin D receptor. Some elderly individuals may also have vitamin D resistance, although the cause for this form is unknown.

Vitamin D resistance may lead to the development of FRACTURES stemming from OSTEOPOROSIS. Children with untreated vitamin D resistance have a rickets-like appearance, with bowed legs and weak limbs, and they may also experience balding (alopecia). Treatment may improve the condition considerably.

Vitamin D resistance syndrome cannot be completely diagnosed by blood tests alone. Researchers performing clinical studies on normal patients as well as those with Vitamin D deficiency and resistance report that measurement of fingernail thickness may correlate with each syndrome.

The treatment of vitamin D resistance is usually supplementation with calcitriol. Some patients are more responsive to supplements of calcium, while others require both calcitriol and calcium supplements.

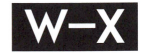

Wermer's syndrome   See MULTIPLE ENDOCRINE NEOPLASIA.

xanthomas   Fatty deposits in the skin that may indicate disorders of triglyceride or cholesterol levels. They typically appear on the elbows, knuckles, Achilles tendon, or other large tendons on extensor surfaces of the body. The cholesterol that makes up these nodules is both inside and outside the cells. Xanthomas are firm to hard and are often slightly painful.

Hard tendon xanthomas are most often seen in type IIa hyperlipidemia (familial hypercholes-terolemia). Tuberous xanthomas are softer, often seen on the buttocks and can also be seen in type IIa, type IIb, or type IV hyperlipidemia. Smaller groupings of yellowish brown to reddish eruptions in a variety of places on the skin are called eruptive xanthomata, which are usually seen in patients with type IIa or type IV hyperlipidemia when the triglyceride levels are greater than 1,000 mg/dl. These xanthomatas will regress and disappear with normalization of the lipid levels. The harder xanthomas can regress with therapy but usually do not regress completely.

APPENDIXES

APPENDIX I
IMPORTANT ORGANIZATIONS
IN THE UNITED STATES

AARP
601 E. Street Northwest
Washington, DC 20049
(888) OUR-AARP
http://www.aarp.org

Academy for Eating Disorders
6728 Old McLean Village Drive
McLean, VA 22101
(703) 556-9222
http://www.aedweb.org

Administration on Aging
Department of Health and Human Services
330 Independence Avenue SW
Washington, DC 20201
(202) 619-0724
http://www.aoa.gov

Agency for Healthcare Research & Quality
   (AHRQ)
Publications Clearinghouse
P.O. Box 8547
Silver Spring, MD 20907
(800) 358-9295
http://www.ahrq.gov

Alcoholics Anonymous
Grand Central Station
P.O. Box 459
New York, NY 10163
http://www.alcoholics-anonymous.org

Alliance for Aging Research
2021 K Street NW
Suite 305
Washington, DC 20006
(202) 293-2856
http://www.agingresearch.org

Alliance of Genetic Support Groups
4301 Connecticut Avenue NW
Suite 104
Washington, DC 20008
(202) 966-5557
http://www.geneticalliance.org

American Academy of Family Physicians
   (AAFP)
11400 Tomahawk Creek Parkway
Leawood, KS 66211
(800) 274-2237
http://www.aafp.org

American Academy of Neurology
1080 Montreal Avenue
St. Paul, MN 55116
(800) 879-1960
http://www.aan.com

American Academy of Ophthalmology
P.O. Box 7424
San Francisco, CA 94120
(415) 561-8500
http://www.aao.org

American Academy of Pediatrics
141 Northwest Point Boulevard
Elk Grove Village, IL 60007
(847) 434-4000
http://www.aap.org

American Academy of Physical Medicine
   and Rehabilitation
One IBM Plaza
Suite 2500
Chicago, IL 60611
(312) 464-9700
http://www.aapmr.org

American Anorexia Bulimia Association
165 West 46 Street, #1108
New York, NY 10036
(212) 575-6200

**American Association of Clinical
Endocrinologists (AACE)**
1000 Riverside Avenue
Suite 205
Jacksonville, FL 32304
(904) 353-7878
http://www.aace.com

American Association of Diabetes Educators
444 North Michigan Avenue, Suite 1240
Chicago, IL 60611
(800) 338-3633
http://www.aadenet.org

**American Autoimmune Related Diseases
Association**
22100 Gratiot Avenue
East Detroit, MI 48021
(586) 776-3900
http://www.aarda.org

American Board of Medical Specialties
47 Perimeter Center East, Suite 500
Atlanta, GA 36346
(800) 776-2378
http://www.abms.org

American Board of Pediatric Surgery
1601 Dolores Street
San Francisco, CA 94110
(415) 826-3200

**American Board of Physician Nutrition
Specialists**
University of Alabama at Birmingham
439 Susan Mott Webb Nutrition Sciences Building
1675 University Boulevard
Birmingham, AL 35294
(205) 934-5564
http://main.uab.edu/ipnec/show.asp?durki=37725

American Cancer Society
1599 Clifton Road NE
Atlanta, GA 30329
(800) 227-2345 or (404) 320-2408
http://www.cancer.org

American Chronic Pain Association
P.O. Box 850
Rocklin, CA 95677
(916) 632-0922
http://www.theacpa.org

**American College of Obstetricians and
Gynecologists (ACOG)**
409 12th Street SW
P.O. Box 96920
Washington, DC 20090
(202) 863-2518
http://www.acog.org

**American College of Physicians, American
Society of Internal Medicine (ACP-ASIM)**
190 N. Independence Mall West
Philadelphia, PA 19106
(800) 523-1546
http://www.acpoline.org

American College of Rheumatology
1800 Century Place
Suite 250
Atlanta, GA 30345
(404) 633-3777
www.rheumatology.org

American College of Sports Medicine
P.O. Box 1440
Indianapolis, IN 46206
(317) 637-9200
http://www.ascm.org/sportsmed

American College of Surgeons (ACS)
633 North St. Clair Street
Chicago, IL 60611
(312) 202-5000
http://www.facs.org

American Diabetes Association (ADA)
1701 North Beauregard Street
Alexandria, VA 22311
(800) 342-2383
http://www.diabetes.org

American Dietetic Association
216 West Jackson Boulevard
Chicago, IL 60606
(312) 899-0040
http://www.eatright.org

American Federation for Aging Research (AFAR)
1414 Sixth Avenue, 18th Floor
New York, NY 10019
(212) 752-2327
http://www.afar.org

American Foundation of Thyroid Patients
P.O. Box 820195
Houston, TX 77282
(281) 496-4460
http://www.thyroidfoundation.org

American Health Assistance Foundation
15825 Shady Grove Road
Suite 140
Rockville, MD 20850
(800) 437-2423
http://www.ahaf.org

American Health Care Association (AHCA)
1201 L Street NW
Washington, DC 20005
(202) 842-4444
http://www.ahca.org

American Heart Association/American Stroke Association
7272 Greenville Avenue
Dallas, TX 75231
(800) AHA-USA1
http://www.americanheart.org

American Hospital Association (AHA)
One North Franklin
Chicago, IL 60606
(312) 422-3000
http://www.aha.org

American Fertility Association
666 Fifth Avenue
Suite 278
New York, NY 10103
(888) 917-3777
http://www.theafa.org

American Institute for Cancer Research
1759 R Street NW
Washington, DC 20009
(800) 843-8114
http://www.aicr.org

American Medical Association
515 North State Street
Chicago, IL 60610
(312) 464-5000
http://www.ama-assn.org

American Medical Women's Association
801 North Fairfax Street
Suite 400
Alexandria, VA 22314
(703) 838-0500
http://www.amwa-doc.org

American Menopause Foundation
350 Fifth Avenue
Suite 2822
New York, NY 10118
(212) 714-2398
http://www.americanmenopause.org

American Mental Health Counselor's Association
801 N. Fairfax Street, Suite 304
Alexandria, VA 22314
(703) 548-6002
http://www.amhca.org

American Nurses Association
600 Maryland Avenue SW
Suite 100 West
Washington, DC 20024
(202) 554-4444
http://www.nursingworld.org

American Obesity Association
1250 24th Street NW, Suite 300
Washington, DC 20037
(800) 98-OBESE
http://www.obesity.org

American Pharmaceutical Association
2215 Constitution Avenue NW
Washington, DC 20037
(202) 628-4410
http://www.aphanet.org

American Physical Therapy Association (APTA)
111 North Fairfax Street
Alexandria, VA 22314
(800) 999-2782, ext. 3395
http://www.apta.org

American Podiatric Medical Association
9312 Old Georgetown Road
Bethesda, MD 20814
(301) 581-9200
http://www.apma.org

American Psychiatric Association
1400 K Street NW
Washington, DC 20005
(202) 682-6000
http://www.psych.org

American Psychological Association
750 First Street NE
Washington, DC 20002
(202) 336-5500
http://www.apa.org

American Society for Bariatric Surgery
7328 West University Avenue, Suite G
Gainesville, FL 32607
(352) 331-4900
http://www.asbs.org

American Society for Bone and Mineral Research
1200 Nineteenth Street NW, Suite 300
Washington, DC 20036
(202) 857-1161
http://www.asbmr.org

American Society for Reproductive Medicine
1209 Montgomery Highway
Birmingham, AL 35216
(205) 978-5000
http://www.asrm.org

American Society of Bariatric Physicians
5453 East Evans Place
Denver, CO 80222
(303) 770-2526
http://www.asbp.org

American Society of Human Genetics
9650 Rockville Pike
Bethesda, MD 20814
(301) 571-1825
http://www.faseb.org/genetics

American Society of Nephrology
1200 Nineteenth Street Northwest, Suite 300
Washington, DC 20039

(202) 857-1190
http://www.asn-online.com

American Society of Ophthalmic Plastic & Reconstructive Surgery
1133 West Morse Boulevard, Suite 201
Winter Park, FL 32789
(407) 647-8839
http://www.asoprs.org

American Thyroid Association
6066 Leesburg Pike, Suite 550
Falls Church, VA 22041
(703) 998-8890
http://www.thyroid.org

American Urological Association
1120 North Charles Street
Baltimore, MD 21201
(410) 727-1100
http://www.auanet.org

Association for Glycogen Storage Disease
P.O. Box 896
Durant, IA 52747
(319) 785-6038
http://www.agsdus.org

Association for Neuro-Metabolic Disorders
5223 Brookfield Lane
Sylvania, OH 43560
(419) 885-1497

Association of American Indian Physicians
1235 Sovereign Row, Suite C-9
Oklahoma City, OK 73108
(405) 946-7651
http://www.aaip.com

Association of Asian Pacific Community Health Organizations
1440 Broadway #510
Oakland, CA 94612
(510) 272-9536
http://www.aapcho.org

Cancer Research Foundation of America
1600 Duke Street, Suite 110
Alexandria, VA 22314
(800) 227-2732
http://www.preventcancer.org

Centers for Disease Control and Prevention (CDC)
1600 Clifton Road
Atlanta, GA 30333
(404) 639-3534
http://www.cdc.gov

Centers for Medicare and Medicaid Services (Formerly the Health Care Financing Administration)
6325 Security Boulevard
Baltimore, MD 21207
(410) 786-3000
http://www.hcfa.gov

Children with Diabetes Foundation
2525 Araphoe Avenue
Suite E4, PMB #506
Boulder, CO 80302
http://www.cwdfoundation.org

Creutzfeldt-Jakob Disease Foundation
P.O. Box 5312
Akron, OH 44334
(800) 659-1991
http://www.cjdfoundation.org

Cushing's Support and Research Foundation, Inc.
65 East India Row 22B
Boston, MA 02110
(617) 723-3824
http://www.csrf.net

Diabetes Action Research and Education Foundation
426 C Street NE
Washington, DC 20002
(202) 333-4520
http://www.diabetesaction.org

Diabetes Exercise and Sports Association
1647 West Bethany Home Road #B
Phoenix, AZ 85015
(800) 898-4322
http://www.diabetes-exercise.org

Disability Rights Education and Defense Fund, Inc.
2212 Sixth Street
Berkeley, CA 94710
(800) 466-4232
http://www.dredf.org

Emergency Nurses Association
915 Lee Street
Des Plaines, IL 60016
(800) 900-9659
http://www.ena.org

Endocrine Society
4350 East West Highway
Suite 500
Bethesda, MD 2081
(301) 941-0200
http://www.endo-society.org

Food and Drug Administration (FDA)
HFE88
5600 Fishers Lane
Rockville, MD 20857
(888) 463-6332
http://www.fda.org

The Genetic Alliance
4301 Connecticut Avenue NW
Suite 404
Washington, DC 20008
(202) 966-5557
http://www.geneticalliance.org

Harvard Eating Disorders Center
55 Fruit Street
YAW 6900
Boston, MA 02114
(617) 726-8470
http://www.hedc.org

H.E.L.P., The Institute for Body Chemistry
P.O. Box 1338
Bryn Mawr, PA 19010
(610) 525-1225

Hepatitis Foundation International
504 Blick Drive
Silver Spring, MD 20904
(800) 891-0707
http://www.hepfi.org

Hormone Foundation
4350 East-West Highway, Suite 500
Bethesda, MD 20814
(800) HORMONE
http://www.hormone.org

Human Growth Foundation
997 Glen Cove Avenue
Glen Head, NY 11545
(800) 451-6434
http://www.hgfound.org

Hypoglycemia Support Foundation, Inc.
3822 Northwest 122nd Terrace
Sunrise, FL 33345
(954) 742-3098
http://www.hypoglycemia.org

Hypoparathyroidism Association, Inc.
2835 Salmon
Idaho Falls, ID 83406
(208) 524-3857
http://www.hypoparathyroidism.org

Impotence World Association
10400 Little Patuxent Parkway
Suite 485
Columbia, MD 21044
(800) 669-1603

**Indian Health Service
  Headquarters**
Diabetes Program
5300 Homestead Road NE
Albuquerque, NM 87110
(505) 248-4182

**International Association for Medical
  Assistance to Travellers**
417 Center Street
Lewiston, NY 14092
(716) 754-4883
http://www.iamat.org

**International Diabetic Athletes
  Association**
1647 West Bethany Home Road #B
Phoenix, AZ 85015
(800) 898-4322
http://www.diabetes-exercise.org

Joslin Diabetes Center
One Joslin Place
Boston, MA 02215
(617) 732-2415
http://www.joslin.harvard.edu

**Juvenile Diabetes Research Foundation
  (JDF) International**
120 Wall Street
19th Floor
New York, NY 10005
(800) 223-1138
http://www.jdf.org

Klinefelter Syndrome and Associates, Inc.
P.O. Box 119
Roseville, CA 95678
(916) 773-1449
http://www.genetic.org/ks

La Leche League International
1400 North Meacham Road
Schaumburg, IL 60173-4840
(847) 519-7730
http://www.lalecheleague.org

Light of Life Foundation
32 Marc Drive
Englishtown, NJ 07726
(732) 972-0461
http://www.lightoflifefoundation.org

Little People of America, Inc.
5289 Northeast Elam Young Parkway
Hillsboro, OR 97124
(888) LPA-2001
http://www.lpaonlne.org

Magic Foundation
6645 West North Avenue
Oak Park, IL 60302
(708) 383-0808
http://www.magicfoundation.org

**March of Dimes Birth Defects
  Foundation**
1275 Mamaroneck Avenue
White Plains, NY 10605
(914) 428-7100
http://www.modimes.org

Medic Alert Foundation
P.O. Box 109
Turlock, CA 95831
(209) 668-3331
http://www.medicalalert.org

Metabolic Information Network
P.O. Box 670847
Dallas, TX 75367
(800) 945-2188

The Myelin Project
1747 Pennsylvania Avenue Northwest, Suite 950
Washington, DC 20006
(202) 452-8994
http://www.myelin.org

National Adrenal Diseases Foundation
505 Northern Boulevard, Suite 200
Great Neck, NY 11021
(516) 487-4992
http://www.medhelp.org/nadf

National Alliance for Hispanic Health
1501 Sixteenth Street NW
Washington, DC 20036
(202) 387-5000
http://www.hispanichealth.org

**National Association of Anorexia Nervosa
and Associated Disorders**
P.O. Box 7
Highland Park, IL 60035
(847) 831-3438
http://www.anad.org

National Cancer Institute
Division of Cancer Epidemiology and Genetics
6120 Executive Boulevard, MSC-7224
Executive Plaza South, 7th Floor
Bethesda, MD 20892
(301) 496-1691
http://dceg.cancer.gov

**National Center for Chronic Disease
Prevention and Health Promotion**
Division of Diabetes Translation
Mail Stop K-10
4770 Buford Highway NE
Atlanta, GA 30341
(877) CDC-DIAB
http://www.cdc.gov/diabetes

**National Center for Complementary and
Alternative Medicine (NCCAM)
Clearinghouse**
National Institutes of Health (NIH)
P.O. Box 8218

Silver Spring, MD 20907
(888) 644-6226
http://www.nccam.nih.gov

**National Center for the Study
of Wilson's Disease**
432 West 58th Street, Suite 614
New York, NY 10091
(212) 523-8717

**National Certification Board
for Diabetes Educators**
330 East Algonquin Road, Suite 4
Arlington Heights, IL 60005
(847) 228-9795
http://www.ncbde.org

**National Clearinghouse for
Alcohol and Drug Information**
11426 Rockville Pike, Suite 200
Rockville, MD 20852
(800) 729-6686
http://www.health.org

**National Coalition for Cancer
Survivorship (NCCS)**
1010 Wayne Avenue, Suite 770
Silver Spring, MD 20910
(877) 622-7937
http://www.cansearch.org

National Council on Aging
300 D Street SW, Suite 801
Washington, DC 20024
(202) 479-1200
http://www.ncoa.org

**National Council on Alcoholism
and Drug Dependence
(NCADD)**
20 Exchange Place, Suite 2902
New York, NY 10005
(800) NCA-CALL (24-hour Affiliate referral) or
      (212) 269-7797
http://www.ncadd.org

**National Diabetes Information
Clearinghouse**
1 Information Way
Bethesda, MD 20892
(800) 860-8747
http://diabetes.niddk.nih.gov

National Digestive Diseases Information Clearinghouse (NDIC)
National Institute of Diabetes and Digestive and Kidney Diseases (NIDDK)
National Institutes of Health (NIH)
2 Information Way
Bethesda, MD 20892
(800) 891-5389
http://digestive.niddk.nih.gov

National Dissemination Center for Children and Youth with Disabilities
P.O. Box 1492
Washington, DC 20013
(800) 695-0285
http://www.nichcy.org

National Easter Seal Society
230 West Monroe Street
Suite 1800
Chicago, IL 60606
(800) 221-6827
http://www.easter-seals.org

National Eating Disorders Organization
603 Stewart Street
Suite 803
Seattle, WA 98101
(800) 931-2237
http://www.nationaleatingdisorders.org

National Eye Health Education Program (NEHEP)
2020 Vision Place
Bethesda, MD 20892
(301) 496-5248
http://www.nei.nih.gov

National Eye Institute
2020 Vision Place
Bethesda, MD 20892
(301) 496-5248
http://www.nei.nih.gov/nehep

National Graves' Disease Foundation
P.O. Box 1969
Brevard, NC 28712
(828) 877-5251
http://www.ngdf.org

National Health Information Center (NHIC)
Office of Disease Prevention and Health Promotion (ODPHP)
Department of Health and Human Services
P.O. Box 1133
Washington, DC 20013
(800) 336-4797
http://www.health.gov/NHIC

National Heart, Lung, and Blood Institute
P.O. Box 30105
Bethesda, MD 20824
(301) 592-8573
http://www.nhlbi.nih.gov

National Institute of Diabetes and Digestive and Kidney Diseases (NIDDK)
National Institutes of Health
Building 31, Room 9A04
31 Center Drive, MSC 2560
Bethesda, MD 20892
(301) 496-3583
http://www.niddk.nih.gov

National Institute of Mental Health
NIMH Public Inquiries
6001 Executive Boulevard
Room 8184, MSC 9663
Bethesda, MD 20892
(301) 443-4513
http://www.nimh.nih.gov

National Institute on Aging
Building 31, Room 5C27
31 Center Drive, MSC 292
Bethesda, MD 20892
(301) 496-1752
http://www.nia.nih.gov

National Institute on Drug Abuse
National Institutes of Health
6001 Executive Boulevard, Room 5213
Bethesda, MD 20892
(301) 443-1124
http://www.nida.nih.gov

National Institutes of Health (NIH)
P.O. Box 8218
Silver Spring, MD 20907
(888) 644-6226
http://www.nccam.nih.gov

National Kidney and Urologic Diseases Information Clearinghouse
3 Information Way
Bethesda, MD 20892
(800) 891-5390

National Kidney Foundation, Inc.
30 East 33rd Street
New York, NY 10016
(800) 622-9010
http://www.kidney.org

National Mental Health Association
1021 Prince Street
Alexandria, VA 22314
(703) 684-7722
http://www.nmha.org

National Neurofibromatosis Foundation
95 Pine Street, 16th Floor
New York, NY 10005
(800) 344-6633
http://www.nf.org

National Oral Health Information Clearinghouse
1 NOHIC Way
Bethesda, MD 20892
(301) 402-3500
http://www.nohic.nidcr.nih.gov

National Organization for Rare Disorders (NORD)
55 Kenosia Avenue
P.O. Box 1968
Danbury, CT 06813-1968
(203) 746-6518
http://www.rarediseases.org

National Osteoporosis Foundation
1232 22nd Street NW
Washington, DC 20037
(202) 223-2226
http://www.nof.org

National Ovarian Cancer Coalition (NOCC)
500 NE Spanish River Boulevard
Suite 8
Boca Raton, FL 33431
(561) 393-0005
http://www.ovarian.org

National Rehabilitation Information Center
4200 Forbes Boulevard
Suite 202
Lanham, MD 20706
(800) 346-2742
http://www.naric.com

National Self-Help Clearinghouse
Graduate School and University Center of the City University of New York
365 Fifth Avenue, Suite 3300
New York, NY 10016
(212) 817-1822
http://www.selfhelpweb.org

National Women's Health Network
514 10th Street NW
Suite 400
Washington, DC 20004
(202) 347-1140
http://www.nwhn.org

Neurofibromatosis, Inc.
9320 Annapolis Road, Suite 300
Lanham, MD 20706
(301) 918-4600
http://www.nfinc.org

North American Menopause Society (NAMS)
P.O. Box 94527
Cleveland, OH 44101
(440) 442-7550
http://www.menopause.org

Office of Minority Health Resource Center
P.O. Box 37337
Washington, DC 20013
(800) 444-6472
http://www.omhrc.gov

Ovarian Cancer National Alliance (OCNA)
910 17th Street NW, Suite 413
Washington, DC 20006
(202) 331-1332
http://www.ovariancancer.org

Overeaters Anonymous
P.O. Box 44020
Rio Rancho, NM 87124
(505) 891-2664
http://www.oa.org

Oxalosis and Hyperoxaluria Foundation
20 E. 19th Street, #12 E
New York, NY 10003
(800) OHF-8699
http://www.ohf.org

Paget Foundation for Paget's Disease of Bone and Related Disorders
120 Wall Street
Suite 1602
New York, NY 10005
(800) 23-PAGET
http://www.paget.org

Pancreatic Cancer Action Network
2221 Rosecrans Avenue
Suite 131
El Segundo, CA 90245
(877) 272-6226
http://www.pancan.org

Pediatric Endocrinology Nursing Society
P.O. Box 2933
Gaithersburg, MD 20886
http://www.pens.org

Pedorthic Footwear Association
7150 Columbia Gateway Drive
Suite G
Columbia, MD 21046
(410) 381-7278
http://www.pedorthics.org

Pituitary Tumor Network Association
P.O. Box 1958
Thousand Oaks, CA 91358
(805) 499-9973
http://www.pituitary.org

Polycystic Ovarian Syndrome Association
P.O. Box 3403
Englewood, CO 80111
(877) 775-PCOS
http://www.pcosupport.org

Prader-Willi Alliance for Research
28 Vesey Street
Suite 2104
New York, NY 10007
(212) 332-0970
http://www.p-war.org

The Foundation for Prader-Willi Research
6407 Bardstown Road
Suite 252
Louisville, KY 40291
(502) 254-9375

President's Council on Physical Fitness and Sports
701 Pennsylvania Avenue NW
Suite 250
Washington, DC 20004
(202) 272-3421
http://www.fitness.gov

RESOLVE: The National Infertility Association
1310 Broadway
Somerville, MA 02144
(888) 623-0744
http://www.resolve.org

Social Security Administration (SSA)
Office of Public Inquiries
Windsor Park Building
6401 Security Boulevard
Baltimore, MD 21235
(800) 772-1213
http://www.ssa.gov

Society for Inherited Metabolic Disorders
Oregon Health Sciences University/L473
3181 Southwest Sam Jackson Park Road
Portland, OR 97201
(503) 494-5400
http://www.simd.org

Society for Neuroscience
11 Dupont Circle NW
Suite 500
Washington, DC 20036
(202) 462-6688
http://www.sfn.org

Substance Abuse and Mental Health Services Administration (SAMSHA)
Department of Health and Human Services
Room 12-105 Parklawn Building
5600 Fishers Lane
Rockville, MD 20857
(800) 729-6686
http://www.samhsa.gov

**ThyCa: Thyroid Cancer Survivors'
Association, Inc.**
P.O. Box 1545
New York, NY 10159
(877) 588-7904
http://www.thyca.org

Thyroid Foundation of America, Inc.
One Longfellow Place
Suite 158
Boston, MA 02114
(800) 832-8321
http://www.allthyroid.org

Thyroid Society for Education and Research
7515 South Main Street
Suite 545
Houston, TX 77030
(800) THYROID

**Transplant Recipients International
Organization, Inc.**
2117 L Street NW, #353
Washington, DC 20037
(202) 293-0980
http://www.trioweb.org

United Leukodystrophy Foundation
2304 Highland Drive
Sycamore, IL 60178
(800) 728-5483
http://www.ulf.org

United Network for Organ Sharing
P.O. Box 2484
Richmond, VA 23218
(804) 330-8500
http://www.unos.org

Veterans Health Administration
810 Vermont Avenue NW
Washington, DC 20420
(202) 273-8490
http://www1.va.gov/health_benefits

Weight-Control Information Network
1 Win Way
Bethesda, MD 20892
(800) WIN-8098
http://www.niddk.nih.gov/health/nutrit/nutrit.htm

Weight Watchers International
175 Crossways Park West
Woodbury, NY 11797
(800) 651-6000
http://www.weightwatchers.com

Wilson's Disease Association International
1802 Brookside Drive
Wooster, OH 44691
(800) 399-0266
http://www.wilsonsdisease.org

APPENDIX II
KEY HEALTH ORGANIZATIONS IN CANADA

Canadian Cancer Society
National Office, Suite 200
10 Alcorn Avenue
Toronto, Ontario M4V 3B1
(416) 961-7223
http://www.cancer.ca

Canadian Diabetes Association
National Life Building
1400-522 University Avenue
Toronto, Ontario M5G 2R5
(800) BANTING
http://www.diabetes.ca

Canadian Institutes of Health Research
410 Laurier Avenue West, Ninth Floor
Address Locator 4209A
Ottawa, Ontario K1A 0W9
(888) 603-4178 (Canada) or 613-941-2672
http://www.cihr.ca

Canadian MedicAlert Foundation
2005 Sheppard Avenue East, Suite 800
Toronto, Ontario M2J 5B4
800-668-1507 (English) or 800-668-6381
  (French)
http://www.medicalert.ca

Canadian Mental Health Association
8 King Street East, Suite 810
Toronto, Ontario M5C 1B5
(416) 484-7750
http://www.cmha.ca

Health Canada
A.L. 0900C2
Ottawa, Ontario K1A 0K9
(613) 957-2991
http://www.hc-sc.gc.ca/english

Heart and Stroke Foundation of Canada
222 Queen Street, Suite 1402
Ottawa, Ontario K1P 5V9
(613) 569-4361
ww2.heartandstroke.ca

Infertility Awareness Association of Canada
2100 Marlowe Avenue, Suite 39
Montreal, Quebec H4A 3L5
(800) 263-2929
http://www.iaac.ca

Osteoporosis Society of Canada
33 Laird Drive
Toronto, Ontario M4G 3S9
(800) 463-6842 (Canada) or (416) 696-2663
http://www.osteoporosis.ca

Thyroid Federation International
797 Princess Street, Suite 304
Kingston, Ontario K7L 1G1
(613) 544-8364
http://www.thyroid-fed.org

Thyroid Foundation International
797 Princess Street, Suite 304
Kingston, Ontario K7L 1G1
(613) 544-8364
http://www.thyroid.ca

APPENDIX III
CHART OF THYROID
MEDICATIONS TO TREAT HYPOTHYROIDISM

Brand Name	Generic Name	Available Dosages	Manufacturer
Armour thyroid	Dessicated pork thyroid (T3 and T4)	Many dosages, ranging from 1/4–5 grains	Forest Pharmaceuticals St. Louis, MO
Cytomel	Liothyronine (T4)	5–50 micrograms	Jones Pharma, Inc. St. Louis, MO
Levoxyl	Levothyroxine (T4)	Many dosages, ranging from 25–300 micrograms	Jones Pharma, Inc. St. Louis, MO
Levothroid	Levothyroxine (T4)	25, 50, 75, 88, 100, 112, 125, 137, 150, 175, 200, 300 micrograms	Forest Pharmaceuticals St. Louis, MO
Synthroid	Levothyroxine (T4)	Many dosages, ranging from 25–300 micrograms	Abbott Laboratories North Chicago, IL
Unithroid	Levothyroxine (T4)	25, 50, 75, 88, 100, 112, 125, 150, 175, 200, 300 micrograms	Watson Pharm. Corona, CA

APPENDIX IV
CHART OF THYROID
MEDICATIONS TO TREAT HYPERTHYROIDISM

Brand Name	Generic Name	Available Dosages	Manufacturer
Generic methimazole	Methimazole	5, 10 milligrams	Many companies
Propylthiouracil (PTU)	Propylthiouracil	50 milligrams	Many companies
Tapazole	Methimazole	5, 10 milligrams	Jones/King Pharm. St. Louis, MO

APPENDIX V
MEDICATIONS TO TREAT DIABETES

I. INSULIN SECRETAGOGUES

	1st Generation	2nd Generation
Sulfonylureas	Tolbutamide	Glyburide/ Micronized Glyburide
	Tolazamide	Glipizide
	Chlorpropramide	Glimepiride
Meglitinide	Repaglinide (Prandin)	
Phenylalanine Derivatives	Nateglinide (Starlix)	
Thiazolidinediones (TZDs)	Rosiglitazone (Avandia) Pioglitazone (Actos)	
Alpha Glucosidase Inhibitors	Acarbose (Precose)	
	Miglitol (Glyset)	
Biguanide	Metformin (Glucophage)	

SULFONYLUREA MEDICATIONS AND TYPICAL DOSING

Generic Name	Trade Name	Number of Daily Doses	Typical Daily Dose
Tolbutamide	Orinase	2–3	500–3000 mg/day
Acetohexamide	Dymelor	1–2	250–500 mg/1–2 a day
Tolazamide	Tolinase	1–2	100–1000 mg/day
Chlorpropamide	Diabinese	1	100–500 mg/day
Glyburide	Diabeta Micronase	1	1.25–20 mg/day
Micronized glyburide	Glynase PresTab	1	1.5–12 mg/day
Glipizide	Glucotrol	1–2	2.5–40 mg/day
Glipizide GITS	Glucotrol XL	1	2.5–20 mg/day
Glimepiride	Amaryl	1	0.5–8 mg/day

SECRETAGOGUE MEDICATIONS AND TYPICAL DOSING

Generic Name	Trade Name	Typical Dosing
Repaglinide	Prandin	1.5–16 mg, 3 or 4/day
Nateglinide	Starlix	180–360 mg/day

TZD MEDICATIONS AND TYPICAL DOSING

Generic Name	Trade Name	Typical Dosing
Rosiglitazone	Avandia	2–8 mg/day, 1–2/day
Pioglitazone	Actos	15–45 mg/day

ALPHA GLUCOSIDE INHIBITOR MEDICATIONS AND TYPICAL DOSING

Generic Name	Trade Name	Typical Doses
Miglitol	Glyset	75–300 mg/day
Acarbose	Precose	75–300 mg/day

APPENDIX VI
13 LITTLE-KNOWN FACTS ABOUT ENDOCRINE DISEASES

1. Some people may initially have an overactive thyroid gland, often due to the autoimmune disease Graves' disease and then later they become hypothyroid (underactive) due to the autoimmune disease known as Hashimoto's thyroiditis. The reverse phenomenon, or the development of Graves' disease after Hashimoto's thyroiditis, can also occur but is seen infrequently.

2. When a person has a serious endocrine disease is not always obvious. Primary hyperparathyroidism is often found by accident when blood work is done for other reasons. The patient may have had kidney stones in the past and now has osteoporosis or a fracture, both potentially related to hyperparathyroidism. If the patient does not share this past medical history with a physician, the diagnosis of hyperparathyroidism might not be considered. Doctors need complete medical information from patients, and they also need to take laboratory tests to help them determine if an endocrine disorder is present.

3. Most endocrine disorders are treatable, although they may not be curable.

4. Infertility may be caused by an underlying endocrine disorder in a man or a woman (and sometimes in both of them). This is most commonly caused by mild elevations of the hormone prolactin due to tiny microadenomas of the pituitary gland that may be as small as one to two millimeters in diameter. Prior to the current imaging of the pituitary that is possible with magnetic resonance imaging, these lesions could not be visualized by the physician.

5. Babies and elderly people can develop treatable endocrine disorders, as can people of any other age.

6. Herbal remedies and supplements may be dangerous because they can boost or weaken the effects of other drugs patients take, such as insulin, thyroid supplements, and so forth. Patients should always check with their doctors before taking any herbal remedy or supplement.

7. Treatments that may work well for one member of the family with diabetes, thyroid disease, or other endocrine disorders may also work well for other members with the same disease, but everyone is different. Sometimes other family members need different medications for their condition to improve.

8. Some thyroid diseases, such as hypothyroidism, are common in the general population.

9. Testing for most forms of thyroid disease with blood tests is relatively simple.

10. Pregnant women have an increased risk of developing thyroid disease, both during pregnancy and immediately afterward.

11. Vitamin D deficiency is extremely common in the elderly and is treatable. Often these patients present with nonspecific aches and pains in the muscles and especially in their wrists and shins. Vitamin D deficiency is usually easily treated with supplemental vitamin D.

12. Gastric bypass surgery for severe obesity clearly has the best track record to date of all the therapies tried for this common and difficult-to-treat disorder.

13. Thyroid medication must be taken on an empty stomach, because various foods and medications, especially iron and other supplements, may decrease the absorption of thyroid hormone and lead to hypothyroidism.

APPENDIX VII
10 LITTLE-KNOWN FACTS ABOUT DIABETES MELLITUS

1. People with diabetes *can* eat foods with sugar (also known as carbohydrates or starches), contrary to popular belief. Many people believe that diabetes means that patients must never eat any cakes, cookies, or related items. The fact is that people with diabetes can eat such foods in moderation. In addition, people with diabetes may actually develop low blood sugar levels (hypoglycemia). When that happens, then they need to consume something with sugar in it in order to treat the hypoglycemia and stay healthy. This is one of the reasons why people with diabetes need to test their blood on a regular basis—to find out whether their glucose levels are too high or too low.

2. Not everyone with diabetes needs insulin. Insulin is required by people with Type 1 diabetes. Some people with Type 2 diabetes, usually after having the disease for many years, will also require insulin as well. Many patients with Type 2 diabetes will do very well with a good nutritional program, exercise, and oral medications.

3. Some women develop diabetes only during pregnancy, which is called *gestational diabetes.* Once they deliver their babies, their blood sugar usually returns to normal. However, these women are at greater risk for developing either Type 1 or Type 2 diabetes later in life. Also, should they get pregnant again, the gestational diabetes will often return.

4. The names of the two primary types of diabetes have been changed in recent years. Type 1 diabetes was once called *juvenile-onset diabetes,* because it is often diagnosed during childhood. The name was changed because the disease is sometimes diagnosed in adulthood. Also, even if diagnosed during childhood, the illness persists throughout life. Type 2 diabetes was previously called *adult-onset diabetes* or *noninsulin-dependent diabetes.* These names were misleading, because adolescents and even children can develop this form of diabetes. Also, some people with Type 2 diabetes do require insulin.

5. People with diabetes have a greater risk of developing many medical complications. However, with good and continuous control of their blood glucose, patients can lead normal and active lives.

6. Everyone with Type 1 diabetes needs insulin. The insulin may be given by injection or via an insulin pump (a small catheter under the skin). Researchers are also testing an inhaled delivery method of insulin.

7. Smoking is very bad for people with diabetes, and it greatly increases the risk that the patient will suffer from complications, including amputations, cancer, heart attack, stroke, and so forth. People with diabetes who smoke should work with their doctors to kick the habit.

8. Many supermarkets and pharmacies sell sugar-free food products for people with diabetes and other individuals. They also sell glucose supplements for when people with diabetes become low in blood sugar.

9. Some schools still fail to acknowledge the need of schoolchildren and adolescents to self-inject insulin, and parents may need to determine school guidelines about medications and actively work to obtain exceptions to them. (Multiple laws and guidelines cover

these issues. Contact the American Diabetes Association for further information.)

10. Some hypoglycemic adults (and children) may appear to be in a drunken state when they are, in fact, in serious need of glucose.

Wearing a medical bracelet can help alert medical experts and other authorities to the presence of diabetes and other chronic medical problems and may also help to increase the probability of fast and effective treatment.

APPENDIX VIII
WEB SITES WITH INFORMATION ON ENDOCRINE DISEASES AND DISORDERS

American Academy of Pediatrics
http://www.aap.org

American Association of Clinical Endocrinologists
http://www.aace.com

American Association of Diabetes Educators
http://www.aadenet.org

American Autoimmune Related Diseases Association
http://www.aarda.org

American Cancer Society
http://www.cancer.org

American Diabetes Association (ADA)
http://www.diabetes.org/

American Dietetic Association
http://www.eatright.org

American Foundation of Thyroid Patients
http://www.thyroidfoundation.org

American Menopause Foundation
http://www.americanmenopause.org

American Obesity Association
http://www.obesity.org

American Society for Reproductive Medicine
http://www.asrm.org

American Society of Human Genetics
http://www.faseb.org/genetics

American Society of Nephrology
http://www.asn-online.com

American Society of Ophthalmic Plastic & Reconstructive Surgery
http://www.asoprs.org

American Thyroid Association
http://www.thyroid.org

Camps for Children with Diabetes
http://www.childrenwithdiabetes.com

Canadian Cancer Society
http://www.cancer.ca

Canadian Diabetes Association
http://www.diabetes.ca

Centers for Disease Control and Prevention
http://www.cdc.gov

Centers for Medicare and Medicaid Services
http://cms.hhs.gov

Children with Diabetes Foundation
http://www.cwdfoundation.org

Department of Veterans Affairs
http://www.va.gov/health/diabetes

Diabetes Action Research and Education Foundation
http://www.diabetesaction.org

Diabetes Exercise and Sports Association
http://www.diabetes-exercise.org

Endocrine Society
http://www.endo-society.org

Gilda Radner Familial Ovarian Cancer Registry
http://www.ovariancancer.com

Health Resources and Services Administration
http://www.hrsa.gov

Hormone Foundation
http://www.hormone.org

Human Growth Foundation
http://www.hgfound.org

Hypoglycemia Support Foundation, Inc.
http://www.hypolglycemia.org

Hypoparathyroidism Association, Inc.
http://www.hypoparathyroidism.org

Indian Health Service
http://www.ihs.gov

International Diabetic Athletes Association
http://www.diabetes-exercise.org

Joslin Diabetes Center
http://www.joslin.harvard.edu

Juvenile Diabetes Research Foundation (JDF) International
http://www.jdf.org

Light of Life Foundation
http://lightoflifefoundation.org

Little People of America, Inc.
http://www.lpaonline.org

March of Dimes Birth Defects Foundation
http://www.modimes.org

National Cancer Institute of Canada (NCIC)
http://www.ncic.cancer.ca

National Coalition for Cancer Survivorship (NCCS)
http://www.canceradvocacy.org

National Diabetes Education Program
http://www.ndep.nih.gov

National Diabetes Information Clearinghouse
http://www.niddk.nih.gov/health/diabetes.ndic.htm

National Digestive Diseases Information Clearinghouse (NDIC)
http://www.niddk.nih.gov

National Easter Seal Society
http://www.easter-seals.org

National Eye Institute
http://www.nei.nih.gov

National Graves' Disease Foundation
http://www.ngdf.org

National Health Information Center (NHIC)
http://www.health.gov/NHIC

National Information Center for Children and Youth with Disabilities
http://www.nichcy.org

National Institute of Diabetes and Digestive and Kidney Diseases
http://www.niddk.nih.gov

National Institute of Mental Health
http://www.nimh.nih.gov

National Institute of Neurological Disorders
http://www.ninds.nih.gov

National Institute on Aging
http://www.nia.nih.gov

National Kidney Foundation, Inc.
http://www.kidney.org

National Oral Health Information Clearinghouse
http://www.nohic.nidcr.nih.gov

National Organization for Rare Disorders (NORD)
http://www.rarediseases.org

National Osteoporosis Foundation
http://www.nof.org

National Ovarian Cancer Coalition (NOCC)
http://www.ovarian.org

National Rehabilitation Information Center
http://www.naric.com

National Self-Help Clearinghouse
http://www.selfhelpweb.org

National Women's Health Network
http://www.womenshealthnetwork.org

North American Menopause Society (NAMS)
http://www.menopause.org

Office of Minority Health Resource Center
http://www.omhrc.gov

Ovarian Cancer National Alliance (OCNA)
http://www.ovariancancer.org

Oxalosis and Hyperoxaluria Foundation
http://www.ohf.org

Paget Foundation for Paget's Disease of Bone and Related Disorders
http://www.paget.org

Pancreatic Cancer Action Network
http://www.pancan.org

Pituitary Tumor Network Association
http://www.pituitary.com

Power of Prevention (A Diabetes Web Site)
www.powerofprevention.com

Prader-Willi Alliance for Research
http://www.pwsresearch.org

Prader-Willi Syndrome Association
http://www.pwsausa.org

RESOLVE: The National Infertility Association
http://www.resolve.org

Society for Neuroscience
http://www.sfn.org

ThyCa: Thyroid Cancer Survivors' Association, Inc.
http://www.thyca.org

Thyroid-Cancer.net
http://www.thyroid-cancer.net

Thyroid Foundation of America, Inc.
http://www.allthyroid.org

Transplant Recipient International Organization
http://www.trio.org

United Network for Organ Sharing
http://www.unos.org

Wilson's Disease Association
http://www.wilsonsdisease.org

APPENDIX IX

FREQUENCIES OF DIABETES AMONG PERSONS 18 YEARS OF AGE AND OLDER, BY SELECTED CHARACTERISTICS: UNITED STATES, 1999

	NUMBERS IN THOUSANDS	
	All Persons 18 and Older	All Persons 18 and Older With Diabetes
Total	199,617	10,755
Sex		
Male	95,565	5,090
Female	104,053	5,666
Age		
18–44 years	108,523	1,806
45–64 years	58,617	4,678
65–74 years	17,806	2,468
75 years and older	14,671	1,803
Race		
Caucasian	163,210	8,177
Black or African American	22,350	1,725
American Indian or Alaska Native	1,202	114
Asian	5,786	221
Native Hawaiian or other Pacific Islander	164	3
Region		
Northeast	38,973	2,242
Midwest	51,107	2,587
South	71,998	4,112
West	37,540	1,814
Sex and Age		
Male:		
18–44 years	53,460	767
45–64 years	28,342	2,289
65 years and older	13,763	2,034
Female:		
18–44 years	55,063	1,039
45–64 years	30,275	2,389
65 years and older	18,714	2,237

Source: Pleis, J. R. and R. Coles. *Summary Health Statistics for U.S. Adults: National Health Interview Survey,* 1999, Series 10, Number 212, National Center for Health Statistics, 2003.

APPENDIX X
PERCENT OF DIABETES AMONG PERSONS 18 YEARS OF AGE AND OVER, BY SELECTED CHARACTERISTICS: 1999

	UNITED STATES, 1999
Total	5.4
Sex	
Male	5.4
Female	5.5
Age	
18–44 years	1.7
45–64 years	8.1
65–74 years	14.1
75 years and older	12.5
Race	
Caucasian	5.1
Black or African American	7.8
American Indian or Alaskan Native	9.5
Asian	3.8
Native Hawaiian or other Pacific Islander	2.0
Region	
Northeast	5.8
Midwest	5.1
South	5.8
West	4.9
Sex and Age	
Male:	
18–44 years	1.4
45–64 years	8.2
65 years and older	15.1
Female:	
18–44 years	1.9
45–64 years	8.0
65 years and older	12.2

Source: Pleis, J. R. and R. Coles. *Summary Health Statistics for U.S. Adults: National Health Interview Survey,* 1999, Series 10, Number 212, National Center for Health Statistics, 2003.

APPENDIX XI

FREQUENCY DISTRIBUTIONS OF BODY MASS INDEX AMONG PERSONS 18 YEARS OF AGE AND OVER, BY SELECTED CHARACTERISTICS: UNITED STATES, 1999

UNITED STATES, 1999

Selected Characteristic	All Persons 18 Years of Age and Older	Underweight	Healthy Weight	Overweight	Obese
Total (number in thousands)	199,617	4,220	79,876	67,974	40,692
Sex					
Male	95,565	830	31,985	40,537	20,306
Female	104,053	3,390	47,891	27,437	20,386
Age					
18–44 years	108,523	2,684	48,049	34,061	20,264
45–64 years	58,617	617	18,831	22,162	14,693
65 years and older	32,477	920	12,997	11,751	5,735
Race and Ethnicity					
Caucasian	163,210	3,537	66,048	56,049	32,159
Black or African American	22,350	327	7,215	7,809	6,105
American Indian or Alaska Native	1,202	12	321	413	439
Asian	5,786	214	3,820	1,198	313
Native Hawaiian or other Pacific Islander	164	3	28	55	74
Hispanic or Latino	20,508	239	7,305	7,683	4,567
Education					
Less than a high school diploma	29,923	678	10,204	10,658	7,390
High school graduate/GED recipient	51,995	767	18,490	18,562	12,398
Some college	46,712	859	17,063	16,620	10,734
Bachelor of Arts, science degree, or professional degree	43,365	799	19,010	16,614	6,571
Family Income					
Less than $20,000	39,756	1,175	16,256	12,372	8,523
$20,000 or more	149,828	2,854	59,880	52,510	30,231
$20,000–34,999	30,471	645	12,012	10,047	7,038
$35,000–$54,999	33,956	632	13,235	11,821	7,633
$55,000–$74,999	23,603	404	9,361	8,396	4,843
$75,000 or more	35,057	746	14,597	13,018	6,006
Marital Status					
Married	116,328	1,782	42,766	42,642	25,200
Widowed	13,483	479	5,518	4,366	2,614
Divorced or separated	20,787	450	8,127	7,095	4,444
Never married	37,300	1,191	18,273	10,067	6,502
Living with a partner	11,085	303	4,975	3,603	1,868

(continues)

**FREQUENCY DISTRIBUTIONS OF BODY MASS INDEX AMONG PERSONS 18 YEARS OF AGE
AND OLDER, BY SELECTED CHARACTERISTICS: UNITED STATES, 1999** *(continued)*

Selected Characteristic	All Persons 18 Years of Age and Older	Underweight	Healthy Weight	Overweight	Obese
Region					
Northeast	38,973	831	15,896	13,261	7,063
Midwest	51,107	961	20,121	17,322	11,166
South	71,998	1,687	27,842	24,581	15,668
West	37,540	742	16,017	12,810	6,795
Sex and Age					
Male:					
18–44 years	53,460	496	19,680	21,647	10,516
45–64 years	28,342	156	7,355	12,900	7,433
65 years and older	13,763	179	4,951	5,990	2,356
Female:					
18–44 years	55,063	2,188	28,369	12,414	9,748
45–64 years	30,275	461	11,476	9,262	7,260
65 years and older	18,714	741	8,046	5,761	3,379

Source: Pleis, J. R. and R. Coles. *Summary Health Statistics for U.S. Adults: National Health Interview Survey,* 1999, Series 10, Number 212, National Center for Health Statistics, 2003.

APPENDIX XII

PERCENT DISTRIBUTIONS OF BODY MASS INDEX AMONG PERSONS 18 YEARS OF AGE AND OVER, BY SELECTED CHARACTERISTICS: UNITED STATES, 1999

			UNITED STATES, 1999		
Selected Characteristic	**Total**	**Underweight**	**Healthy Weight**	**Overweight**	**Obese**
Sex					
Male	100.0	0.9	34.2	43.3	21.7
Female	100.0	3.4	48.3	27.7	20.6
Age					
18–44 years	100.0	2.6	45.7	32.4	19.3
45–64 years	100.0	1.1	33.4	39.4	26.1
65 years and older	100.0	2.9	41.4	37.4	18.3
Race and Ethnicity					
Caucasian	100.0	2.2	41.9	35.5	20.4
Black or African American	100.0	1.5	33.6	36.4	28.5
American Indian or Alaska Native	100.0	1.0	27.1	34.9	37.0
Asian	100.0	3.9	68.9	21.6	5.6
Native Hawaiian or other Pacific Islander	100.0	2.0	17.6	34.3	46.1
Hispanic or Latino					
Education					
Less than a high school diploma	100.0	2.3	35.3	36.8	25.5
High school graduate/GED recipient	100.0	1.5	36.8	37.0	24.7
Some college	100.0	1.9	37.7	36.7	23.7
Bachelor of Arts, science degree, or professional degree	100.0	1.9	45.3	37.2	15.6
Family Income					
Less than $20,000	100.0	3.1	42.4	32.3	22.2
$20,000–$34,999	100.0	2.2	40.4	33.8	23.7
$35,000–$54,999	100.0	1.9	39.7	35.5	22.9
$55,000–$74,999	100.0	1.8	40.7	36.5	21.1
$75,000 or more	100.0	2.2	42.5	37.9	17.5
Marital status					
Married	100.0	1.6	38.1	37.9	22.4
Widowed	100.0	3.7	42.5	33.6	20.1
Divorced or separated	100.0	2.2	40.4	35.3	22.1
Never married	100.0	3.3	50.7	27.9	18.0
Living with a partner	100.0	2.8	46.3	33.5	17.4
Region					
Northeast	100.0	2.2	42.9	35.8	19.1
Midwest	100.0	1.9	40.6	34.9	22.5
South	100.0	2.4	39.9	35.2	22.5
West	100.0	2.0	44.0	35.2	18.7

(continues)

PERCENT DISTRIBUTIONS OF BODY MASS INDEX AMONG PERSONS 18 YEARS OF AGE AND OLDER, BY SELECTED CHARACTERISTICS: UNITED STATES: 1999 *(continued)*

Selected Characteristic	Total	Underweight	Healthy Weight	Overweight	Obese
Sex and Age					
Male:					
18–44 years	100.0	0.9	37.6	41.4	20.1
45–64 years	100.0	0.6	26.4	46.3	26.7
65 years and older	100.0	1.3	36.7	44.4	17.5
Female:					
18–44 years	100.0	4.2	53.8	23.5	18.5
45–64 years	100.0	1.6	40.3	32.5	25.5
65 years and older	100.0	4.1	44.9	32.1	18.8

Source: Pleis, J. R. and R. Coles. *Summary Health Statistics for U.S. Adults: National Health Interview Survey,* 1999, Series 10, Number 212, National Center for Health Statistics, 2003.

APPENDIX XIII

DIABETES DEATHS, RATES PER 100,000

DEATHS DUE TO DIABETES, BY SEX, 2001

State	Total Number	Total Rate*	Male Number	Male Rate*	Female Number	Female Rate*
Alabama	1,344	29.3	609	33.2	735	26.6
Alaska	80	22.7	41	20.6	39	23.2
Arizona	1,057	20.1	535	23.0	522	17.7
Arkansas	756	25.8	347	28.3	409	23.7
California	6,395	21.4	3,049	23.7	3,346	19.5
Colorado	667	18.7	307	20.1	360	17.5
Connecticut	759	19.6	348	22.7	411	17.2
Delaware	218	27.1	94	27.6	124	26.0
District of Columbia	209	37.0	82	36.8	127	37.5
Florida	4,631	22.0	2,344	25.8	2,287	18.9
Georgia	1,475	21.9	684	24.1	791	19.8
Hawaii	173	13.3	93	15.8	80	11.1
Idaho	318	26.2	141	26.3	177	25.7
Illinois	3,092	25.4	1,380	28.1	1,712	23.3
Indiana	1,677	27.7	763	31.1	914	25.2
Iowa	709	20.1	310	22.4	399	18.4
Kansas	721	25.0	327	28.1	394	23.2
Kentucky	1,099	27.1	491	29.9	608	25.1
Louisiana	1,734	41.7	688	39.4	1,046	42.5
Maine	398	26.9	186	31.0	212	24.2
Maryland	1,458	29.2	689	33.4	769	26.1
Massachusetts	1,422	20.2	656	24.0	766	17.7
Michigan	2,655	26.9	1,169	28.7	1,486	25.4
Minnesota	1,213	24.3	612	30.2	601	20.0
Mississippi	661	24.1	263	24.1	398	24.1
Missouri	1,535	25.5	714	29.2	821	22.8
Montana	229	23.2	98	23.1	131	23.0
Nebraska	400	21.2	175	23.3	225	20.2
Nevada	322	17.6	180	19.6	142	14.9
New Hampshire	291	23.6	157	30.3	134	18.4
New Jersey	2,556	28.5	1,190	33.1	1,366	25.3
New Mexico	538	31.4	266	35.5	272	27.9
New York	3,844	19.4	1,770	22.3	2,074	17.3
North Carolina	2,181	27.8	964	30.0	1,217	26.0
North Dakota	196	25.7	87	27.6	109	24.1
Ohio	3,750	31.4	1,670	34.7	2,080	28.9
Oklahoma	1,065	29.5	450	29.6	615	28.9
Oregon	1,011	27.9	466	30.4	545	26.0
Pennsylvania	3,826	25.7	1,696	28.4	2,130	23.6
Rhode Island	265	21.7	120	25.2	145	19.3
South Carolina	1,088	27.5	497	29.8	591	25.4
South Dakota	212	24.2	94	26.2	118	22.8
Tennessee	1,746	30.6	786	33.3	960	28.3

(continues)

DEATHS DUE TO DIABETES, BY SEX, 2001 *(continued)*

State	Total		Male		Female	
	Number	Rate*	Number	Rate*	Number	Rate*
Texas	5,456	31.6	2,445	33.5	3,011	30.0
Utah	509	31.9	235	33.9	274	30.6
Vermont	155	24.1	67	24.5	88	23.7
Virginia	1,613	24.5	741	26.9	872	22.3
Washington	1,403	25.1	687	28.6	716	22.2
West Virginia	802	37.6	358	40.6	444	34.6
Wisconsin	1,337	23.3	663	28.8	674	19.6
Wyoming	120	25.5	56	28.2	64	23.6
United States	71,371	25.2	32,840	28.0	38,531	23.0

*Deaths per 100,000
Source: Centers for Disease Control and Prevention. *The Burden of Chronic Diseases and Their Risk Factors: National and State Perspectives.* U.S. Department of Health and Human Services, February 2004.

APPENDIX XIV

INCIDENCE OF INVASIVE CANCERS OF THE ENDOCRINE SYSTEM

Males, 2000				
Primary Site	All Races	Caucasian	African American	Asian/Pacific Islander
All sites, all forms of cancer	560,533	483,519	52,985	11,037
Pancreas	12,229	10,510	1,290	297
Testes	6,267	5,833	194	101
Thyroid	4,200	3,726	229	147
Other endocrine, including thymus	757	628	75	37

Note: Racial information was not available in some cases.
Source: U.S. Cancer Statistics Working Group. *United States Cancer Statistics: 2000 Incidence.* Department of Health and Human Services, Centers for Disease Control and Prevention and National Cancer Institute, 2003.

Females, 2000				
Primary Site	All Races	Caucasian	African American	Asian/Pacific Islander
All sites, all forms of cancer	533,647	465,477	46,569	11,894
Pancreas	12,891	10,931	1,508	322
Ovary	20,188	17,989	1,352	493
Thyroid	13,019	11,114	932	624
Other endocrine, including thymus	677	534	96	27

Note: Racial information was not available in some cases
Source: U.S Cancer Statistics Working Group. *United States Cancer Statistics: 2000 Incidence.* Department of Health and Human Services, Centers for Disease Control and Prevention and National Cancer Institute, 2003.

APPENDIX XV
STATE CANCER REGISTRIES

ALABAMA

Alabama Statewide Cancer Registry
Alabama Department of Public Health
P.O. Box 303017
Montgomery, AL 36130
(334) 206-5552
http://www.adph.org/cancer_registry

ALASKA

Alaska Cancer Registry
3601 C Street, Suite 540
P.O. Box 240249
Anchorage, AK 99524
(907) 269-8000
http://www.epi.hss.state.ak.us

ARIZONA

Arizona Cancer Registry
Arizona Department of Health Services
1740 West Adams Room 410
Phoenix, AZ 85007
(602) 542-7308
http://www.hs.state.az.us/phs/phstats/acr/index.htm

ARKANSAS

Arkansas Central Cancer Registry
Arkansas Department of Health
Division of Chronic Disease/Disability Prevention
4815 West Markham Street, Slot 7
Little Rock, AR 72295
(501) 661-2392
http://www.healthyarkansas.com/arkcancer/
    arkcancer.html

CALIFORNIA

California Department of Human Services
Cancer Surveillance Section

1700 Tribute Road, Suite 100
Sacramento, CA 95815
(916) 779-0303
http://www.ccrcal.org/index.htm

COLORADO

Colorado Department of Public Health and Environment
Colorado Central Cancer Registry
PPD-CR-A5
4300 Cherry Creek Drive South
Denver, CO 80246
(303) 692-2542
http://www.cdphe.state.co.us/pp/cccr.cccrhom.asp

CONNECTICUT

Connecticut Tumor Registry
410 Capitol Avenue
P.O. Box 340308 MS #13-TMR
Hartford, CT 06134
(860) 509-7163
http://www.dph.state.ct.us/OPPE/hptumor.htm

DELAWARE

Delaware Department of Health and Social Services
Division of Public Health
P.O. Box 637
Dover, DE 19903
(302) 739-5617
http://www.state.de.us/dhss/dph

DISTRICT OF COLUMBIA

District of Columbia Cancer Registry
District of Columbia Department of Health
825 North Capitol Street NE
Room 3145

Washington, DC 20002
(202) 442-5910
http://www.dchealth.dc.gov/services/special_pro-
    grams/cancer_control/index.shtm

FLORIDA

Florida Cancer Data System
University of Miami School of Medicine
P.O. Box 016960 (D4-11)
Miami, FL 33101
(305) 243-4600
http://fcds.med.miami.edu

GEORGIA

Georgia Department of Human Services
Division of Public Health/Cancer Control Section
Two Peachtree Street NW
14th Floor, 14.283
Atlanta, GA 30303
(404) 657-1943
http://www.ph.dhr.state.ga.us/programs/cancer

HAWAII

Hawaii Tumor Registry
1236 Lauhala Street
Honolulu, HI 96813
(808) 586-9750
http://planet-hawaii.com/htr

IDAHO

Idaho Hospital Association
Cancer Data Registry of Idaho
615 North Seventh Street
Boise, ID 83702
(208) 338-5100
http://www.idcancer.org

ILLINOIS

Illinois State Cancer Registry
Illinois Department of Public Health
605 West Jefferson Street
Springfield, IL 62761
(217) 785-1873
http://www.idph.state.il.us/about/epi/cancer.htm

INDIANA

Indiana State Department of Health
State Cancer Registry
Two North Meridian Street
Section 7-D
Indianapolis, IN 46204
(317) 233-7158
http://www.in.gov/isdh/dataandstast/cancer.htm

IOWA

State Health Registry of Iowa
250 FB Building
Iowa City, IA 52242
(319) 335-8609
http://www.public-health.uiowa.edu/shri

KANSAS

Kansas Cancer Registry
University of Kansas Medical Center
3901 Rainbow Boulevard
Kansas City, KS 66160
(913) 588-2744
http://www.kumc.edu/som/kcr

KENTUCKY

Kentucky Cancer Registry
2365 Harrodsburg Road
Suite A230
Lexington, KY 40504
(859) 219-0773
http://www.kcr.uky.edu

LOUISIANA

Louisiana Tumor Registry
Louisiana State University Health Sciences
    Center—New Orleans
1600 Canal Street
Suite 1104
New Orleans, LA 70112
(504) 568-4283
http://www.lcltfb.org/registry.html

MAINE

Maine Cancer Registry
Division of Family and Community Health

Bureau of Health
Key Bank Plaza
Fourth Floor
11 State House Station
Augusta, ME 04333
(207) 287-5272
http://www.state.me.us/dhs/bohdcfh/mcr/index2.
html

MARYLAND

Maryland Cancer Registry
Maryland Department of Health and Mental
    Hygiene
201 West Preston Street
Baltimore, MD 21201
(410) 767-4055
http://www.fha.state.md.us/cancer/registry

MASSACHUSETTS

Massachusetts Department of Public Health
Massachusetts Cancer Registry
250 Washington Street
Sixth Floor
Boston, MA 02108
(617) 624-5618
http://www.state.ma.us.dph/bhsre/mcr/canreg.htm

MICHIGAN

Michigan Cancer Surveillance Program
Division for Vital Records and Health Statistics
Michigan Department of Community Health
3423 North Martin Luther King, Jr. Boulevard
Lansing, MI 48909
(517) 335-8702
http://www.michigan.gov/mdch

MISSISSIPPI

Mississippi Department of Health
P.O. Box 1700
Jackson, MS 39215
(601) 576-7411
http://www.cancer.msdh.state.ms.us

MISSOURI

Missouri Cancer Registry
Health Management and Informatics

324 Clark Hall
University of Missouri—Columbia
Columbia, MO 65211
(573) 882-7775

MONTANA

Montana Central Tumor Registry
Montana Department of Public Health and
    Human Services
Health Policy and Services Division
Cogswell Building
P.O. Box 202952
Helena, MT 59620
(406) 444-6786
http://www.dphhs.state.mt.us

NEBRASKA

**Nebraska Department of Health and Human
Services Regulation and Licensure**
Public Health Assurance Division
Data Management Section
301 Centennial Mall South
Lincoln, NE 68509
(402) 471-0147
http://www/hhs.state.ne.us/ced/cancer

NEVADA

Nevada State Cancer Registry
3811 West Charleston Boulevard
Suite 208
Las Vegas, NV 89102
(702) 486-6260, ext. 224
http://health2k.state.nv.us/cancer

NEW HAMPSHIRE

New Hampshire State Cancer Registry
P.O. Box 186
Hanover, NH 03755
(603) 653-1032
http://cancer.dartmouth.edu/nhcr

NEW JERSEY

Cancer Epidemiology Services
New Jersey State Department of Health and
    Senior Services
P.O. Box 369

Trenton, NJ 08625
(609) 588-3500
http://www.state.nj.us/health/cancer/statistics.htm

NEW MEXICO

New Mexico Tumor Registry
2325 Camino de Salud, NE
Albuquerque, NM 87131
(505) 272-5541
http://hsc.unm.edu/epiccpro

NEW YORK

New York State Cancer Registry
New York State Department of Health
Corning Tower, Room 536
Empire State Plaza
Albany, NY 12237
(518) 474-2255
http://www.health.state.ny.us/nysdoh/cancer/can-
cer.htm

NORTH CAROLINA

North Carolina Central Cancer Registry
North Carolina Department of Health and Human
    Services
State Center for Health Statistics
1908 Mail Service Center
Raleigh, NC 27699
(919) 715-4558
http://www.schs.state.nc.us/dphmoved.html

NORTH DAKOTA

North Dakota Department of Health
Division of Health Promotion and Education
600 East Boulevard Avenue
Department 301
Bismarck ND 58505
(701) 328-2419
http://www.health.state.nd.us/cancerregistry

OHIO

Ohio Department of Health
Bureau of Health Surveillance, Information, and
    Operational Support
P.O. Box 118
Columbus, OH 43266

(614) 466-5350
http://www.odh.state.oh.us/ODHPrograms/CI_SU
    RV/ci_sur1.htm

OKLAHOMA

Oklahoma Central Cancer Registry
Chronic Disease Service
Oklahoma Department of Health
1000 Northeast Tenth Street
Oklahoma City, OH 73117
(405) 271-4072, ext. 57123
http://www.health.state.ok.us/program/cds/can-
    cereg.html

OREGON

Oregon State Cancer Registry
Department of Human Services
800 Northeast Oregon Street
Suite 730
Portland, OR 97232
(503) 731-4858
http://www.ohd.hr.state.or.us/oscar/index.cfm

PENNSYLVANIA

Pennsylvania Cancer Registry
Division of Statistical Registries
Pennsylvania Department of Health
555 Walnut Street
Sixth Floor
Harrisburg, PA 17101
(717) 783-2548
http://www.health.state.pa.us/stats

PUERTO RICO

Departamento de Salud de Puerto Rico
Registro Central de Puerto Rico
P.O. Box 70184
San Juan, PR 00927
(787) 274-7866

RHODE ISLAND

Rhode Island Department of Health
3 Capitol Hill
Providence, RI 02908
(401) 222-1172
http://www.health.ri.gov/disease/cancer/canreg.htm

SOUTH CAROLINA

**South Carolina Department of Health and
  Environmental Control**
PHSIS/SCCCR
2600 Bull Street
Columbia, SC 29201
(803) 898-3626
http://www.scdhec.gov/cancer/cancer-registry.htm

SOUTH DAKOTA

South Dakota Cancer Registry
Office of Health Promotion, Health and Medical
  Services
Department of Health
615 East Fourth Street
Pierre, SC 57501
(605) 773-5740
http://www.state.sd.us/doh/stats

TENNESSEE

Tennessee Cancer Registry
Cordell Hull Building
Sixth Floor North
425 Fifth Avenue North
Nashville, TN 37247
(615) 253-5937
http://www.mtmc.org/cancer/registry.htm

TEXAS

Texas Cancer Registry
Bureau of Epidemiology
Texas Department of Health
1100 West 49th Street
Austin, TX 78756
(512) 458-7523
http://www.tdh.state.tx.us/tcr

UTAH

Utah Cancer Registry
546 Chipeta Way, Suite 410
Salt Lake City, UT 84108
(801) 581-8407
http://www.uuhsc.utah.edu/ucr

VERMONT

Vermont Cancer Registry
Vermont Department of Health
P.O. Box 70
108 Cherry Street
Burlington, VT 05402
(802) 863-7644
http://www.healthvermonters.info

VIRGINIA

Virginia Cancer Registry
Virginia Department of Health
P.O. Box 2448
Room 114
Richmond, VA 23218
(804) 786-1668
http://www.vdh.state.va.us/epi/cancer/index.asp

WASHINGTON

Washington State Cancer Registry
Department of Health
7211 Cleanwater Lane
Building 10
Olympia, WA 98504
(360) 236-3676
http://www.doh.wa.gov

WEST VIRGINIA

**West Virginia Department of Health and
  Human Resources**
Bureau for Public Health
West Virginia Cancer Registry
350 Capitol Street
Room 126
Charleston, WV 25301
(304) 558-6421
http://www.wvdhhr.org/bph/oeh/sdc/cancerrep.htm

WISCONSIN

**Wisconsin Department of Health and Family
  Services**
Bureau of Health Information
Division of Health Care Financing
P.O. Box 309

Madison, WI 53701
(608) 266-8926
http://www.dhfs.state.wi.us/wcrs/index.htm

WYOMING

Wyoming Cancer Surveillance Program
Wyoming Central Tumor Registry

6101 Yellowstone Road
Room 259A
Cheyenne, WY 82002
(307) 777-3477
http://wdhfs.tate.wy.us/cancer

APPENDIX XVI
DIABETES RESEARCH AND TRAINING CENTERS AND ENDOCRINOLOGY RESEARCH CENTERS IN THE UNITED STATES

Note: These organizations are supported by the National Institute on Diabetes and Digestive and Kidney Diseases (NIDDK). They perform important basic and clinical research and also provide information on diabetes.

DIABETES RESEARCH AND TRAINING CENTERS (DRTCS)

ALBERT EINSTEIN COLLEGE OF MEDICINE DRTC

Director, Prevention and Control Division
Diabetes Research and Training Center
701 Belfer Building
Albert Einstein College of Medicine
1300 Morris Park Avenue
Bronx, NY 10461
(718) 430-2908

INDIANA UNIVERSITY DRTC

Indiana University School of Medicine
The National Institute for Fitness and Sport
Room 122
250 North University Boulevard
Indianapolis, IN 46202
(317) 278-0905

UNIVERSITY OF CHICAGO DRTC

Howard Hughes Medical Institute
University of Chicago
5841 South Maryland Avenue, MC 1028
Room N-216
Chicago, IL 60637
(773) 702-1334

UNIVERSITY OF MICHIGAN DRTC

Michigan Diabetes Research and Training Center
1331 E. Ann St. Room 5111
University of Michigan Medical School
Ann Arbor, MI 48109
(734) 763-5730
http://www.med.umich.edu/mdrtc

VANDERBILT UNIVERSITY DRTC

Division of Diabetes, Endocrinology & Metabolism
715 PRB
2220 Pierce Avenue
Nashville, TN 37232
(615) 936-1649
http://medschool.mc.vanderbilt.edu/vdc/html/drtc.htm

WASHINGTON UNIVERSITY DRTC

Division of Health Behavior Research
Washington University
4444 Forest Park Avenue
St. Louis, MO 63108
(314) 286-1900
http://medicine.wustl.edu/~drtc

DIABETES ENDOCRINOLOGY AND RESEARCH CENTERS (DERCS)

Joslin Diabetes Center DERC
Harvard Medical School
One Joslin Place
Boston, MA 02215

(617) 732-2635
http://www.joslinresearch.org/HomeDir/home.htm

Massachusetts General DERC
Diabetes Unit
Department of Molecular Biology
Wellman 8
50 Blossom Street
Boston, MA 02114
(617) 726-6909

University of Colorado DERC
Barbara Davis Center for Childhood Diabetes
4200 East 9th Avenue
Box B-140
Denver, CO 80262
(303) 315-8197
http://www.uchsc.edu/misc/diabetes/bdc.html

University of Iowa DERC
Department of Internal Medicine
VA Medical Center
Iowa City, IA 52246
(319) 338-0581, extension 7625

University of Massachusetts Medical School DERC
373 Plantation Street, Suite 218

Worcester, MA 01605
(508) 856-3800
http://www.umass.edu/derc

University of Pennsylvania DERC
Division of Endocrinology, Diabetes and
   Metabolism
611 Clinical Research Building
415 Curie Boulevard
Philadelphia, PA 19104
(215) 898-0198
http://www.uphs.upenn.edu/pdc

University of Washington DERC
Box 358285
DVA Puget Sound Health Care System
1660 S. Columbian Way
Seattle, WA 98108
(206) 764-2688

Yale University School of Medicine DERC
Box 208020
333 Cedar Street
Fitikin 1
Section of Endocrinology
New Haven, CT 06520
(203) 785-4183

BIBLIOGRAPHY

Abraham, Jame, and Carmen J. Allegra, eds. *Bethesda Handbook of Clinical Oncology.* Philadelphia, Pa.: Lippincott Williams & Wilkins, 2001.

Abugassa, Salem, et al. "Bone Mineral Density in Patients with Chronic Hypoparathyroidism." *Journal of Clinical Endocrinology & Metabolism* 76, no. 6 (1993): 1,617–1,621.

Achermann, John C., et al. "Genetic Causes of Human Reproductive Disease." *Journal of Clinical Endocrinology & Metabolism* 87, no. 6 (2002): 2,447–2,454.

Adamec, Christine, and William L. Pierce. *The Encyclopedia of Adoption,* 2d ed. New York: Facts On File, Inc., 2000.

Adams, Robert, et al. "Prompt Differentiation of Addison's Disease From Anorexia Nervosa During Weight Loss and Vomiting." *Southern Medical Journal* 91, no. 2 (February 1998): 208–211.

Adan, L., et al. "Adult Height in 24 Patients Treated for Growth Hormone Deficiency and Early Puberty." *Journal of Clinical Endocrinology & Metabolism* 82, no. 1 (1997): 229–233.

Adashi, Eli, and Jon D. Ahennebold. "Single-Gene Mutations Resulting in Reproductive Dysfunction in Women." *New England Journal of Medicine* 340, no. 9 (1999): 709–718.

Adrogue, Horacio, J., M.D., and Nicolaos E. Masias, M.D. "Hypernatremia." *New England Journal of Medicine* 342, no. 20 (May 18, 2000): 1,493–1,499.

Adrogue, Horacio, J., M.D., and Nicolaos E. Masias, M.D. "Hyponatremia." *New England Journal of Medicine* 342, no. 21 (May 25, 2000): 1,581–1,589.

Alexander, Erik K., M.D., et al. "Natural History of Benign Solid and Cystic Thyroid Nodules." *Annals of Internal Medicine* 138, no. 4 (February 2003): 315–318.

Althof, Stanley, E. "Quality of Life and Erectile Dysfunction." *Urology* 59, no. 6 (2002): 803–810.

Altman, Robert, and Michael J. Sarg. *The Cancer Dictionary.* New York: Facts On File, Inc., 2000.

American Academy of Pediatrics, Section on Endocrinology and Committee on Genetics. "Technical Report: Congenital Adrenal Hyperplasia." *Pediatrics* 106, no. 6 (December 2000): 1,511–1,518.

American Diabetes Association. "Economic Costs of Diabetes in the U.S. in 2002." *Diabetes Care* 26, no. 3 (March 2003): 917–932.

American Diabetes Association and National Institute of Diabetes and Digestive and Kidney Diseases. "The Prevention or Delay of Type 2 Diabetes." *Diabetes Care* 25, no. 4 (April 2002): 742–749.

Ammer, Christine. *The New A to Z of Women's Health.* 4th ed. New York: Facts On File, Inc., 2000.

Amos, Aaron, and J. William Roberts. "Cushing's Syndrome Associated with a Pheochromocytoma." *Urology* 52, no. 2 (1998): 331–335.

Arafah, Baha M., M.D. "Increased Need for Thyroxine in Women with Hypothyroidism During Estrogen Therapy." *New England Journal of Medicine* 344, no. 23 (June 7, 2001): 1,743–1,749.

Ariyasu, Hiroyuki, et al. "Stomach Is a Major Source of Circulating Ghrelin, and Feeding State Determines Plasma Ghrelin-Like Immunoreactivity Levels in Humans." *Journal of Clinical Endocrinology & Metabolism* 86, no. 10 (2001): 4,753–4,758.

Arlt, W., et al. "Dehydroepiandrosterone Replacement in Women with Adrenal Insufficiency." *New England Journal of Medicine* 341, no. 14 (September 30, 1999): 1,013–1020.

Arslanian, Silva, and Chittiwat Suprasongsin. "Testosterone Treatment in Adolescents with Delayed Puberty: Changes in Body Composition, Protein, Fat, and Glucose Metabolism." *Journal of Clinical Endocrinology & Metabolism* 82, no. 10 (1997): 3,213–3,220.

Athyros, V. G., et al. "Atorvastatin Versus Four Statin-Fibrate Combinations in Patients with Familial Combined Hyperlipidemia." *Journal of Cardiovascular Risk* 9, no. 1 (2002): 33–39.

August, Gilbert P., M.D., et al. "Adult Height in Children with Growth Hormone Deficiency Who Are Treated with Biosynthetic Growth Hormone: The National Cooperative Growth Study Experience." *Pediatrics* 102, no. 2 (Supplement; 1998): 512–516.

August, Phyllis. "Initial Treatment of Hypertension." *New England Journal of Medicine* 348, no. 7 (2003): 610–617.

Azizi, F., et al. "Thyroid Function and Intellectual Development of Infants Nursed by Mothers Taking Methimazole." *Journal of Clinical Endocrinology & Metabolism* 85, no. 9 (2000): 3,233–3,238.

Bagatell, Carrie J., and William J. Bremner. "Androgens in Men—Uses and Abuses." *New England Journal of Medicine* 334, no. 11 (March 14, 1996): 707–714.

Bakris, George L., et al. "Preserving Renal Function in Adults with Hypertension and Diabetes: A Consensus Approach." *American Journal of Kidney Diseases* 36, no. 3 (September 2000): 646–661.

Barbieri, R. L. "Metformin for the Treatment of Polycystic Ovary Syndrome." *Obstetrics & Gynecology* 101, no. 4 (2003): 785–793.

Bardsley, Joan K., and Maureen Passaro. "ABCs of Diabetes Research." *Clinical Diabetes* 20, no. 1 (2002): 5–8.

Baris, D., et al. "Acromegaly and Cancer Risk: A Cohort Study in Sweden and Denmark." *Cancer Causes and Control* 13, no. 5 (2002): 395–400.

Bartalena, Luigi, Aldo Pinchera, and Claudio Marcocci. "Management of Graves' Ophthalmopathy: Reality and Perspectives." *Endocrine Reviews* 21, no. 2 (2000): 168–199.

Basaria, Shehzad, Justin T. Wahlstrom, and Adrian S. Dobs. "Anabolic-Androgenic Steroid Therapy in the Treatment of Chronic Diseases." *Journal of Clinical Endocrinology & Metabolism* 86, no. 11 (2001): 5,108–5,117.

Baskin, H. Jack, M.D., et al. "American Association of Clinical Endocrinologists Medical Guidelines for Clinical Practice for the Evaluation and Treatment of Hyperthyroidism and Hypothyroidism." *Endocrine Practice* 8, no. 6 (November/December 2002): 457–469.

Bauer, Douglas C., M.D., et al. "Risk for Fracture in Women with Low Serum Levels of Thyroid-Stimulating Hormone." *Annals of Internal Medicine* 134, no. 7 (2001): 561–568.

Bauer, Douglas, M.D., et al. "Use of Statins and Fracture: Results of 4 Prospective Studies and Cumulative Meta-Analysis of Observational Studies and Controlled Trials." *Archives of Internal Medicine* 164, no. 2 (January 2004): 146–152.

Becker, Anne E., M.D., et al. "Eating Disorders." *New England Journal of Medicine* 340, no. 14 (April 8, 1999): 1,092–1,098.

Bernini, G. P., et al. "Sixty Adrenal Masses of Large Dimensions: Hormonal and Morphologic Evaluation." *Urology* 51, no. 6 (1998): 920–925.

Beuschlein, Felix, et al. "Acromegaly Caused by Secretion of Growth Hormone by a Non-Hodgkin's Lymphoma." *New England Journal of Medicine* 342, no. 25 (June 22, 2000): 1,871–1,876.

Bilezikian, John P. "Management of Hypercalcemia." *Journal of Clinical Endocrinology & Metabolism* 77, no. 6 (1993): 1,445–1,449.

Blomgren, Kerstein B., et al. "Obesity and Treatment of Diabetes with Glyburide May Both Be Risk Factors for Acute Pancreatitis." *Diabetes Care* 25, no. 2 (February 2002): 298–302.

Boonen, S., J. Aerssens, and J. Dequeker. "Age-Related Endocrine Deficiencies and Fractures of the Proximal Femur. I. Implications of Growth Hormone Deficiency in the Elderly." *Journal of Endocrinology* 149, no. 1 (1996): 7–12.

Boonen, S., J. Aerssens, and J. Dequeker. "Age-Related Endocrine Deficiencies and Fractures of the Proximal Femur. II. Implications of Vitamin D Deficiency in the Elderly." *Journal of Endocrinology* 149, no. 1 (1996): 13–17.

Bove, Lisa Anne. "Restoring Electrolyte Balance: Calcium & Phosphorus." *RN* 59, no. 3 (March 1996): 47–51.

Brandi, Maria Luisa, et al. "Guidelines for Diagnosis and Therapy of MEN Type 1 and Type 2." *Journal of Clinical Endocrinology and Metabolism* 86, no. 12 (2001): 5,658–5,671.

Braunstein, G. D. "Diagnosis and Treatment of Gynecomastia." *Hospital Practice* (Office Edition) 28, no. 10A (1993): 37–46.

Bray, George, A., M.D. "Risks of Obesity." *Endocrinology and Metabolism Clinics of North America* 32, no. 4 (2003): 787–804.

Briet, Judy M., et al. "Neonatal Thyroxine Supplementation in Very Preterm Children: Developmental Outcome Evaluated at Early School Age." *Pediatrics* 107, no. 4 (April 2001): 712–718.

Brito, V. N., M. C. Batista, et al. "Diagnostic Value of Fluorometric Assays in the Evaluation of Precocious Puberty." *Journal of Clinical Endocrinology & Metabolism* 84, no. 10 (1999): 3,539–3,544.

Brix, Thomas Hieberg, et al. "Cigarette Smoking and Risk of Clinically Overt Thyroid Disease." *Archives of Internal Medicine* 160, no. 5 (March 13, 2000): 661–666.

Brugh, Victor M., III, H. Merrill Matschke, and Larry I. Lipshultz "Male Factor Infertility." *Endocrinology and Metabolism Clinics of North America* 32, no. 3 (2003): 689–707.

Brzezinski, Amnon. "Melatonin in Humans." *New England Journal of Medicine* 336, no. 3 (January 16, 1997): 186–195.

Burke, James P., et al. "A Quantitative Scale of Acanthosis Nigricans." *Diabetes Care* 22, no. 10 (October 1999): 1,655–1,659.

Burman, Pia, E. Martin Ritzen, and Ann Christin Lindgren. "Endocrine Dysfunction in Prader-Willi

Syndrome: A Review with Special Reference to GH." *Endocrine Reviews* 22, no. 6 (2001): 787–799.

Calle, Eugenia E., et al. "Overweight, Obesity and Mortality from Cancer in a Prospectively Studied Cohort of U.S. Adults." *New England Journal of Medicine* 348, no. 17 (April 24, 2003): 1,625–1,638.

Camacho, Pauline M., and Arcot A. Dwarkanathan. "Sick Euthyroid Syndrome." *Postgraduate Medicine* 105, no. 4 (April 1999): 215–228.

Canaris, Gay J., et al. "The Colorado Thyroid Disease Prevalence Study." *Archives of Internal Medicine* 160, no. 4 (2000): 526–534.

Carmi, Doron, et al. "Growth, Puberty, and Endocrine Functions in Patients with Sporadic or Familial Neurofibromatosis Type 1: A Longitudinal Study." *Pediatrics* 103, no. 6 (June 1999): 1,257–1,262.

Carney, J. A., et al. "The Complex of Myxomas, Spotty Pigmentation, and Endocrine Overactivity." *Medicine* (Baltimore) 64, no. 4 (July 1985): 270–283.

Carpenter, Thomas O., M.D. "Oncogenic Osteomalacia—A Complex Dance of Factors." *New England Journal of Medicine* 348, no. 17 (April 24, 2003): 1,705–1,708.

Carpenter, Thomas O., et al. "24-25-Dihydroxyvitamin D Supplementation Corrects Hyperparathyroidism and Improves Skeletal Abnormalities in X-Linked Hypophosphatemic Rickets: A Clinical Research Center Study." *Journal of Clinical Endocrinology & Metabolism* 81, no. 6 (1996): 2,381–2,388.

Carrel, Aaron L., et al. "Benefits of Long-Term GH Therapy in Prader-Willi Syndrome: A 4-Year Study." *Journal of Clinical Endocrinology & Metabolism* 87, no. 4 (2002): 1,581–1,585.

Carrel, A. L., et al. "Growth Hormone Improves Body Composition, Fat Utilization, Physical Strength and Agility in Prader-Willi Syndrome." *Journal of Pediatrics* 134, no. 2 (1999): 215–221.

Cherry, Daniel K., Catharine W. Burt, and David A. Woodwell. "National Ambulatory Medical Care Survey: 2001 Summary." Division of Health Care Statistics, Centers for Disease Control and Prevention, no. 337 (August 11, 2003).

Chopra, Inder J. "Euthyroid Sick Syndrome: Is It a Misnomer?" *Journal of Clinical Endocrinology & Metabolism* 82, no. 2 (1997): 329–334.

Chrousos, George P. "The Hypothalmic-Pituitary-Adrenal Axis and Immune-Mediated Inflammation." *New England Journal of Medicine* 332, no. 20 (1995): 1,351–1,362.

Clark, Robin E., Judith Freeman Clark, and Christine Adamec. *The Encyclopedia of Child Abuse*, 2d ed. New York: Facts On File, Inc., 2001.

Cohen, Pinchas, et al. "Effects of Dose and Gender on the Growth and Growth Factor Response to GH in GH-Deficient Children: Implications for Efficacy and Safety." *Journal of Clinical Endocrinology & Metabolism* 87, no. 1 (2002): 90–98.

Colton, Patricia A., et al. "Eating Disturbances in Young Women with Type 1 Diabetes Mellitus: Mechanisms and Consequences." *Psychiatric Annals* 29, no. 4 (April 1, 1999): 213–218.

Cook, David M. "Shouldn't Adults with Growth Hormone Deficiency Be Offered Growth Hormone Replacement Therapy?" *Annals of Internal Medicine* 137, no. 3 (2002): 197–201.

Cooper, James W., ed. *Diabetes Mellitus in the Elderly.* New York: The Haworth Press, 1999.

Corcoran, Colleen and Steven Grinspoon. "Treatments for Wasting in Patients with the Acquired Immunodeficiency Syndrome." *New England Journal of Medicine* 340, no. 22 (June 3, 1999): 1,740–1,750.

Corpas, Emiliano, S. Mitchell Harman, and Marc R. Blackman. "Human Growth Hormone and Human Aging." *Endocrine Reviews* 14, no. 1 (1993): 20–39.

Coutant, Regis, et al. "Growth and Adult Height in GH-Treated Children with Nonacquired GH Deficiency and Idiopathic Short Stature: The Influence of Pituitary Magnetic Resonance Imaging Findings." *Journal of Clinical Endocrinology & Metabolism* 86, no. 10 (2001): 4,649–4,654.

Crossen, Margon H., et al. "Endocrinologic Disorders and Optic Pathway Gliomas in Children with Neurofibromatosis Type 1." *Pediatrics* 100, no. 4 (October 1997): 667–670.

Cummings, D. E., et al. "Plasma Ghrelin Levels after Diet-Induced Weight Loss or Gastric Bypass Surgery." *New England Journal of Medicine* 346, no. 21 (2002): 1,623–1,630.

Damcott, Coleen M., Paul Sack, and Alan R. Shuldiner. "The Genetics of Obesity." *Endocrinology and Metabolism Clinics of North America* 32, no. 4 (2003): 761–786.

Danesh-Meyer, H. V., et al. "Surgical and Radiation Therapy Lowers Intraocular Pressure in Patients with Graves' Ophthalmopathy." *Ophthalmology* 108 (2001): 145–150.

David Allerheilegen. "Hyperparathyroidism," *American Family Physician.* Available online. URL: http://www.aafp.org/afp/980415ap/allerhei.html. Downloaded on April 15, 1998.

Davidson, Nancy E., and Kathy J. Helzlsouer. "Good News About Oral Contraceptives." *New England Journal of Medicine* 346, no. 26 (June 27, 2002): 2,078–2,079.

Davies, M. J., N. T. Raymond, J. L. Day, et al. "Impaired Glucose Tolerance and Fasting Hyperglycemia Have Different Characteristics." *Diabetes Medicine* 17, no. 6 (2000): 433–440.

Dayan, Colin M., and Gilbert H. Daniels. "Chronic Autoimmune Thyroiditis." *New England Journal of Medicine* 35, no. 2 (July 11, 1996): 99–107.

DeBella, Kimberly, Jacek Szudek, and Jan Marshall Friedman. "Use of the National Institutes of Health Criteria for Diagnosis of Neurofibromatosis 1 in Children." *Pediatrics* 105, no. 3 (March 2000): 608–614.

DeBoer, H., et al. "Clinical Aspects of Growth Hormone Deficiency in Adults." *Endocrine Review* 16, no. 1 (February 1995): 63–86.

Delmas, Pierre D., and Pierre J. Meunier. "The Management of Paget's Disease of Bone." *New England Journal of Medicine* 336, no. 8 (February 20, 1997): 558–566.

Demers, Lawrence M., and Carole A. Spencer. *Laboratory Medicine Practice Guidelines: Laboratory Support for the Diagnosis and Monitoring of Thyroid Disease*. National Academy of Clinical Biochemistry, 2002. Available online. URL: http://www.nacb.org/lmpg/thyroid_lmpg-pub.stm. Downloaded January 15, 2004.

De Smet, Peter A. "Herbal Remedies." *New England Journal of Medicine* 347, no. 25 (December 19, 2002): 2,046–2,056.

Diamanti-Kandarakis, Evanthia, et al. "Increased Endothelin-1 Levels in Women with Polycystic Ovary Syndrome and the Beneficial Effect of Metformin Therapy." *Journal of Clinical Endocrinology & Metabolism* 86, no. 10 (2001): 4,666–4,673.

Dixon, John B., Maureen E. Dixon, and Paul E. O'Brien. "Depression in Association with Severe Obesity." *Archives in Internal Medicine* 163 (September 22, 2003): 2,058–2,065.

Drake, W. M., et al. "Optimizing GH Therapy in Adults and Children." *Endocrine Reviews* 22, no. 4 (2001): 425–450.

Dwivedi, Rohit, and Michael J. Econs. *NORD Guide to Rare Disorders: The National Organization for Rare Disorders*. Philadelphia, Pa.: Lippincott Williams & Wilkins, 2003.

Eastell, Richard. "Treatment of Postmenopausal Osteoporosis." *New England Journal of Medicine* 338, no. 1 (March 12, 1998): 736–746.

Emanuele, Mary Ann, and Nicholas V. Emanuele. "Alcohol's Effects on Male Reproduction." *Alcohol Health & Research World* 22, no. 3 (1998): 195–201.

Engster, Erica A., and Antoinette M. Moran. *Endocrine Physiology*. Madison, Conn.: Fence Creek Publishing, 1998.

Engster, Erica A., and Ora H. Pescovitz. "Gigantism." *Journal of Clinical Endocrinology & Metabolism* 84, no. 12 (1999): 4,379–4,383.

Facchini, Francesco S., et al. "Insulin Resistance as a Predictor of Age-Related Diseases." *Journal of Clinical Endocrinology & Metabolism* 86, no. 8 (August 2001): 3,574–3,578.

Faroq, I. Sadaf, et al. "Clinical Spectrum of Obesity and Mutations in the Melanocortin 4 Receptor Gene." *New England Journal of Medicine* 348, no. 12 (March 20, 2003): 1,085–1,095.

Fearon, K. C. H., et al. "Effect of a Protein and Energy Dense N-3 Fatty Acid Enriched Oral Supplement on Loss of Weight and Lean Tissue in Cancer Cachexia: A Randomised Double Blind Trial." *Gut* 52 no. 10 (2003): 1,479–1,486.

Finkelstein, Eric A., Ian C. Fiebelkorn, and Guijing Wang. "State-Level Estimates of Annual Medical Expenditures Attributable to Obesity." *Obesity Research* 12 (2004): 18–24.

Fisher, Joseph N. "Management of Thyrotoxicosis." *Southern Medical Journal* 95, no. 5 (2002): 493–505.

Fleisch, Herbert. "Bisphosphanates: Mechanisms of Action." *Endocrine Reviews* 19, no. 1 (1998): 80–100.

Francomano, Clair, A. "The Genetic Basis of Dwarfism." *New England Journal of Medicine* 332, no. 1 (January 5, 1995): 58–59.

Franklyn, J. A., et al. "Mortality After the Treatment of Hyperthyroidism with Radioactive Iodine." *New England Journal of Medicine* 338, no. 11 (March 12, 1998): 712–718.

Franks, Stephen. "Assessment and Management of Anovulatory Infertility in Polycystic Ovary Syndrome." *Endocrinology and Metabolism Clinics of North America* 32, no. 3 (2003): 639–651.

Franks, Stephen. "Polycystic Ovary Syndrome." *New England Journal of Medicine* 333, no. 13 (September 28, 1995): 853–861.

Fried, V. M., et al. "Chartbook on Trends in the Health of Americans." Available online. URL: http://www.cdc.gov/nchs/hus.htm. Downloaded on April 24, 2004.

Frindik, J. Paul, and Joyce Baptista. "Adult Height in Growth Hormone Deficiency: Historical Perspective and Examples from the National Cooperative Growth Study." *Pediatrics* 104, no. 4 (October 1999): 1,000–1,004.

Frohman, L. A. "Controversy About Treatment of Growth Hormone-Deficient Adults: A Commentary." *Annals of Internal Medicine* 137, no. 3 (2002): 202–204.

Gallagher, J. C., et al. "Combination Treatment with Estrogen and Calcitriol in the Prevention of Age-Related Bone Loss." *Journal of Clinical Endocrinology & Metabolism* 86, no. 8 (2001): 3,618–3,628.

Ganguly, Arunabha. "Primary Aldosteronism." *New England Journal of Medicine* 339, no. 25 (December 17, 1998): 1,828–1,834.

Garfinkel, D., et al. "Improvement of Sleep Quality in Elderly People by Controlled-Release Melatonin." *Lancet* 346, no. 8974 (1995): 541–544.

Garrapa, Gabriella, et al. "Body Composition and Metabolic Features in Women with Adrenal Incidentaloma or Cushing's Syndrome." *Journal of Clinical Endocrinology & Metabolism* 86, no. 11 (2001): 5,301–5,306.

Gasperi, M., et al. "Nodular Goiter is Common in Patients with Acromegaly." *Journal of Endocrinological Investigation* 25, no. 3 (2002): 240–245.

Gharib, Hossein, et al. "American Association of Clinical Endocrinologists Medical Guidelines for Clinical Practice for Growth Hormone Use in Adults and Children—2003 Update." *Endocrine Practice* 9, no. 1 (January/February 2003): 64–76.

Gibril, Fathia, et al. "Prospective Study of the Natural History of Gastrinoma in Patients with MEN1: Definition of an Aggressive and a Nonaggressive Form." *Journal of Endocrinology & Metabolism* 86, no. 11 (2001): 5,282–5,293.

Gilliland, F. D., et al. "Prognostic Factors for Thyroid Carcinomas: A Population Based Study of 15,698 Cases from the Surveillance, Epidemiology and End Results (SEE) Program 1973–1991." *Cancer* 79, no. 3 (1997): 564–573.

Glaser, Nicole, et al. "Risk Factors for Cerebral Edema in Children with Diabetic Ketoacidosis." *New England Journal of Medicine* 344, no. 4 (January 25, 2001): 264–269.

Gmyrek, Glenn A., et al. "Bilateral Laparoscopic Adrenalectomy as a Treatment for Classic Congenital Adrenal Hyperplasia Attributable to 21-Hydroxylase Deficiency." *Pediatrics* 109, no. 2 (February 2002). Available online. URL: http://pediatrics.aappublications.org/cgi/content/full/109/2/e28?maxtoshow=&HITS=10&hits=10&RESULTFORMAT=&author1=gmyrek&searchid=1093707875788_2272&stored_search=&FIRSTINDEX=0&sortspec=relevance&journalcode=pediatrics. Downloaded January 15, 2004.

Gold, D. T., et al. "Paget's Disease of Bone and Quality of Life." *Journal of Bone Mineral Research* 11, no. 12 (1996): 1,897–1,904.

Grady, D., et al. "Cardiovascular Disease Outcomes During 6.8 Years of Hormone Therapy: Heart and Estrogen/Progestin Replacement Study Follow-up (HERS II)." *Journal of the American Medical Association* 288 (2002): 49–57.

Griffin, James E., and Sergio R. Ojeda, eds. *Textbook of Endocrine Physiology,* 4th ed. New York: Oxford University Press, 2000.

Grindik, J. Paul, and Joyce Baptista. "Adult Height in Growth Hormone Deficiency: Historical Perspective and Examples from the National Cooperative Growth Study." *Pediatrics* 104, no. 4 (October 1999): 1,000–1,004.

Gott, Vincent L., et al. "Replacement of the Aortic Root in Patients with Marfan's Syndrome." *New England Journal of Medicine* 340, no. 17 (April 29, 1999): 1,307–1,313.

Greenspan, Susan L., and Francis S. Greenspan. "The Effect of Thyroid Hormone on Skeletal Integrity." *Annals of Internal Medicine* 130, no. 9 (1999): 750–758.

Grino, P. B., et al. "Androgen Resistance Associated with a Qualitative Abnormality of the Androgen Receptor and Responsive to High Dose Androgen Therapy." *Journal of Clinical Endocrinology & Metabolism* 68, no. 3 (1989): 578–584.

Grinspoon, Steven, and Marie Gelato. "Editorial: The Rational Use of Growth Hormone in HIV-Infected Patients." *Journal of Clinical Endocrinology & Metabolism* 86, no. 8 (2001): 3,478–3,479.

Grodstein, Francine, Thomas B. Clarkson, and JoAnn E. Manson. "Understanding the Divergent Data on Postmenopausal Hormone Therapy." *New England Journal of Medicine* 348, no. 7 (February 13, 2003): 645–650.

Guha, Bhuvana, Guha Krishnaswamy, and Alan Peiris. "The Diagnosis and Management of Hypothyroidism." *Southern Medical Journal* 95, no. 5 (2002): 475–480.

Guise, Theresa A., and Gregory R. Mundy. "Cancer and Bone." *Endocrine Reviews* 19, no. 1 (1998): 18–54.

Gruber, Christian J., et al. "Production and Actions of Estrogens." *New England Journal of Medicine* 346, no. 5 (January 31, 2002): 340–352.

Guay, Andre T., et al. "American Association of Clinical Endocrinologists Medical Guidelines for Clinical Practice for the Evaluation and Treatment of Male Sexual Dysfunction: A Couple's Problem—2003 Update." *Endocrine Practice* 9, no. 1 (January/February 2003): 77–95.

Guzick, David S. "Sperm Morphology, Motility, and Concentration in Fertile and Infertile Men." *New England Journal of Medicine* 345, no. 19 (November 8, 2001): 1,388–1,393.

Haddad, J. G. "Vitamin D—Solar Rays, the Milky Way, or Both?" *New England Journal of Medicine* 326, no. 18 (1992): 1,213–1,215.

Haden, Susan T., et al. "Alternations in Parathyroid Dynamics in Lithium-Treated Subjects." *Journal of Clinical Endocrinology & Metabolism* 82, no. 9 (1997): 2,844–2,848.

Hahn, Tina M., Kenneth C. Copeland, and Savio L. C. Woo. "Phenotypic Correction of Dwarfism by Constitutive

Expression of Growth Hormone." *Endocrinology* 137, no. 11 (1996): 4,988–4,993.

Hansen, Michele, et al. "The Risk of Major Birth Defects After Intracytoplasmic Sperm Injection and In Vitro Fertilization." *New England Journal of Medicine* 346, no. 10 (March 7, 2002): 725–730.

Hansen, P., T. Bax, and L. Swanstrom. "Laparoscopic Adrenalectomy: History, Indications, and Current Techniques for a Minimally Invasive Approach to Adrenal Pathology." *Endoscopy* 29, no. 4 (1997): 309–314.

Hanson, J. A., et al. "Computed Tomography Appearance of the Thymus and Anterior Mediastinum in Active Cushing's Syndrome." *Journal of Clinical Endocrinology & Metabolism* 84, no. 2 (1999): 602–605.

Harman, S. Mitchell, et al. "Longitudinal Effects of Aging on Serum Total and Free Testosterone Levels in Healthy Men." *Journal of Clinical Endocrinology & Metabolism* 86, no. 2 (2001): 724–731.

Headley, Carol M. "Hungry Bone Syndrome Following Parathyroidectomy." *ANNA Journal* 25, no. 3 (June 1998): 283–289.

Heaney, Robert P., and Connie M. Weaver. "Calcium and Vitamin D." *Endocrinology and Metabolism Clinics of North America* 32, no. 1 (2003): 181–194.

Hitchcock, Polly, and Jacqueline A. Pugh, "Management of Overweight and Obese Adults." *British Journal of Medicine* 325 (October 5, 2002): 757–761.

Hoffman, E. "Chvostek Sign." *Amerian Journal of Surgery* 96, no. 1 (1958): 33–37.

Holm, Ingrid A., et al. "Mutational Analysis and Genotype-Phenotype Correlation of the PHEX Gene in X-Linked Hypophosphatemic Rickets." *Journal of Clinical Endocrinology & Metabolism* 86, no. 8 (2001): 3,889–3,899.

Homocysteine Studies Collaboration. "Homocysteine and Risk of Ischemic Heart Disease and Stroke: A Meta-Analysis." *Journal of the American Medical Association* 288, no. 16 (2002): 2,015–2,022.

Horvath, Tamas L., et al. "Minireview: Ghrelin and the Regulation of Energy Balance—A Hypothalmic Perspective." *Endocrinology* 142, no. 10 (2001): 4,163–4,169.

Hosam, K. Kamel. "Hypothyroidism in the Elderly." Available online. URL: http://www.mmhc.com/cg/articles/ CG9911/kamel.html. Downloaded on November 14, 2003.

Hsing, Ann W., et al. "Risk Factors for Adrenal Cancer: An Exploratory Study." *International Journal of Cancer* 65, no. 4 (1996): 432–436.

Hu, Frank B. "Television Watching and Other Sedentary Behaviors in Relation to Risk of Obesity and Type 2 Diabetes Mellitus in Women." *Journal of the American Medical Association* 289, no. 14 (April 9, 2003): 1,785–1,791.

Hull, M. G., et al. "Population Study of Causes, Treatment, and Outcome of Infertility." *British Medical Journal* 291, no. 6,510 (1985): 1,693–1,697.

Hundahl, S. A., et al. "Two Hundred Eighty-Six Cases of Parathyroid Carcinoma Treated in the U.S. Between 1985–1995: A National Cancer Data Base Report. The American College of Surgeons Commission on Cancer and the American Cancer Society." *Cancer* 86, no. 3 (August 1, 1999): 538–544.

Imrie, Helen, et al. "Evidence for a Graves' Disease Susceptibility Locus at Chromosome Xp11 in a United Kingdom Population." *Journal of Clinical Endocrinology & Metabolism* 86, no. 2 (2001): 626–630.

Isley, William L. "Growth Hormone Therapy for Adults: Not Ready for Prime Time." *Annals of Internal Medicine* 137, no. 3 (2002): 190–196.

Jain, Tarun, Bernard L. Harlow, and Mark D. Hornstein. "Insurance Coverage and Outcomes of In Vitro Fertilization." *New England Journal of Medicine* 347, no. 9 (August 29, 2002): 661–666.

Kalmijn, S., et al. "Subclinical Hyperthyroidism and the Risk of Dementia. The Rotterdam Study." *Clinical Endocrinology* 53, no. 6 (2000): 733–737.

Kalro, Brinda N. "Impaired Fertility Caused by Endocrine Dysfunction in Women." *Endocrinology and Metabolism Clinics of North America* 32, no. 3 (2003): 573–592.

Kandel, Joseph, and Christine Adamec. *The Encyclopedia of Senior Health and Well-Being.* New York: Facts On File, Inc., 2003.

Kane, Robert L., Joseph G. Ouslander, and Itamar B. Abrass. *Essentials of Clinical Geriatrics,* 4th ed. New York: McGraw-Hill, 1999.

Kaplowitz, Paul B., Sharon E. Oberfield, and the Drug and Therapeutics and Executive Committees of the Lawson Wilkins Pediatric Endocrine Society. "Reexamination of the Age Limit for Defining When Puberty is Precocious in Girls in the United States: Implications for Evaluation and Treatment." *Pediatrics* 104, no. 4 (October 1999): 936–941.

Kaufman, David W., et al. "Recent Patterns of Medication Use in the Ambulatory Adult Population of the United States: The Slone Study." *Journal of the American Medical Association* 287, no. 3 (2002): 337–344.

Kelly, Chris C. J., et al. "Low Grade Chronic Inflammation in Women with Polycystic Ovarian Syndrome." *Journal of Clinical Endocrinology & Metabolism* 86, no. 6 (2001): 2,453–2,455.

Khavinson, Vladimir, and Vyacheslav Morozov. "Peptides of Pineal Gland and Thymus Prolong Human Life."

Neuroendocrinology Letters 24, no. 3 and 4 (June/August 2003): 233–240.

Khaw, Kay-Tee, et al. "Prediction of Total and Hip Fracture Risk in Men and Women by Quantitative Ultrasound of the Calcaneus: EPIC-Norfolk Prospective Population Study." *Lancet* 363, no. 9,404 (January 17, 2004): 197–200.

Kjos, Siri L., and Tomas A. Buchanan. "Gestational Diabetes Mellitus." *New England Journal of Medicine* 341, no. 23 (December 2, 1999): 1,749–1,756.

Klein, Irwin, and Kaie Ojamaa. "Thyroid Hormone and the Cardiovascular System." *New England Journal of Medicine* 344, no. 7 (February 15, 2001): 501–509.

Klein, S. M., and C. R. Carcia. "Asherman Syndrome: A Critique and Current Review." *Fertility and Sterility* 24, no. 9 (1973): 722–735.

Klinger, H. Cristoph, et al. "Pheochromocytoma." *Urology* 57, no. 6 (2001): 1,025–1,032.

Klump, K. L., et al. "Genetic and Environmental Influences on Anorexia Nervosa in a Population-Based Twin Sample." *Psychological Medicine* 31, no. 4 (2001): 737–740.

Kotler, Donald P. "Cachexia." *Annals of Internal Medicine* 133, no. 8 (2000): 622–634.

Kovacs, Christopher S., and Henry M. Kronenbergy. "Maternal-Fetal Calcium and Bone Metabolism During Pregnancy, Puerperium, and Lactation." *Endocrine Reviews* 18, no. 6 (1997): 832–872.

Kunz, D., et al. "Melatonin in Patients with Reduced REM Sleep Duration: Two Randomized Controlled Trials." *Journal of Clinical Endocrinology & Metabolism* 89, no. 1 (2004): 128–134.

Kurzrock, Eric A., et al. "Klinefelter Syndrome and Precocious Puberty: A Harbinger for Tumor." *Urology* 60, no. 3 (2002): 515xiv–515xv.

Ladenson, Paul W. "American Thyroid Association Guidelines for Detection of Thyroid Dysfunction." *Archives of Internal Medicine* 160, no. 11 (June 12, 2000): 1,573–1,575.

Lamberg-Allardt, C., et al. "Low Serum 25-Hydroxyvitamin D Levels and Secondary Hyperparathyroidism in Middle-Aged White Strict Vegetarians." *American Journal of Clinical Nutrition* 58, no. 5 (1998): 684–689.

Lange, Paul H., and Christine Adamec. *Prostate Cancer for Dummies.* New York: Wiley Publishing, 2003.

Langer, Oded, et al. "A Comparison of Glyburide and Insulin in Women with Gestational Diabetes Mellitus." *New England Journal of Medicine* 343, no. 16 (October 19, 2000): 1,134–1,138.

Lauretti, S., et al. "Etiological Diagnosis of Primary Adrenal Insufficiency Using an Original Flowchart of Immune and Biochemical Markers." *Journal of Clinical Endocrinology & Metabolism* 83, no. 9 (1998): 3,163–3,168.

Layman, Lawrence C., et al. "Delayed Puberty and Hypogonadism Caused by Mutations in the Follicle-Stimulating Hormone β-Subunit Gene." *New England Journal of Medicine* 337, no. 9 (August 28, 1997): 607–611.

Lazar, L., et al. "Sexual Precocity in Boys Accelerated Versus Slowly Progressive Puberty Gonadotropin-Suppressive Therapy and Final Height." *Journal of Clinical Endocrinology & Metabolism* 86, no. 9 (2001): 4,127–4,132.

Lechan, Ronald M., and Jeffrey B. Tatro, "Editorial: Hypothalamic Melanocortin Signaling in Cachexia." *Endocrinology* 142, no. 8 (2001): 3,288–3,291.

Leger, J., et al. "Influence of Severity of Hypothyroidism and Inadequacy of Treatment Limit School Achievement in Children with Congenital Hypothyroidism." *Acta Paediatrics* 90 (2001): 1,249–1,256.

Lepage, R., et al., "Hypocalcemia Induced During Major and Minor Abdominal Surgery in Humans." *Journal of Clinical Endocrinology & Metabolism* 84, no. 8 (1999): 2,654–2,658.

Lerman, Steven E., Irene M. McAleer, and George W. Kaplan. "Sex Assignment in Cases of Ambiguous Genitalia and Its Outcome." *Urology* 55, no. 1 (2000): 8–12.

LeRoux, Carel, Abeda Mulla, and Karim Meeran. "Pituitary Carcinoma as a Cause of Acromegaly." *New England Journal of Medicine* 345, no. 22 (November 29, 2001): 1,645–1,646.

Levenson, David I., and Kevin Al Ohayon. "A Practical Analysis of Calcium Supplements." *Alternative Therapies in Women's Health Archives* 2 (April 1, 2000): 28–31.

Levin, Nikka A., and Kenneth E. Greer. "Cutaneous Manifestations of Endocrine Disorders." *Dermatology Nursing* 13, no. 3 (June 1, 2001): 185–196.

Lidegaard O., B. Edstrom, and S. Kreiner. "Oral Contraceptives and Venous Thromboembolism: A Five-Year National Case-Control Study." *Contraception* 65, no. 3 (March 2002): 187–196.

Lindholm, J., et al. "Incidence and Late Prognosis of Cushing's Syndrome: A Population-Based Study." *Journal of Clinical Endocrinology & Metabolism* 86, no. 1 (2001): 117–123.

Lips, Paul. "Vitamin D Deficiency and Secondary Hypoparathyroidism in the Elderly: Consequences for Bone Loss and Fractures and Therapeutic Implications." *Endocrine Reviews* 22, no. 4 (2001): 477–501.

Lobo, Rogerio A., and Enrico Carmina. "The Importance of Diagnosing the Polycystic Ovary Syndrome." *Annals of Internal Medicine* 132, no. 12 (2000): 989–993.

Lockshin, Michael D. "Endocrine Origins of Rheumatic Disease." *Postgraduate Medicine* 111, no. 4 (April 2002): 87–92.

Lucas, A., et al. "Postpartum Thyroid Disease Is Not Associated with Postpartum Depression." *Clinical Endocrinology* 55, no. 6 (2001): 809–814.

Lue, Tom F. "Erectile Dysfunction." *New England Journal of Medicine* 342, no. 24 (June 15, 2000): 1,802–1,813.

Lupo, Virginia R., and Catherine B. Niewoehner. *Endocrine Pathophysiology.* Madison, Conn.: Fence Creek Publishing, 1998.

Lyritis, G. P., et al. "Analgesic Effects of Salmon Calcitonin in Osteoporotic Vertebral Fractures: A Double-Blind Placebo Controlled Case Study." *Calcification Tissue International* 49, no. 6 (December 1991): 369–372.

MacLennan A., et al. "Oral Oestrogen Replacement Therapy Versus Placebo for Hot Flushes." (Cochrane Review) in *The Cochrane Library* 3 (2002). Oxford: Update Software. Available online. Downloaded January 4, 2004.

Maghnie, Mohamad, et al. "Central Diabetes Insipidus in Children and Young Adults." *New England Journal of Medicine* 343, no. 14, (October 5, 2000): 998–1,007.

Marcus, Amy Dockser. "Finding a Cheaper Way to Make a Baby." *Wall Street Journal* (March 6, 2004): D1.

Marcus, Donald M., and Arthur P. Grollman. "Botanical Medicines—The Need for New Regulations." *New England Journal of Medicine* 347, no. 25 (December 19, 2002): 2,073–2,075.

Marks, Daniel L., and Roger D. Cone. "Central Melanocortins and the Regulation of Weight During Acute and Chronic Disease." *Recent Progress in Hormone Research* 56 (2001): 359–376.

Marshall, Keri. "Polycystic Ovary Syndrome: Clinical Considerations." *Alternative Medicine Review* 6, no. 3 (2001): 272–292.

Marx, Stephen J. "Hyperparathyroid and Hypoparathyroid Disorders." *New England Journal of Medicine* 343, no. 25 (December 21, 2000): 1,863–1,875.

Mather, K. J., C. L. Chik, and B. Corenblum. "Maintenance of Serum Calcium by Parathyroid Hormone-Related Peptide During Lactation in a Hypoparathyroid Patient." *Journal of Clinical Endocrinology & Metabolism* 84, no. 2 (1999): 424–427.

Matthaei, Stephan, et al. "Pathophysiology and Pharmacological Treatment of Insulin Resistance." *Endocrine Reviews* 21, no. 6 (2000): 585–618.

McCanlies, Erin, et al. "Hashimoto's Thyroiditis and Insulin-Dependent Diabetes Mellitus: Differences Among Individuals With and Without Abnormal Thyroid Function." *Journal of Clinical Endocrinology & Metabolism* 83, no. 5 (1998): 1,548–1,551.

McDermott, Michael T. *Endocrine Secrets.* Philadelphia, Pa.: Hanley & Belfus, Inc., 2002.

McKane, W. Roland, et al. "Mechanism of Renal Calcium Conservation with Estrogen Replacement Therapy in Women in Early Menopause—A Clinical Research Center Study." *Journal of Clinical Endocrinology & Metabolism* 80, no. 12 (1995): 3,458–3,464.

Mechanick, Jeffrey I., et al. "American Association of Clinical Endocrinologists Medical Guidelines for the Clinical Use of Dietary Supplements and Nutraceuticals." *Endocrine Practice* 9, no. 5 (September/October 2003): 417–470.

Mehler, Philip S. "Diagnosis and Care of Patients with Anorexia Nervosa in Primary Care Settings." *Annals of Internal Medicine* 134, no. 11 (2001): 1,048–1,059.

Meunier, Pierre, J., et al. "The Effects of Strontium Ranelate on the Risk of Vertebral Fracture in Women with Postmenopausal Osteoporosis." *New England Journal of Medicine* 350, no. 5 (January 29, 2004): 459–468.

Midyett, L. Kurt, Wayne V. Moore, and Jill D. Jacobson. "Are Pubertal Changes in Girls Before Age 8 Benign?" *Pediatrics* 111, no. 1 (January 2003): 47–51.

Miller, K. K., and G. H. Daniels. "Lithium Therapy Can Cause Silent Thyroiditis and Hyperthyroidism." *Clinical Endocrinology* 55, no. 4 (2001): 501–508.

Milliner, Dawn S., et al. "Results of Long-Term Treatment with Orthophosphate and Pyridoxine in Patients with Primary Hyperoxaluria." *New England Journal of Medicine* 331, no. 23 (December 8, 1994): 1,553–1,558.

Minocha, Anil, and Christine Adamec. *The Encyclopedia of Digestive Diseases and Disorders.* New York: Facts On File, Inc., 2004.

Modan, Baruch, et al. "Parity, Oral Contraceptives, and the Risk of Ovarian Cancer Among Carriers and Noncarriers of BRCA1 or BRCA2 Mutation." *New England Journal of Medicine* 345, no. 4 (July 26, 2001): 235–240.

Mokdad, Ali H., et al. "Prevalence of Obesity, Diabetes, and Obesity-Related Health Risk Factors, 2001." *Journal of the American Medical Association* 289, no. 1 (January 1, 2003): 76–79.

Molitch, Mark E. *NORD Guide to Rare Diseases.* Philadelphia, Pa.: Lippincott Williams & Wilkins, 2003.

Moreno, Jose C., et al. "Inactivating Mutations in the Gene for Thyroid Oxidase 2 (THOX2) and Congenital

Hypothyroidism." *New England Journal of Medicine* 347, no. 2 (July 11, 2002): 95–102.

Moro, Mirella, et al. "The Desmopressin Test in the Differential Diagnosis Between Cushing's Disease and Pseudo-Cushing States." *Journal of Clinical Endocrinology & Metabolism* 85, no. 10 (2000): 3,569–3,574.

Mortensen, J. D., L. B. Woolner, and W. A. Bennett. "Gross and Microscopic Findings in Clinically Normal Thyroid Glands." *Journal of Clinical Endocrinology & Metabolism* 15, no. 10 (1955): 1,270–1,280.

Moser, H. W., et al. "Adrenoleukodystropy: Survey of 303 Cases: Biochemistry, Diagnosis, and Therapy." *Annals of Neurology* 16, no. 6 (1984): 628–641.

Moss, Scot E., Ronald Klein, and Barbara Klein. "Prevalence and Risk Factors for Dry Eye Syndrome." *Archives of Ophthalmology* 118, no. 9 (September 2000): 1,264–1,268.

Nabel, Elizabeth G. "Cardiovascular Disease." *New England Journal of Medicine* 349, no. 1 (July 3, 2003): 60–72.

Nachtigall, Lisa B., et al. "Adult-Onset Idiopathic Hypogonatatropic Hypogonadism—A Treatable Form of Male Infertility." *New England Journal of Medicine* 336, no. 6 (February 6, 1997): 410–415.

Narayan, K. M. Venkat, et al. "Lifetime Risk for Diabetes Mellitus in the United States." *Journal of the American Medical Association* 290, no. 14 (October 8, 2003): 1,884–1,890.

National Cancer Institute of Canada. *Canadian Cancer Statistics 2003*. Toronto, Ont.: National Cancer Institute of Canada, 2003.

National Center on Addiction and Substance Abuse at Columbia University. *Food for Thought: Substance Abuse and Eating Disorders*. National Center on Addiction and Substance Abuse at Columbia University, New York 2003.

National Cholesterol Education Program. "Third Report of the National Cholesterol Education Program (NCEP) Expert Panel on Detection, Evaluation, and Treatment of High Blood Cholesterol in Adults (Adult Treatment Panel III)." NIH Publication No. 02-5215, September 2002.

National Heart, Lung, and Blood Institute. "JNC 7 Express: The Seventh Report of the Joint National Committee on Prevention, Detection, Evaluation, and Treatment of High Blood Pressure." National Institutes of Health, National Heart, Lung, and Blood Institute, National High Blood Pressure Education Program, NIH Publication No. 03-5233, May 2003.

Neal, J. Matthew. *How the Endocrine System Works*. Williston, Vt.: Blackwell Publishing, 2002.

New, Maria I., et al. "Prenatal Diagnosis for Congenital Adrenal Hyperplasia in 532 Pregnancies." *Journal of Clinical Endocrinology & Metabolism* 86, no. 12 (2001): 5,651–5,657.

Newell-Price, John, et al. "The Diagnosis and Differential Diagnosis of Cushing's Syndrome and Pseudo-Cushing's States." *Endocrine Reviews* 19, no. 5 (1998): 647–672.

Ng, L., and J. M. Libertino. "Adrenocortical Carcinoma: Diagnosis, Evaluation, and Treatment." *Journal of Urology* 169, no. 1 (2003): 5–11.

Niewoehner, Catherine B. *Endocrine Pathophysiology*. Madison, Conn.: Fence Creek Publishing, 1998.

Nijenhuis, Marga, et al. "Familial Neurohypophysial Diabetes Insipidus in a Large Dutch Kindred: Effect of the Onset of Diabetes on Growth in Children and Cell Biological Defects of the Mutant Vasopressin Prohormone." *Journal of Clinical Endocrinology & Metabolism* 86, no. 7 (2001): 3,410–3,420.

Nike M. M. L., et al. "High Prevalence of Testicular Adrenal Rest Tumors, Impaired Spermatogenesis, and Leydig Cell Failure in Adolescent and Adult Males with Congenital Adrenal Hyperplasia." *Journal of Clinical Endocrinology & Metabolism* 86, no. 12 (2001): 5,721–5,728.

Obuobie, K., et al. "McCune-Albright Syndrome: Growth Hormone Dynamics in Pregnancy." *Journal of Clinical Endocrinology & Metabolism* 86, no. 6 (2001): 2,456–2,458.

O'Connor, Hugh, and Adam Magos. "Endometrial Resection for the Treatment of Menorrhagia." *New England Journal of Medicine* 335, no. 3 (July 18, 1996): 151–156.

Oelkers, Wolfgang. "Adrenal Insufficiency." *New England Journal of Medicine* 335, no. 16 (October 17, 1996): 1,208–1,212.

Oerter, Karen E., et al. "Increased Final Height in Precocious Puberty After Long-Term Treatment with LHRH Agonists: The National Institutes of Health Experience." *Journal of Clinical Endocrinology & Metabolism* 86, no. 10 (2001): 4,711–4,716.

Overgaard, K., et. al. "Effect of Salcatonin Given Intranasally on Bone Loss and Fracture Rates in Established Osteoporosis." *British Medical Journal* 305, no. 6,853 (September 5, 1992): 556–561.

———. "Effect of Salcatonin Given Intranasally on Early Postmenopausal Bone Loss." *British Medical Journal* 299, no. 6,697 (August 19, 1989): 477–479.

Pacak, Karel, et al. "A 'Pheo' Lurks: Novel Approaches for Locating Occult Pheochromocytoma." *Journal of Clinical Endocrinology & Metabolism* 86, no. 8 (2001): 3,641–3,646.

Panzer, A., and M. Vijoen. "The Validity of Melatonin as an Oncostatic Agent." *Journal of Pineal Research* 22, no. 4 (1997): 184–202.

Paulus, L. A., et al. "Bone Density in Non-Insulin Dependent Diabetes Mellitus." *Annals of Internal Medicine* 122, no. 6 (March 15, 1995): 409–414.

Pearce, Elizabeth N., Alan P. Farwell, and Lewis E. Braverman. "Thyroiditis." *New England Journal of Medicine* 348, no. 26 (June 26, 2003): 2,646–2,655.

Pearlman, Brian L. "The New Cholesterol Guidelines: Applying Them in Clinical Practice." *Postgraduate Medicine* 11, no. 2 (August 2002): 13–26.

Petak, Steven M. "American Association of Clinical Endocrinologists Medical Guidelines for Clinical Practice for the Evaluation and Treatment of Hypogonadism in Adult Male Patients—2002 Update." *Endocrine Practice* 8, no. 6 (November/December 2002): 439–456.

Petit, William A. Jr., and Christine Adamec. *The Encyclopedia of Diabetes*. New York: Facts On File, Inc., 2002.

Plotkin, Horacio, et al. "Pamidronate Treatment of Severe Osteogenesis Imperfecta in Children Under 3 Years of Age." *Journal of Clinical Endocrinology & Metabolism* 85, no. 5 (2000): 1,846–1,850.

Pollock, M. Anne, et al. "Thyroxine Treatment in Patients with Symptoms of Hypothyroidism but Thyroid Function Tests Within the Reference Range: Randomised Double Blind Placebo Controlled Crossover Trial." *British Medical Journal* 323, no. 7318 (October 20, 2001): 891–895.

Porterfield, Susan P. *Endocrine Physiology,* 2d ed. St. Louis, Mo.: Mosby, Inc., 2001.

Quigley, Charmian A., et al. "Growth Hormone and Low Dose Estrogen in Turner Syndrome: Results of a United States Multi-Center Trial to Near-Final Height." *Journal of Clinical Endocrinology & Metabolism* 87, no. 5 (2002): 2,033–2,041.

Raffaele, Virdis, et al. "Precocious Puberty in Girls Adopted from Developing Countries." *Archives of Disease in Childhood* 78, no. 2 (1998): 162–164.

Ray, J. G. "Metal-analysis of Hyperhomocysteinemia as a Risk Factor for Venous Thromboembolic Disease." *Archives of Internal Medicine* 158, no. 19 (October 26, 1998): 2,101–2,106.

Reaven, Gerald M. "Importance of Identifying the Overweight Patient Who Will Benefit the Most by Losing Weight." *Annals of Internal Medicine* 138, no. 5 (2003): 420–423.

Reichler, H., H. P. Koeffler, and A. W. Norman. "The Role of the Vitamin D Endocrine System in Health and Disease." *New England Journal of Medicine* 320, no. 15 (1989): 980–991.

Rewers, Arleta. "Predictors of Acute Complications in Children with Type 1 Diabetes." *Journal of the American Medical Association* 287, no. 19 (May 15, 2002): 2,511–2,518.

Ringe, J. D., H. Faber, and A. Dorst. "Alendronate Treatment of Established Primary Osteoporosis in Men: Results of a 2-Year Prospective Study." *Journal of Clinical Endocrinology & Metabolism* 86, no. 11 (2001): 5,252–5,255.

Rivkees, Scott A., and John D. Crawford. "Dexamethasone Treatment of Virilizing Congenital Adrenal Hyperplasia: The Ability to Achieve Normal Growth." *Pediatrics* 106, no. 4 (October 2000): 767–773.

Rivkees, Scott A., Charles Sklar, and Michael Freemark, "The Management of Graves' Disease in Children, with Special Emphasis on Radioiodine Treatment." *Journal of Clinical Endocrinology and Metabolism* 83, no. 11 (1998): 3,767–3,777.

Roberts, Helen E., et al. "Population Study of Congenital Hypothyroidism and Associated Birth Defects, Atlanta, 1979–1992." *American Journal of Medical Genetics* 71, no. 1 (July 11, 1997): 29–32.

Ronzio, Robert A. *The Encyclopedia of Nutrition and Good Health.* New York: Facts On File, Inc., 1997.

Rovet, Joanne F., and Robert Ehrlich. "Psychoeducational Outcome in Children with Early-Treated Congenital Hypothyroidism." *Pediatrics* 105, no. 3 (March 2000): 515–522.

Rubin, Mishaela R., and John P. Bilezikian. "New Anabolic Therapies in Osteoporosis." *Endocrinology and Metabolism Clinics of North America* 32, no. 1 (2003): 285–307.

Saenger, P., et al. "Recommendations for the Diagnosis and Management of Turner Syndrome." *Journal of Clinical Endocrinology & Metabolism* 86, no. 7 (2001): 3,061–3,069.

Saenger, Paul. "Turners Syndrome." *New England Journal of Medicine* 335, no. 23 (December 5, 1996): 1,749–1,754.

Salvatori, Roberto, et al. "Familial Dwarfism due to a Novel Mutation of the Growth Hormone-Releasing Hormone Receptor Gene." *Journal of Clinical Endocrinology & Metabolism* 84, no. 3 (1999): 917–923.

Samaha, Frederiak F., et al. "A Low Carbohydrate Diet as Compared with a Low-Fat Diet in Severe Obesity." *New England Journal of Medicine* 348, no. 21 (May 22, 2003): 2,074–2,081.

Sandberg, Ake Andren, and Anders Borgstrom. "Early Prediction of Severity in Acute Pancreatitis. Is it Possible?" *Journal of the Pancreas* 3, no. 5 (September 2002): 116–125.

Sanders, Leonard R. "Hypercalcemia." In *Endocrine Secrets,* 3d ed. Philadelphia, Pa.: Hanley & Belfus, Inc., 2002.

Sawka, Anna M., et al. "Primary Aldosteronism: Factors Associated with Normalization of Blood Pressure After Surgery." *Annals of Internal Medicine* 135, no. 4 (August 21, 2001): 258–261.

Schauer, P. R., et al. "Effect of Laparoscopic Roux-en Y Gastric Bypass on Type 2 Diabetes Mellitus." *Annals of Surgery* 238, no. 4 (2003): 467–485.

Schillinger, Dean, et al. "Closing the Loop: Physicians Communication with Diabetic Patients Who Have Low Health Literacy." *Archives of Internal Medicine* 163, no. 1 (January 13, 2003): 83–90.

Schlette, J. A. "Prolactinoma." *New England Journal of Medicine* 349, no. 21 (2003): 2,035–2,041.

Schoenborn, Charlotte A., Patricia F. Adams, and Patricia M. Barnes. "Body Weight Status of Adults: United States, 1997–98." *Advance Data from Vital and Health Statistics* no. 330 (September 6, 2002): 1–16.

Sedlmeyer, Ines L., and Mark R. Palmert. "Delayed Puberty: Analysis of a Large Case Series from an Academic Center." *Endocrine Care* 87, no. 4 (2002): 1,613–1,620.

Segen, Joseph C., and Joseph Stauffer. *The Patient's Guide to Medical Tests.* New York, N.Y.: Facts On File, Inc., 1998.

Seikaly, M. G., et al. "The Effect of Recombinant Human Growth Hormone in Children with X-Linked Hypophosphatemia." *Pediatrics* 100 (1997): 879–884.

Selevan, Sherry G., et al. "Blood Lead Concentration and Delayed Puberty in Girls." *New England Journal of Medicine* 348, no. 16 (April 17, 2003): 1,527–1,536.

Sellmeyer, Deborah E., and Carl Grunfeld, "Endocrine and Metabolic Disturbances in Human Immunodeficiency Virus Infection and the Acquired Immune Deficiency Syndrome." *Endocrine Reviews* 17, no. 5 (1996): 518–532.

Shane, Elizabeth. "Parathyroid Carcinoma." *Journal of Clinical Endocrinology & Metabolism* 86, no. 2 (2001): 485–493.

Sheehan, H. L. "The Recognition of Chronic Hypopituitarism Resulting from Postpartum Pituitary Necrosis." *American Journal of Obstetrics and Gynecology* 111, number 6 (November 1971): 852–854.

Shohat, M., et al. "Short-Term Recombinant Human Growth Hormone Treatment Increases Growth Rate in Achondroplasia." *Journal of Clinical Endocrinology & Metabolism* 81, no. 11 (1996): 4,033–4,037.

Shoup, M., et. al. "Prognostic Indicators of Outcomes in Patients with Distant Metastases from Differentiated Thyroid Carcinoma." *Journal of the American College of Surgery* 197, no. 2 (August 2003): 191–197.

Shrimpton, Roger, et al. "Worldwide Timing of Growth Faltering: Implications for Nutritional Interventions." *Pediatrics* 107, no. 5 (May 2001). Available online.

URL: http://pediatrics.aappublications.org/cgi/content/full/107/5/e75. Downloaded December 1, 2003.

Sih, Rahmawati, et al. "Testosterone Replacement in Older Hypogonadal Men: A 12-Month Randomized Controlled Trial." *Journal of Clinical Endocrinology & Metabolism* 82, no. 6 (1997): 1,661–1,667.

Silverberg, Shonni J., et al. "A 10-Year Prospective Study of Primary Hyperparathyroidism With or Without Parathyroid Surgery." *New England Journal of Medicine* 341, no. 17 (October 21, 1999): 1,249–1,255.

Silverman, Stuart L. "Calcitonin." *Endocrinology and Metabolism Clinics of North America* 32, no. 1 (2003): 273–284.

Siris, E. S. "Epidemiological Aspects of Paget's Disease: Family History and Relationship to Other Medical Conditions." *Seminars in Arthritis and Rheumatism* 23, no. 4 (1994): 222–225.

Sjoberg, R. J., Simcic, and G. S. Kidd. "The Clonidine Suppression Test for Pheochromcytoma: A Review of Its Utility and Pitfalls." *Archives of Internal Medicine* 152, no. 6 (1992): 1,193–1,197.

Sklar, C., et al. "Abnormalities of the Thyroid in Survivors of Hodgkin's Disease: Data from the Childhood Cancer Survivor Study." *Journal of Clinical Endocrinology & Metabolism* 85, no. 9 (2000): 3,227–3,232.

Slominski, Andrzej, and Jacobo Wortsman. "Neuro-endocrinology of the Skin." *Endocrine Review* 21, no. 5 (2000): 457–487.

Smyth, Cynthia M., and William J. Bremner. "Klinefelter Syndrome." *Archives of Internal Medicine,* 158, no. 12 (June 22, 1998): 1,309–1,314.

Snyder, Peter J., et al. "Effects of Testosterone Replacement in Hypogonadal Men." *Journal of Clinical Endocrinology & Metabolism* 85, no. 8 (2000): 2,670–2,677.

Soulie, Michel, et al. "Retroperitoneal Laparoscopic Adrenalectomy: Clinical Experience in 52 Procedures." *Urology* 56, no. 6 (2000): 921–925.

Speiser, Phyllis W., and Perrin C. White. "Congenital Adrenal Hyperplasia." *New England Journal of Medicine* 349, no. 8 (August 21, 2003): 776–788.

Stein, Emily, and Elizabeth Shane. "Secondary Osteoporosis." *Endocrinology and Metabolism Clinics of North America* 32, no. 1 (2003): 115–134.

Stein, Evan A. "Efficacy and Safety of Lovastatin in Adolescent Males with Heterozygous Familial Hypercholesterolemia: A Randomized Controlled Trial." *Journal of the American Medical Association* 281, no. 2 (January 13, 1999): 137–144.

Steinberg, William, and Scott Tenner. "Acute Pancreatitis." *New England Journal of Medicine* 330, no. 17 (April 28, 1994): 1,198–1,210.

Stikkelbroeck, Nike M., et al. "High Prevalence of Testicular Adrenal Tumors, Impaired Spermatogenesis, and Leydig Cell Failure in Adolescent and Adult Males with Congenital Adrenal Hyperplasia." *Journal of Clinical Endocrinology & Metabolism* 86, no. 12 (2001): 5,721–5,728.

Stock, John L., et al. "Autosomal Dominant Hypoparathyroidism Associated with Short Stature and Premature Osteoarthritis." *Journal of Clinical Endocrinology & Metabolism* 84, no. 9 (1999): 3,036–3,040.

Stouthard, J. M. L., et al. "Effects of Acute and Chronic Interleukin-t Administration on Thyroid Hormone Metabolism in Humans." *Journal of Clinical Endocrinology & Metabolism* 79, no. 5 (1994): 1,342–1,346.

Stratakis, Constantine A., Lawrence S. Kirschner, and J. Aidan Carney. "Clinical and Molecular Features of the Carney Complex: Diagnostic Criteria and Recommendations for Patient Evaluation." *Journal of Clinical Endocrinology & Metabolism* 87, no. 9 (2001): 4,041–4,046.

Stuart, C. A., et al. "Hyperinsulinemia and Acanthosis Nigricans in African Americans." *Journal of the National Medical Association* 89, no. 8 (August 1997): 523–527.

Sturm, Roland. "Increases in Clinical Severe Obesity in the United States, 1986–2000." *Archives in Internal Medicine* 163, no. 18 (October 13, 2003): 2,146–2,148.

Supit, Edwin J., and Alan N. Peiris. "Interpretation of Laboratory Thyroid Function Tests for the Primary Care Physician." *Southern Medical Journal* 95, no. 5 (2002): 481–485.

Surks, M. I., et al. "Subclinical Thyroid Disease: Scientific Review and Guidelines for Diagnosis and Management." *Journal of the American Medical Association* 291, no. 2 (January 13, 2004): 228–238.

Surks, Martin I., and Ruben Sievert. "Drugs and Thyroid Function." *New England Journal of Medicine* 333, no. 25 (1995): 1,688–1,694.

Szudek, J., P. Birch, and J. M. Friedman. "Growth in North American White Children with Neurofibromatosis I (NF 1)." *Journal of Medical Genetics* 37, no. 12 (2000): 933.

Tan, G. H., and H. Gharib. "Thyroid Incidentalomas: Management Approaches to Nonpalpable Nodules Discovered Incidentally on Thyroid Imaging." *Annals of Internal Medicine* 126, no. 3 (1997): 226–231.

Tanner, T. M. *Growth at Adolescence with a General Consideration of the Effects of Hereditary and Environmental Factors Upon Growth and Maturation from Birth to Maturity.* 2d ed. Springfield, Ill.: Charles C. Thomas, 1962.

Ten, Svetlana, Maria New, and Noel MacLaren. "Addison's Disease 2001." *Journal of Clinical Endocrinology & Metabolism* 86, no. 7 (2001): 2,909–2,922.

Tetiker, Tamer, Murat Sert, and Mustafa Kocak. "Efficacy of Indapamide in Central Diabetes Insipidus." *Archives of Internal Medicine* 159, no. 17 (1999): 2,085–2,087.

Thearle, Marie, and Louis J. Aronne. "Obesity and Pharmacologic Therapy." *Endocrinology and Metabolism Clinics of North America* 32, no. 4 (2003): 1,005–1,024.

Therrell, Bradford L., Jr., et al. "Results of Screening 1.9 Million Texas Newborns for 21-Hydroxylase-Deficient Congenital Adrenal Hyperplasia." *Pediatrics* 101, no. 4 (April 1998): 583–590.

Thomas, Melissa K. "Hypovitaminosis D in Medical Inpatients." *New England Journal of Medicine* 338, no. 12 (March 19, 1998): 777–783.

Toft, Andrew D. "Subclinical Hypothyroidism." *New England Journal of Medicine* 345, no. 7 (August 16, 2001): 512–516.

Tohme, J. F., and J. P. Bilezikian. "Hypocalcemic Emergencies." *Endocrinology and Metabolism Clinics of North America* 22, no. 2 (1993): 363–375.

Tordoff, Michael G. "Calcium: Taste, Intake, and Appetite." *Physiological Reviews* 81, no. 4 (October 1, 2001): 1,567–1,597.

Trainer, Peter J., et al. "Treatment of Acromegaly with the Growth Hormone-Receptor Antagonist Pegvisomant." *New England Journal of Medicine* 342, no. 16 (April 20, 2000): 1,171–1,177.

Tritos, Nicholas A. "Kallmann Syndrome and Idiopathic Hypogonadotropic Hypogonadism." Available online. URL: http://www.emedicine.com/med/topic1216.htm. Downloaded on November 26, 2003.

Travis, Lois B., et al. "Risk of Second Malignant Neoplasms Among Long-Term Survivors of Testicular Cancer." *Journal of the National Cancer Institute* 89, no. 19 (October 1, 1997): 1,429–1,439.

Tseng, A. Jr., et al. "Gynecomastia in Testicular Cancer Patients: Prognostic and Therapeutic Implications." *Cancer* 56, no. 10 (1985): 2,534–2,538.

Tsilchorozidou, T., C. Overton, and G. S. Conway. "The Pathophysiology of Polycystic Ovary Syndrome." *Clinical Endocrinology* 60, no. 1 (2004): 1–17.

Tuomilehto, Jaako, et al. "Prevention of Type 2 Diabetes Mellitus by Changes in Lifestyle Among Subjects with Impaired Glucose Tolerance." *New England Journal of Medicine* 344, no. 18 (May 3, 2001): 1,343–1,350.

Turkington, Carol, and Jeffrey S. Dover. *Skin-Deep: An A-Z of Skin Disorders, Treatments, and Health.* Updated ed. New York: Facts On File, Inc., 1998.

Turner, H. H. "A Syndrome of Infantilism, Congenital Webbed Neck, and Cubitus Vagus." *Endocrinology* 28, no. 23 (1938): 566–574.

Tyler, Kenneth L. "Cretzfeldt-Jakob Disease." *New England Journal of Medicine* 348, no. 8 (February 20, 2003): 681–682.

Umpierrez, Guillermo E. "Euthyroid Sick Syndrome." *Southern Medical Journal* 95, no. 5 (2002): 506–513.

United States Cancer Statistics Working Group. *United States Cancer Statistics: 2000 Incidence.* Atlanta, Ga.: Department of Health and Human Services, Centers for Disease Control and Prevention and National Cancer Institute, 2003.

Urbano, Frank L. "Signs of Hypocalcemia: Chvostek's and Trousseau's Signs." *Hospital Physician* 36, no. 3 (March 2000): 43–45.

Utiger, Robert. "Treatment of Acromegaly." *New England Journal of Medicine* 342, no. 16 (April 20, 2000): 1,210–1,211.

Vajo, Zoltan, Clair A. Francomano, and Douglas J. Wilkin. "The Molecular and Genetic Basis of Fibroblast Growth Receptor 3 Disorders: The Acondroplasia Family of Skeletal Dysplasias, Muenke Craniosynostotis, and Crouzon Syndrome with Acanthosis Nigricans." *Endocrine Reviews* 21, no. 1 (2000): 23–39.

Vance, Mary Lee. "Hypopituitarism." *New England Journal of Medicine* 330, no. 23 (June 9, 1994): 1,651–1,662.

Vander, J. B., E. A. Gaston, and T. R. Dawber. "The Significance of Non-Toxic Thyroid Nodules. Final Report of a 15-Year Study of the Incidence of Thyroid Malignancy." *Annals in Internal Medicine* 69, no. 3 (1968): 537.

Vassilopoulou-Sellin, R., and P. M. Schwartz. "Adrenocortical Carcinoma: Clinical Outcome at the End of the 20th Century." *Cancer* 92, no. 5 (2001): 1,113–1,121.

Veldman, R. Groote, and A. E. Meinders. "On the Mechanism of Alcohol-Induced Pseudo-Cushing's Syndrome." *Endocrine Reviews* 17, no. 3 (996): 262–268.

Vermeulen, E. G., C. D. Stehouwer, J. W. Twisk, et al. "Effect of Homocysteine-Lowering Treatment with Folic Acid Plus Vitamin B6 on Progression of Subclinical Atherosclerosis: A Randomized, Placebo-Controlled Trial." *Lancet* 355, no. 9,203 (2000): 517–522.

Vlaeminck-Guillen, Virginie, et al. "Pseudohypoparathyroidism Ia and Hypercalcitoneinemia." *Journal of Clinical Endocrinology & Metabolism* 86, no. 7 (2001): 3,091–3,096.

Vliet, G. V., et al. "Sudden Death in Growth Hormone-Treated Children with Prader-Willi Syndrome." *Journal of Pediatrics* 144, no. 1 (2004): 129–131.

Vogiatzi, Maria G., and John L. Kirkland. "Frequency and Necessity of Thyroid Function Tests in Neonates and Infants with Congenital Hypothyroidism." *Pediatrics* 100, no. 3 (September 1997): E6.

Weber, Karl T. "Aldosterone in Congestive Heart Failure." *New England Journal of Medicine* 345, no. 23 (December 6, 2001): 1,689–1,697.

Weetman, Anthony P. "Graves' Disease." *New England Journal of Medicine* 343, no. 17 (October 26, 2000): 1,236–1,248.

Whitaker, Robert C., et al. "Predicting Obesity in Young Adulthood from Childhood and Parental Obesity." *New England Journal of Medicine* 337, no. 13 (September 25, 1997): 869–873.

Whyte, Michael P., M.D., et al. "Oseoprotegerin Deficiency and Juvenile Paget's Disease." *New England Journal of Medicine* 347, no. 3 (July 15, 2002): 175–184.

William D. Knopp, Matthew E. Bohm, and James C. McCoy. "Hypothyroidism Presenting as Tendinitis." Available online. URL: http://www.physsportsmed.com/issues/1997/01jan/knopp.htm. Downloaded on January 20, 2004.

Woodhouse, C. R. J. "Sexual Function in Boys Born with Exstrophy, Myelomeningocele, and Micropenis." *Urology* 52, no. 1 (1998): 3–11.

Wren, A. M., et al. "Ghrelin Enhances Appetite and Increases Food Intake in Humans." *Journal of Clinical Endocrinology & Metabolism* 86, no. 12 (2001): 5,992–5,995.

Wright, Charlotte M., et al. "Effect of Community Based Management in Failure to Thrive: Randomised Controlled Trial." *British Medical Journal* 317, no. 7158 (August 29, 1998): 571–574.

Writing Group for the Women's Health Initiative Investigtors. "Risks and Benefits of Estrogen Plus Progestin in Healthy Postmenopausal Women." *Journal of the American Medical Association* 288, no. 3 (July 17, 2002): 321–333.

Wu, Tiejian, Pauline Mendola, and Germaien M. Buck. "Ethnic Differences in the Presence of Secondary Sex Characteristics and Menarche Among U.S. Girls: The Third National Health and Nutrition Examination Survey: 1988–1994." *Pediatrics* 110, no. 4 (October 2002): 752–757.

Wynbrandt, James, and Mark D. Ludman. *The Encyclopedia of Genetic Disorders and Birth Defects,* 2d ed. New York: Facts On File, Inc., 2000.

Yang, Sharon, and Pamela Taxel. "Osteoporosis in Older Men: An Emerging Clinical Problem." *Clinical Geriatrics* 10, no. 8 (August 2002): 28–37.

Yeh, Shing-Shing and Michael W. Schuster. "Geriatric Cachexia: The Role of Cytokines." *American Journal for Clinical Nutrition* 70, no. 2 (August 1999): 183–197.

Yeung, S. Jim, et al. "Use of Long-Term Intravenous Phosphate Infusion in the Palliative Treatment of Tumor-Induced Osteomalacia." *Journal of Clinical Endocrinology & Metabolism* 85, no. 2 (2000): 549–555.

Young, W. F. "Pheochromocytoma and Primary Aldosteronism: Diagnostic Approaches." *Endocrinology and Metabolism Clinics of North America* 26, no. 4 (1997): 801–827.

Zenel, J. R. Jr. "Failure to Thrive: A General Pediatrician's Perspective." *Pediatric Review* 18, no. 11 (1997): 371–378.

Zini, Armand, Kristine Garrels, and Donna Phang. "Antioxidant Activity in the Semen of Fertile and Infertile Men." *Urology* 55, no. 6 (2000): 922–926.

Zipfel, Stephan, et al. "Osteoporosis in Eating Disorders: A Follow-Up Study of Patients with Anorexia and Bulimia Nervosa." *Journal of Clinical Endocrinology & Metabolism* 86, no. 11 (2001): 5,227–5,233.

INDEX

subclinical thyroid disorders 212

thyroid cancer 208, 225–226

thyroid-stimulating immunoglobulin 223

thyroid storm **232–233**

thyroidectomy 213, **226**
  Graves' disease 105, 226
  hyperthyroidism 124
  hypocalcemia after 125, 219
  hypoparathyroidism after 226
  radioiodine therapy after 208, 225
  tetany after 219
  thyroid cancer 213, 225, 226
  thyroid-stimulating hormone 208

thyroiditis **227–230**
  differential diagnosis 105
  drug-induced 229
  fibrous 230
  goiter 104
  Hashimoto's **109–110**. See also Hashimoto's thyroiditis
  hyperthyroidism 123, 124
  painful subacute 228
  painless lymphocytic or sporadic 228, 233
  palpation-induced 230
  postpartum 137, 200, 228, 233
  radioiodine uptake test 207
  suppurative 229

Thyrolar (liotrix tablets) **233**

thyrotoxicosis **233**
  amiodarone-induced 229
  apathetic 77, 124
  elderly 77, 79, 124
  Graves' disease 104, 232, 233
  hyperphosphatemia 123
  iodine-induced **145**
  osteoporosis 79
  postpartum thyroiditis 228, 233

thyroid storm 232–233
triiodothyronine levels 234

thyrotropin-releasing hormone 221, 232

thyroxine 114, 227, **233–234**
  blood test 220, 222–223, 233–234
  desiccated preparations 57, 153, 222
  euthyroid sick syndrome 85
  Hashimoto's thyroiditis 110, 222
  hyperthyroidism 124, 222
  hypothyroidism 134, 136, 137, 222, 234
  secondary 211
  therapy 18, 135, 136, 137, 153, 159, 161
  levothyroxine formulation **153**. See also levothyroxine
  liotrix tablets 233
  postpartum pituitary necrosis 200
  reverse T3 208–209
  subclinical disorders 212

topiramate in obesity 174

triglycerides **92–93, 124–125**
  dysbetalipoproteinemia, familial 91
  hyperlipidemia, familial combined 90
  hypertriglyceridemia **124–125,** 192–193
  familial **92–93,** 124
  insulin resistance syndrome 145
  pancreatitis 92, 192–193
  polycystic ovary syndrome 198

triiodothyronine 227, 233, **234**
  blood test 220, 221–222
  desiccated preparations 57, 222
  euthyroid sick syndrome 85
  hyperthyroidism 124, 222, 234
  hypothyroidism 136, 137, 222

liotrix tablets 233
reverse T3 **208–209**
subclinical disorders 212

Trousseau-von Bonsdorff test 234

Trousseau's sign 46, **234**
  hypocalcemia 46, 126, 130, 219, 234
  hypoparathyroidism 130
  tetany 219

tuberculosis, adrenal insufficiency in 6, 12

Turner syndrome **234–235**
  amenorrhea 22
  delayed puberty 56
  estrogen 84, 235
  follicle-stimulating hormone 95
  menopause symptoms 114
  osteoporosis 180, 235
  short stature 70, 234, 235
  thyroid disorders 109, 234, 235

Turner Syndrome Society 235

type 1 diabetes mellitus **236**. See also diabetes mellitus

type 2 diabetes mellitus 60, 63–64, **236–238**
  acanthosis nigricans 1
  aldosterone levels 17
  cholesterol levels 44, 124, 238
  elderly 76, 77–78
  gastric surgery for weight loss 97
  genetic factors 99, 236
  and gestational diabetes 100, 101, 238
  glucose blood levels 35, 237, 238
  glucose tolerance test 175, 176, 237
  hypertriglyceridemia 124
  infertility 139
  insulin resistance 114, 144, 236
  insulin therapy 142, 238
  Klinefelter syndrome 151
  medications 63–64, 237–238